Current Concepts in Erythropoiesis

Current Concepts in Erythropoiesis

Edited by

C. D. R. Dunn

Research Associate Professor
Division of Experimental Biology
Baylor College of Medicine
Houston, Texas

A Wiley Medical Publication

JOHN WILEY & SONS

Chichester · New York · Brisbane · Toronto
Singapore

Library of Congress Cataloging in Publication Data:
Main entry under title:

Curent concepts in erythropoiesis.

  (A Wiley medical publication)
  Includes index.
  1. Erythropoiesis.   I. Dunn, C. D. R.   II. Series.
  QP96.C87   1983   599'.0142   82-13389

ISBN 0 471 90033 8

British Library Cataloguing in Publication Data:

Current concepts in erythropoiesis.
  (A Wiley medical publication)
  1. Erythropoiesis
  I. Dunn, C. D. R.
  612'.111   QP96

ISBN 0 471 90033 8

Typeset by Activity, Salisbury, Wilts.,
and printed by The Pitman Press, Bath.

Contributors

Chapter numbers given in parentheses

A. ANAGNOSTOU, (10) *University of Illinois at the Medical Center, Chicago, IL 60616, U.S.A.*

J. CARO, (1) *Department of Medicine, Cardeza Foundation for Hematologic Research, Jefferson Medical College of Thomas Jefferson University, Philadelphia, PA 19107, U.S.A.*

A. COVELLI, (14) *Instituto Pathologia Medica, 2nd Faculty, University of Naples, Naples, Italy*

A. C. EAVES, (7) *Terry Fox Laboratories, B. C. Cancer Research Center, 601 West 10th Avenue, Vancouver, B.C., V5Z 1L3, Canada*

C. J. EAVES, (7) *Terry Fox Laboratories B.C. Cancer Research Center, 601 West 10th Avenue, Vancouver, B.C., V5Z 1L3, Canada*

A. ERSLEV, (1) *Department of Medicine, Cardeza Foundation for Hematologic Research, Jefferson Medical College of Thomas Jefferson University, Philadelphia, PA 19107, U.S.A.*

J. W. FISHER, (8) *Department of Pharmacology, Tulane University School of Medicine, 1430 Tulane Avenue, New Orleans, LA 70112, U.S.A.*

W. FRIED, (10) *Department of Medicine, Michael Reese Hospital & Medical Center, 29th Street & Ellis Avenue, Chicago, IL 60616, U.S.A.*

D. R. GOODMAN, (3) *Department of Philosophy, University of California, Berkeley, CA 94720, U.S.A.*

J. W. GOODMAN, (3) *Biology & Medicine Division, Building 74, Lawrence Berkeley Laboratory, University of California, Berkeley, CA 94720, U.S.A.*

A. GIULIANI, (14) *Laboratorio Pathologia non Infettiva, Istituto Superiore di Sanita, Viale Regina Elena, 299, 00161 Rome, Italy*

P. C. JOHNSON, (12) *Medical Research Branch, Mail Code SD3, Lyndon B. Johnson Space Center, National Aeronautics & Space Administration, Houston, TX 77058, U.S.A.*

J. B. JONES, (6) *Department of Medical Biology, University of Tennessee Memorial Center, 1924 Alcoa Highway, Knoxville, TN 37920, U.S.A.*

K. KIRSCH, (11) *Institute of Physiology, Free University of Berlin, West Berlin, Germany*

R. D. LANGE, (6) *Department of Medical Biology, University of Tennessee Memorial Center, 1924 Alcoa Highway, Knoxville, TN 37920, U.S.A.*

M. LANIADO, (11) *Institute of Physiology, Free University of Berlin, West Berlin, Germany*

G. MASTROBERARDINO, (14) *Instituto Pathologia Medica, 2nd Faculty, University of Naples, Naples, Italy*

F. MAVILIO, (14) *Laboratorio Pathologia non Infettiva, Istituto Superiore di Sanita, Viale Regina Elena, 299, 00161 Rome, Italy*

K. MERCOLA, (15) *Division of Hematology/Oncology, Department of Medicine, U.C.L.A. School of Medicine, Los Angeles, CA 90024, U.S.A.*

A. R. MIGLIACCIO, (14) *Istituto Pathologia Medica, 2nd Faculty, University of Naples, Naples, Italy*

G. MIGLIACCIO, (14) *Istituto Pathologia Medica, 2nd Faculty, University of Naples, Naples, Italy.*

F. C. MONETTE, (2) *Department of Biology, Boston University, 2 Cummington Street, Boston, MA 02115, U.S.A.*

M. OGAWA, (4) *Division of Hematology, Department of Medicine, Medical University of South Carolina, 80 Barre Street, Charleston, SC 29401, U.S.A.*

C. PESCHLE, (14) *Laboratorio Pathologia non Infettiva, Istituto Superiore di Sanita, Viale Regina Elena, 299, 00161 Rome, Italy*

P. N. PORTER, (4) *Division of Hematology, Department of Medicine, Medical University of South Carolina, 80 Barre Street, Charleston, SC 29401, U.S.A.*

H. W. RADTKE, (8) *Department of Nephrology, University Hospital, Frankfurt, West Germany*

A. B. REGE, (8) *Department of Pharmacology, Tulane University School of Medicine, 1430 Tulane Avenue, New Orleans, LA 70112, U.S.A.*

L. RÖCKER, (11) *Institute of Physiology, Free University of Berlin, West Berlin, Germany*

B. M. SCHER, (13) *Department of Microbiology, Cancer Chemotherapy Foundation Laboratory, Mount Sinai School of Medicine of City University of New York, New York, NY 10029, U.S.A.*

W. SCHER, (13) *Department of Medicine, Cancer Chemotherapy Foundation Laboratory, Mount Sinai School of Medicine of City University of New York, New York, NY 10029, U.S.A.*

S. F. WALLNER, (10) *Medical Services Division, Veterans Administration Hospital, 1055 Clermont Street, Denver, CO 80220, U.S.A.*

S. WAXMAN, (13) *Department of Medicine, Cancer Chemotherapy Foundation Laboratory, Mount Sinai School of Medicine of City University of New York, New York, NY 10029, U.S.A.*

H. E. WICHMANN, (5) *Medizinische Universitätsklinik, Joseph-Stelzmann-Strasse 9, D5000 Köln 41, West Germany*

Contents

Preface

The object of this volume is to bring together a series of up-to-date, provocative reviews for the specialist reader. Undoubtedly the subject matter of the contributions reflects, to a certain extent, the interests of the editor but hopefully this has been minimized by the selection of topics in either rapidly moving areas (such as our growing interest in the manipulation of the genetics of the erythron) or those in which it is perhaps time to bring the information together, stand away from it for a while and re-assess the direction of future activities (e.g., the anemia of chronic disorders. Contributions aimed at both these over-all objectives can be found in this volume.

The scene is set in the introductory chapter by Drs Erslev and Caro in which the status of many of the subjects covered later in the book are addressed. Thus, Dr Monette's contribution explores in depth the cell kinetics of the erythron particularly of those cells which, perhaps loosely, are often designated the erythrocytic committed stem cells. The discussion of regulatory aspects of erythropoiesis are continued by Drs J. W. and D. R. Goodman (who bring together many of the often contradictory observations on the role of 'lymphocytes' in erythropoiesis) and by Drs Porter and Ogawa who provide a status report on burst-promoting activity. In something of a change of pace, Dr Wichmann looks at the regulation of erythropoiesis in mathematical terms and it is obvious that this approach can be particularly rewarding when combined with an active biological research program. There is no doubt that mathematics has, as Wichmann points out, provided some new insights into the significance of changes in, for example, the oxyhemoglobin dissociation curve at altitude, and in the role of alterations in the operating point of 'feedback circuits' which may be the underlying cause of such diseases as cyclic hematopoiesis.

Wichmann's chapter is followed by a series of reports on four different disease entities in which considerable progress has been made in the recent past. It is obvious that although cycling of granulocytes and their progeny in cyclic hematopoiesis has received most attention, cycling of erythrocytic elements is a frequent occurrence. As Drs Lange and Jones note, it now seems possible to identify one particular day of the cycle in cyclic hematopoiesis (at least in the dog) where a major event(s) occurs. An understanding of this event, and how it leads to cycling of the peripheral blood elements will almost certainly lead to a greater understanding of the regulation of hematopoiesis in the normal steady state. Drs A. C. and C. J. Eaves cogently discuss the contributions of *in vitro* culture techniques to our understanding of polycythemia vera and weigh the relative merits of progenitor cell 'hypersensitivity' to erythropoietin compared to completely 'erythropoietin-independent' growth. The approach to the recognition of spermine as an important erythrocytic inhibitor which appears to be responsible for the anemia of chronic renal failure is summarized in the chapter by Dr Fisher and his colleagues. The fourth clinical hematological problem in this series, the anemia of chronic disorders, is discussed by Dr Wallner. Many data are consistent with the concept that this anemia is due to inadequate production of erythropoietin although other pathologies can still not be completely excluded. It is of interest that the conclusion that erythropoietin titers in the anemia of chronic disorders are inappropriate is often based on a comparison of the titers seen in 'simple' iron deficiency anemia. As Drs Erslev and Caro note the size of these changes are a little hard to understand given their large magnitude in comparison to the relatively small maximum increase in red blood cell production. Dr Wallner brings up the possibility that the anemia of chronic disorders may be due, at least in part, to nutritional factors. This subject is reviewed in more detail by Drs Fried and Anagnostou. There is little doubt that even relatively minor changes in diet can have a marked, and often unappreciated effect, on erythropoiesis. Nutritional status has also been shown to modify the pathology of 'sports anemia'. Some semblance of order to the published literature on the effects of exercise on the hematopoietic system is provided in the chapter by Dr Röcker and his colleagues. It is appropriate from several viewpoints that this monograph includes a chapter by Dr Johnson on the so-called 'anemia of space flight'. Not only has this been linked to changes in the nutritional and exercise status of the crew, but Dr Johnson has been involved from the outset, in the determination of the erythrocytic status of the American crews returning from space flight. As the U.S.A. enters the 'Shuttle' era it is fitting that the mechanism of the consistent decrease in red blood cell mass be discussed by someone so intimately involved in the program.

The concluding three chapters provide, in many ways, a look into the future in that they discuss various aspects of the genetic control of erythropoiesis and its potential modification. Dr Scher and colleagues outline what is known regarding nuclear events during differentiation of murine erythroleukemia cells. The current status of a more specific genetic event (the switch from fetal to adult hemoglobin synthesis and its possible reversal) is summarized by Dr Peschle and colleagues. Finally, Dr Mercola outlines what it may be possible to achieve from an experimental and clinical viewpoint, when genetic manipulation of the erythron becomes routine. It is likely that one of the major advances in this area is going to be in the preparation of monoclonal antibodies to erythropoietin which will no doubt open the way to radioimmunoassays for the hormone which, as Drs Erslev and Caro note, is likely to bring erythropoietin much more into clinical medicine than it is currently.

Many people deserve thanks and gratitude for putting this book together. The authors in particular put up with considerable harassment from the editor in all the efforts to meet one deadline or another. I am exceedingly grateful to them for their tolerance. Considerable gratitude is also due to Ms S. Gabriel and, particularly, Ms L. Gibson, who gave so freely of their own time in assisting with all the editorial work. Special thanks are due to Ms J. Treleaven who designed the cover.

In so far as is possible, the nomenclature and abbreviations in this volume have been made consistent by the editor. The choice of terminology and abbreviations was dictated almost entirely by those used most frequently by the contributing authors. I have modified other contributions only from the point of view of consistency and no endorsement of the particular form used in this volume is intended.

Houston, Texas   C. D. R. Dunn
May 1982

Current Concepts in Erythropoiesis
Edited by C. D. R. Dunn
© 1983 John Wiley & Sons Ltd.

CHAPTER 1

Pathophysiology of erythropoietin

A. J. ERSLEV and J. CARO
Cardeza Foundation for Hematologic Research
Thomas Jefferson University
Philadelphia, U.S.A.

Contents

I. INTRODUCTION

Erythropoietin (EPO) is a renal hormone designed to
cell mass (RCM) to the need for oxygen in the tis
identified in 1953 (1) but prior to that numerous inve
Deflandre (2) through Gordon and Dubin (3), Krur
and Hodgson *et al.* (6) had provided data which ma
question of techniques rather than concept. Since
avalanche of papers and hypotheses and many

1

moments of euphoria felt that EPO might be a general stimulus for growth and differentiation. Recent studies, however, have relegated its action to a corner in the ever expanding galaxy of stem cells, an important but still quite limited area. Nevertheless, its crucial position in the basic feedback circuit which maintains the RCM at an optimal size has not been challenged.

'Feedback control' is a recent electronic term for the mechanism which maintains an optimal environment—in this case, for cellular function. The need for such a mechanism was dimly envisioned by Claude Bernard more than a century ago when he emphasized the importance of a constant *milieu intérieur* (7). Paul Bert, his most celebrated pupil and successor to the chair of physiology at the Faculté des Sciences in Paris, failed to grasp the principle that continuous adjustments to the environment are required in order to maintain such intrinsic constancy. Paul Bert was a true renaissance figure who after having trained as an engineer, lawyer, and physician became a respiratory physiologist and uncompromising anti-royalist and ended his life as the President General of Indochina. His main scientific interest was directed at studying the effect of low barometric pressure on body functions and he is often called the father of aviation medicine. In this venture, he was supported both financially and scientifically by a less glamorous but most observant physician, Dennis Jourdanet (Figure 1). Dr Jourdanet, in response to the quest of Napolean III for a French empire in the New World, had moved to the highlands of Mexico to practice medicine. There, he became impressed by the fact that many of his Mexican patients not only looked as if they had 'chloro-anemia', which could be accounted for by their yellow complexion, but also had anemic symptoms such as weakness, shortness of breath, and lightheadedness. Nevertheless, the number of their red blood corpuscles was not decreased. In 1863, Jourdanet published a book entitled *Anemia of Altitude* in which he proposed that anemic symptoms were caused by a lack of oxygen in blood and that such anoxemia could be due to not enough red corpuscles or not enough oxygen (8). He furthermore observed that at high altitudes, the blood of his surgical patients flowed slowly down the operating table, was extremely dark and contained many more than the normal number of red corpuscles. Dr Bert in discussing these observations in his book *The Barometric Pressure* emphasized that such an increase in red corpuscles would tend to compensate for the low atmospheric oxygen pressure (9). Most remarkably however, he refused to believe that this was an acquired adjustment. It was not until Viault in 1890 observed an increase in his own red corpuscles after a stay at Morococha at 15,000 ft (10) that erythrocytosis was recognized as part of acclimatization to high altitudes.

During the following decades, the mechanism responsible for this adjust-ment in the size of the RCM was speculated on by Miescher and by Carnot and Andre. Friedrich Miescher, the famous Swiss discoverer of DNA, had contracted tuberculosis and lived out his life in an alpine sanatorium. Here, he

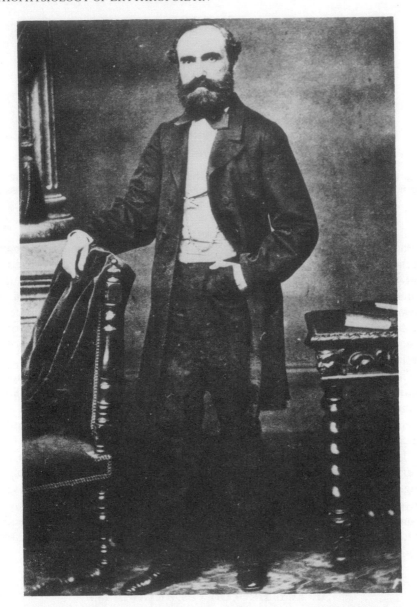

Figure 1. Dr Dennis Jourdanet. By courtesy of the Wellcome Trustees

became fascinated by the presumed healing and stimulating effect of altitudes on the body and he proposed that low oxygen pressure in the bone marrow was equally stimulating on the activity of red blood cell (RBC) precursors (11).

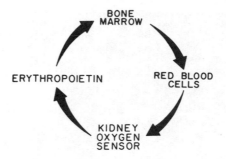

Figure 2. Basic feedback control systems which adjust the size of the red cell mass to the needs for oxygen by the tissues. Reproduced with permission from *Exp. Hemat.*, **Suppl. 8**, 1980

Paul Carnot and Mlle Deflandre on the other hand used experimental methods and, based on some questionable studies some years later, proposed that the stimulation of the RBC precursors was indirect *via* a circulating hematopoietin released somewhere else by low oxygen pressure (2). However, Miescher's hypothesis was generally accepted until the middle of the twentieth century when studies on parabiotic rats (5) and studies on the effect of 'anemic' plasma on normal rabbits (1,6) established the Carnot and Deflandre hypothesis as the correct one.

These studies provided the basic framework for a feedback circuit aimed at controlling the size of the RCM. It operates between the bone marrow and an oxygen sensor, later found to be located primarily in the kidney (12), and it is mediated by RBC bound oxygen in one direction and hematopoietin, now called EPO, in the opposite (Figure 2) (13).

The elucidation of this circuit has provided further insight into the many interlocking mechanisms which maintain normal oxygen transfer from the lungs to the tissues and into the pathogenesis of a number of anemias and polycythemias. The following discussion of these will be selective, aimed at pathophysiologic concepts rather than at biochemical pathways and be divided into considerations of EPO *per se*, its renal and extra-renal production, and its effect on the bone marrow.

II. ERYTHROPOIETIN METABOLISM

Erythropoietin is a single chain acidic glycoprotein with an apparent molecular weight of 39,000 and a carbohydrate content of about 10%. It has been purified to identity and in biologic terms has an activity of 70,000 units per mg protein or about one unit per 14 ng or per 0.35 picomole (14). Initially, one unit of biologic activity was defined as the erythropoietic effect of 5 μM $CoCl_2$ in a fasted rat but is now defined as the erythrocytic activity of a standard unit made from concentrated urinary EPO and maintained at the Bureau of Standards, National Institutes for Medical Research, London, England.

Erythrocytic activity has been measured in many ways but the bench mark assay for EPO is the bioassay in a mouse in which endogenous EPO has been reduced or eliminated by hypertransfusion or previous exposure to hypoxia (15). The baseline erythrocytic activity in such mice is extremely low and when measured in terms of radio-iron utilization, one unit of EPO will increase utilization from less than 0.5% to almost 15%. This assay will measure EPO concentrations between 50 mU and 5,000 mU per mouse with reasonable accuracy and has shown the expected relationship between the degree of anemia and concentration of EPO. However, the assay fails below an injected dose of 50 mU leaving a gap at the levels covering patients with mild anemias and normal individuals. Fortunately, EPO is quite heat resistant and it is possible to prepare a low protein but EPO-containing plasma extract by heating plasma to 100 °C for 5 min (16). When this extract is concentrated and assayed, it has been possible to fill in the less than 50 mU gap and determine that the EPO concentration in normal plasma is about 8 mU with a range of 5–18 mU/ml (Figure 3).

In vitro assays using iron uptake or CFU-E production of cultured erythrocytic cells from bone marrow or fetal livers have given a variety of values for normal plasma but most in the range of 40 mU/ml or below (17). The long awaited development of a radioimmune assay (RIA) is now at hand and the values for normal plasma have been reported to be in the range of 14–20 mU/ml (18,19). Since the immunologic and biologic activities of EPO appear to go in tandem, this RIA with its ease of performance and small sample requirements will undoubtedly be the assay of the future and greatly enhance our information about EPO metabolism.

The biologic half-life of EPO in rats is about 90 min and is similar for other small rodents (20). If desialated, its half-life is reduced to a few minutes since it, like many other desialated proteins, is removed by the monocyte–macrophage system (21). However, its biologic activity is unchanged when measured by *in vitro* assay systems. The half-life of EPO in humans has not been established but is probably shorter than the 24-hr reported in some earlier papers (2). EPO is slowly excreted in the urine and urine from normal individuals contains from 1 to 4 units per liter (23). In anemic individuals, the 24-hr urinary excretion may increase to many thousands of units providing a valuable source of EPO for purification and further use. However, the excreted amount is probably only a fraction of the amount produced since the renal clearance rate in dogs and humans has been found to be as low as 0.1–0.7 ml/min. (24). Both liver (25) and kidney (26) tissue have been claimed to be involved in the degradation of EPO *in vivo* but supporting data are not convincing.

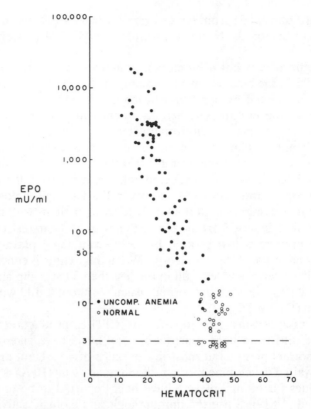

Figure 3. Erythropoietin titers in plasma from patients with anemia uncomplicated by infection or renal damage and from normal individuals

III. ERYTHROPOIETIN PRODUCTION

A. Renal biosynthesis

Cellular hypoxia is obviously the initiating event in the production of EPO but the exact location and identification of the cells responsible for translating oxygen pressure into hormone synthesis are still unknown. The early study by Jacobson and co-workers in 1957 (12) established the kidney as the key organ in the biosynthesis of EPO and all subsequent observations have supported this concept. Direct isolation of EPO from renal tissue, however, was not accomplished in a convincing manner until 1965 when Contrera and associates reported on the successful extraction of the hormone from kidneys of rats exposed to hypoxia (27). Unfortunately, shortly afterwards, these results were re-interpreted by the same group as suggesting that the kidney produces an activating enzyme rather than EPO molecules and that this enzyme activates a circulating erythropoietinogen made presumably by the liver (28). Despite some misgivings, this concept was generally accepted until perfusion studies of isolated hypoxic kidneys showed direct renal synthesis of EPO (29). These results led to a renewed search for EPO in renal extracts. In 1981, Fried and co-workers provided convincing evidence for the presence of EPO in extracts of kidneys obtained from rats exposed to severe hypoxia (30), and subsequent papers have supported their data (31,32).

Studies in our laboratory have revealed that renal tissue from rats challenged by severe hypoxia may contain up to 9,000 mU EPO per g of tissue (Table 1). The yield is best if the extraction is carried out using 50% normal plasma or 5% bovine serum albumin, probably reflecting the well known need of EPO for a protein medium in order to maintain stability (33). There is a measurable increase in EPO content of renal extracts after a 2 hr exposure to hypoxia, reaching a maximum after 6 hr exposure. It then levels off or even decreases despite a continued rise in plasma concentration over the next 24 hr (Figure 4). This decrease may be caused by the 2,3–DPG adjustment of oxygen carrying capacity which occurs after hypoxia but is first noticed as a decrease in plasma titers after 24–48 hr exposure to hypoxia (see Chapter 5 for further consideration of this point).

Within the kidney, the site of production appears to be the cortex since extracts of the medulla and intermediary layers have less activity than the cortex (Table 2). This location of the synthesizing cells conforms with old data on the site of EPO production (34). However, the cortex with its extensive blood supply and relatively low oxygen consumption would seem to be a poor location for an oxygen sensor. Because of the vascular system in the kidney and the borderline hypoxia present in the medulla, it seems more attractive to have the oxygen sensor located in the medulla from where it could control cortical biosynthesis *via* a short range releasing hormone. However, perfusion of isolated normal kidneys in our laboratory with renal extracts from hypoxic kidneys did not result in the activation of EPO synthesis. Furthermore, extra-renal EPO synthesis by the liver is also regulated by oxygen tension despite the absence of a vascular system as intricate as that of the kidney. Consequently, it seems more reasonable to believe that the oxygen tension in the cortical EPO-synthesizing cells themselves regulate hormone production. Maybe the flat oxygen dissociation curve at the high oxygen tension in the cortex provides a sufficiently sensitive probe of small changes in the oxygen saturation of hemoglobin and, in turn, of the need for oxygen by the tissues.

In any case, the concentration of EPO in plasma appears to be a sensitive guide to the presence or absence of general tissue hypoxia. So far, the cumbersome and crude bioassay technique has limited its usefulness for this purpose. Nevertheless, it did very convincingly show that the left-sided shift to the oxygen dissociation curve in a patient with hemoglobin Minneapolis, a

Table 1. Erythropoietin in plasma and kidneys after hypoxia and other erythropoietic stresses

HYPOXIA		EPO	
Preparatory hypoxia (18–24 hr)	Initiating hypoxia (4–6 hr)	Plasma (mU/ml)	Kidney (mU/g)
Bled (25 ml/kg)	—	472 (9)	—
Bled (35 ml/kg)	—	728 (10)	—
CoCl$_2$ (250 mM/kg)	—	218 (3)	163 (3)
Phenyl hydrazine (60 mg/kg)	—	452 (12)	688 (2)
0.4 atmos		3465 (5)	844 (4)
—	0.4 Atmos (4 hr)	1041 (10)	1095 (7)
—	0.4 Atmos (6 hr)	1700 (6)	1329 (3)
Bled (25 ml/kg)	0.4 Atmos (4 hr)	2800 (6)	1233 (6)
CoCl$_2$ (250 mM/kg)	0.4 Atmos (4 hr)	3150 (2)	5750 (2)
Phenyl hydrazine (60 mg/kg)	0.4 Atmos (6 hr)	3323 (11)	3000 (1)
Phenyl hydrazine (60 mg/kg) + T$_3$ (5 µg/kg)	0.4 Atmos (6 hr) + T$_3$ (5 µg/kg)	9183 (3)	9117 (3)

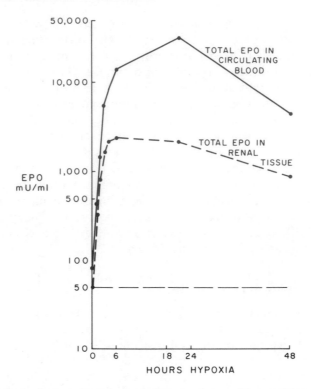

Figure 4. Erythropoietin content in total plasma volume of the rat (about 8 ml) and in total renal mass (about 2 g) after varying lengths of exposure to 0.4 atmos

Table 2. Erythropoietin in kidneys after 4-hour hypoxic hypoxia

| | EPO in mU/0.2 g* | |
Cortex	Middle	Medulla
221 (4)†	123 (4)	55 (4)

*Limit of sensitivity: 50 mU
†Number of preparations and assays

so-called 'human llama', was of advantage for tissue oxygenation at high altitudes (35). The ease and accuracy of RIA for EPO will probably result in the addition of EPO titers to the measurement of pulmonary function studies and arterial gas tensions in the evaluation of patients with cardio-pulmonary disorders.

The steep relationship between EPO titers and hematocrit and presumably tissue tension of oxygen is a little difficult to explain. Both immunologic and biologic assays have shown the same relationship with a 4 log increase in titers at only a 1 log decrease in hematocrit. Since such a decrease rarely causes more than a single log increase in the rate of RBC production and since EPO responsive stem cells (CFU-E) are very sensitive to small amounts of EPO, the large increase in titers appears inappropriate. However, EPO not only differentiates late erythrocytic stem cells, CFU-E, to erythroblasts but also recruits new CFU-E from intermediate erythrocytic stem cells, BFU-E, and it is possible that such recruitment requires more EPO than mere differentiation. It is also possible that the effectiveness of EPO is less at low tissue tensions of oxygen than at normal tensions. Many years ago, Stohlman and Brecher suggested that the action of EPO is influenced by the degree of erythrocytic cellularity (22), a suggestion not supported by more recent studies. However, the concept that some metabolic or cellular consequence of a low tissue tension of oxygen affects the action of EPO may be valid and could explain the discrepancy between a moderate increase in the rate of RBC production and an extreme increase in EPO titers.

B. Extra-renal biosynthesis

Although long suspected, the reality of extra-renal EPO production was first established during the last decade (36). The source appears to be the liver but whether hepatocytes or Kupffer cells has not been determined. Kupffer cells have been shown to attract crude antibodies to EPO (37) and the monocyte–macrophage system in general is involved in the production of colony stimulating factors. Nevertheless, stimulation and expansion of the monocyte–macrophage system does not lead to increased extra-renal EPO production (38) while predominant hepatocyte regeneration after partial hepatectomy or after chemical and viral damage does (39,40). Quantitation of extra-renal and renal EPO production after severe anemia show a parallel relationship to hematocrit (Figure 5). Attempts to increase the yield of extra-renal production have so far been unsuccessful (41) but the potential is there and needs to be explored.

Liver extracts and liver concentrates in distinction to renal extracts have so far not yielded measurable EPO. Taking into account that extra-renal EPO in rats constitutes only about 10–15% of total EPO production and that the liver is about six-times larger than the kidneys, attempts have been made to assay concentrated extracts of livers from nephrectomized hypoxic rats. However, the yield has been insignificant. Protease degradation of EPO does not seem to be the explanation since hepatic tissue mixed with renal tissue fails to reduce the renal yield of EPO. Since perfusion of isolated livers from rats exposed to hypoxia yields considerable amounts of EPO, the liver unquestionably can produce EPO and the issue may well be whether it is synthesized in a form more labile than that synthesized by the kidney. In a circulating serum-bound form, extra-renal EPO behaves very much like renal

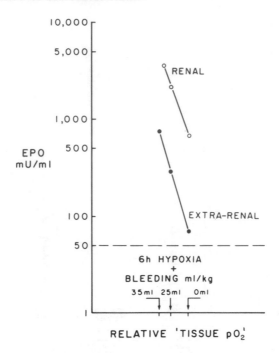

Figure 5. Extra-renal (as determined in nephrectomized rats) and renal erythro-poietin production in rats exposed to blood loss of 24 hr duration and hypoxia of 6 hr duration (38). Reproduced with permission from *Exp. Hemat.,* **Supp. 8**, 1980

EPO but if it does so before it becomes solidly serum-bound needs to be determined.

Studies by Lucarelli, Zanjani, and others (42,43) have shown that fetal production of EPO is not dependent on kidneys and presumably is entirely extra-renal. Indirect studies indicate little if any transplacental passage of EPO from mother to fetus and the source is probably the fetal liver. At time of delivery, there is a switch from hepatic to renal production. (This switch occurs slowly with full renal participation first achieved at day 28 in newborn rats.) Although this change has been believed to occur slowly during post-natal life, recent studies have shown full renal participation in EPO production even at the first week of life (58).

An altered production of EPO can in most, if not all pathologic conditions, be related to adjustments in the feedback circuit which controls oxygen delivery to the tissues. Studies of EPO in such conditions have provided not only clues to their pathophysiology but also in some cases information of diagnostic and therapeutic importance. This has been true especially for the polycythemias and for the anemias of renal failure and chronic disease. (see Chapters 7, 8, and 9).

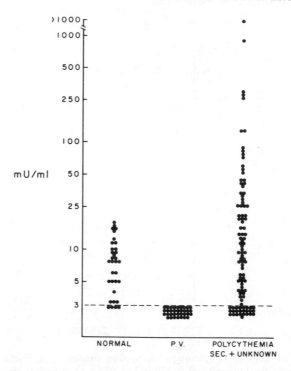

Figure 6. Erythropoietin titers of plasma from normal individuals, patients with polycythemia vera as established by the diagnostic criteria used by the Polycythemia Vera Study Group and patients with hematocrits above 53%

C. Erythropoietin in polycythemia vera

Due to auto-transfusions from an autonomous bone marrow, the level of EPO in patients with polycythemia vera should be low or absent. Using bioassay of plasma extracts concentrated 40–100 times (16), we were able to confirm this by finding no measurable EPO in all of 31 cases in whom the diagnosis was established according to the criteria of the Polycythemia Vera Study Group. In an attempt to test whether or not EPO should be a diagnostic criterion for polycythemia vera, plasma from 101 patients with hematocrits in excess of 53% and recognized as being either secondary to tissue hypoxia or EPO-producing tumors or undiagnosed have been similarly assayed (Figure 6). Of these, 75, including all cases with established tissue hypoxia, had elevated titers while 26 had non-measurable titers. These latter may represent cases of early polycythemia vera or essential erythrocytosis but prolonged follow-up is needed to answer this question. It is of interest, however, that of the elevated titers found in 75 cases, in 61 cases they were below 50 mU and would not have been detected by the routine bioassay in polycythemic mice.

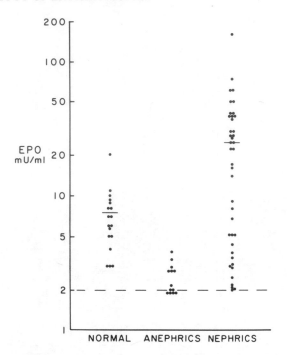

Figure 7. Erythropoietin titers of normal individuals, nephric patients with renal failure and anphric patients

D. Erythropoietin in chronic renal disease

Renal failure has been shown in most cases to be associated with an anemia. This anemia is caused at least in part by inadequate production of EPO. However, the potential for EPO production is preserved, extra-renal in anephrics and renal from remnants in patients with renal disease. If anemic or hypoxic stimulation is severe enough, this preserved ability to produce EPO is turned on and maintains a reduced level of hemoglobin. Measurements of the level of EPO necessary for the maintenance of this reduced level has disclosed in many cases the presence of higher-than-normal amounts of EPO which in turn suggests the presence of an erythrocytic inhibitor (Figure 7). The studies published by Radke and co-workers indicate strongly that this inhibitor is spermine (44).

E. Erythropoietin in chronic disease

Patients with chronic debilitating diseases are usually mildly anemic despite normal renal function. In most cases, the anemia seems causally related to low EPO production (Figure 8) although trapped iron in the monocyte–mac-

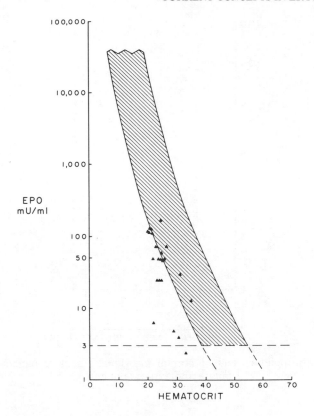

Figure 8. Erythropoietin titers of patients with chronic non-renal disorders and low hematocrit. The shaded area encompasses erythropoietin titers of patients with anemias not caused by renal failure or chronic disease

rophage system may play a role. This reduction in EPO has been puzzling but recent observations in starved rats and measurements of thyroid function in patients with chronic disease have produced a clue.

Starvation causes a sudden decrease in the production of renal and extra-renal EPO, a production restored by caloric supplementation using a 25% sucrose solution in lieu of drinking water (45) (Figure 9). Concomitantly, the levels of T3 are reduced by starvation and restored to normal by glucose supplementation. Furthermore, T3 administration returns renal and extra-renal EPO production to normal. These studies suggest that the reduction in EPO in starvation is caused by the development of a functionally hypothyroid condition with a protective decrease in metabolic activities and demands for oxygen. Since many chronic inflammations and infections also are associated with low T3 and T4 levels (46), it seems possible that one aspect of the pathogenesis of the anemia in these patients is a functional and protective hypothyroidism.

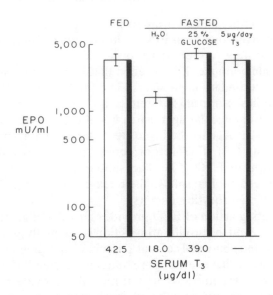

Figure 9. T_3 and erythropoietin production in response to hypoxia of starved rats

IV. ERYTHROPOIETIN ACTION

EPO is a hormone necessary for the transformation of erythrocytic progenitor cells into erythroblasts. These undifferentiated but EPO-responsive progenitor cells are called CFU-E. Although they belong to the hierarchy of stem cells, their capacity for self-renewal is probably extremely limited and in the absence of EPO as after hypertransfusion they disappear promptly from the bone marrow and spleen (37). Consequently, they must be recruited from an earlier stem cell, the so called intermediate BFU-E. When exposed to EPO *in vitro*, these BFU-E will first proliferate for a day or two and mature to CFU-E and then, if EPO is still present in the culture medium, differentiate to clones of hemoglobin-containing erythroblasts (47). In contrast, it appears as if the stimulus for proliferation and differentiation *in vivo* runs concurrently since brief exposure to the short-lived EPO in hypertranfused mice still leads both to proliferation and differentiation (48).

The youngest erythrocytic progenitor cells, so called early BFU-E will also respond to EPO by a wave of proliferation. However, these cells are responsive to other factors such as burst promoting activity (BPA) or factor (BPF) released by lymphocytes and macrophages, and their kinetics is poorly understood (49). It seems likely that they are primarily regulated by feedback signals from the local microenvironment but the presence of a long range EPO-mediated feedback from the RCM cannot be ruled out. At the other end of erythrocytic development, EPO has been claimed to enhance erythroblastic maturation and proliferation (50), shorten medullary transit time (51), and promote early release of reticulocytes (52). These actions, however, have been difficult to identify and separate from the effect of increased population pressure in the marrow due to an EPO-induced influx of proerythroblasts (see Chapters 2, 3, and 4 for further discussion).

As a polypeptide hormone, it is assumed that EPO acts via surface receptors and intracellular secondary messengers. The presence of receptors has been inferred from studies of trypsinized stem cells (53) and from the fact that EPO coupled with macromolecular aggregates is still capable of inducing stem cell differentiation (54). Agents believed to activate adenylcyclases such as adrenergic agonists (55), thyroid hormones (56), and possibly androgens, enhance the action of EPO (57). The subsequent intracellular pathway is speculative but presumably results in the release of messenger RNA coded for still unknown key erythrocytic elements.

The differentiating action of EPO provides a model of great interest in our studies of ontogeny and the proliferating action is of equally great interest in our studies of normal and abnormal cellular growth. Consequently, the fascination with EPO may not only have rewards in a better understanding and treatment of disorders involving oxygen transport but may also provide vital information about normal and abnormal growth and development.

V. ACKNOWLEDGMENT

Supported in part by NIH Grant 04612 and Grant 29780.

VI. REFERENCES

1. Erslev, A. J. (1953). 'Humoral regulation of red cell production', *Blood*, **8**, 349–357.
2. Carnot, P., and Deflandre, C. (1906). 'Sur l'activité hématopoietique des serum su cours de la regeneration du sang', *Acad. Sci. M.*, **3**, 384.
3. Gordon, A. S., and Dubin, M. (1934). 'On the alleged presence of "hemopoietine" in the blood serum of rabbits either rendered anemic or subjected to low pressure', *Am. J. Physiol.*, **107**, 704–708.
4. Krumdieck, N. (1943). 'Erythropoietic substance in the serum of anemic animals', *Proc. Soc. Exp. Biol. Med.*, **54**, 14.
5. Reissmann, K. R. (1950). 'Studies on the mechanism of erythropoietin stimulation in parabiotic rats during hypoxia', *Blood*, **5**, 372–380.
6. Hodgson, G., Toha, J., and Gonzalez, E. (1952). 'Efecto de la inyección de orina de conejos sangrados repetidamente sobre la velocidad de regeneración de la hemoglobina en conejos anemizados', *Bol. Soc. Biol. Concepción*, **27**, 47.
7. Bernard, C. (1865). *An Introduction to the Study of Experimental Medicine*, (Translated by H. C. Greene), Henry Schuman, Inc., U.S.A. (1949).
8. Jourdanet, D. (1863). *De l'Anémie des Altitudes et de l'Anemia en Général dans ses Rapports avecla Pression de l'Atmosphere*, Paris, Bailliere, pp. 44.
9. Bert, P. (1878). *La Pression Barométrique: Recherches de Physiologie Expérimentale*. Paris, Masson. pp. 1168, (Translated by M. A. Hitchcock, and F. A. Hitchcock, Columbus, College Book Co. (1943), pp. 1055.
10. Viault, F. (1890). 'Sur l'augmentation considérable du nombre des globules ranges dans le sang chez les habitants des hautes plateaux de l'amerique du sud', *C. R. Acad. Sci., (Paris)*, **119**, 917–918.

11. Miescher, F. (1893). 'Über die beziehungen zwischen meereshohe und beschaffenheit des blutes', *Coor. Bltt. Schweizer Aerzte*, **24**, 809–830.
12. Jacobson, L. O., Goldwasser, E., Fried, W., and Plzak, L. (1957). 'Role of the kidney in erythropoiesis', *Nature*, **179**, 633–634.
13. Erslev, A. J. (1971). 'Feedback circuits in the control of stem cell differentiation', *Am. J. Path.*, **65**, 629–639.
14. Miyake, T., Kung, C. K.-H., and Goldwasser, E. (1977). 'Purification of human erythropoietin', *J. Biol. Chem.*, **252**, 5558–5564.
15. Erslev, A. J. (1977). 'Erythropoietin assay', in *Hematology* (Eds. W. J. Williams, E. Beutler, A. J. Erslev, and M. Lichtman) McGraw-Hill, New York, pp. 1616.
16. Erslev, A. J., Caro, J., Kansu, E., Miller, O. P., and Cobbs, E. (1979). 'Plasma erythropoietin in polycythemia', *Am. J. Med.*, **66**, 243–247.
17. Dunn, C. D. R., and Lange, R. D. (1980). 'Erythropoietin titers in normal human serum: An appraisal of assay techniques', *Exp. Hemat.*, **8**, 231–235.
18. Goldwasser, E., and Sherwood, J. B. (1981). 'Radioimmunoassay of erythropoietin', *Br. J. Haemat.*, **48**, 359–363.
19. Garcia, J. F., Sherwood, J. B., and Goldwasser, E. (1979). 'Radioimmune assay of erythropoietin', *Blood Cells*, **5**, 405–419.
20. Erslev, A. J. (1957). 'Observations on the nature of the erythropoietic factor. II. Erythropoietic activity of serum and bone marrow after time limited exposure to anemic and hypoxic anoxia', *J. Lab. Clin. Med.*, **50**, 543–549.
21. Goldwasser, E., Kung, C.K.-H. and Eliason, J. F. (1974). 'On the mechanism of erythropoietin-induced differentiation. XIII. The role of sialic acid in erythropoietic action', *J. Biol. Chem.*, **249**, 4202–4206.
22. Stohlman, F., Jr., and Brecher, G. (1959). 'Humoral regulation of erythropoiesis. V. Relationship of plasma erythropoietin level to bone marrow activity', *Proc. Soc. Exp. Biol. Med.*, **100**, 40–43.
23. Adamson, J. W., Alexanian, R., Martinez, C., and Finch, C. A. (1966). 'Erythropoietin excretion in normal man', *Blood*, **28**, 354–364.
24. Rosse, W. F., and Waldman, T. A. (1964). 'The metabolism of erythropoietin in patients with anemia due to deficient erythropoiesis', *J. Clin. Invest.*, **43**, 1348–1354.
25. Alpen, E. L. (1962). 'The metabolic fate of erythropoietin', in *Erythropoiesis* (Eds. L. O. Jacobson and M. Doyle) Grune and Stratton, New York, pp. 134–141.
26. Naets, J. P., and Wittek, M. (1974). 'Role of the kidney in the catabolism of erythropoietin in the rat', *J. Lab. Clin. Med.*, **84**, 99–106.
27. Contrera, J. F., Camiscoli, J. F., Weintraub, A. H., and Gordon, A. S. (1965). 'Extraction of erythropoietin from kidneys of hypoxic and phenylhydrazine treated rats', *Blood*, **25**, 809–816.
28. Contrera, J. F., Gordon, A. S., and Weintraub, A. H. (1966). 'Extraction of an erythropoietin-production factor from a particulate fraction of rat kidney', *Blood*, **28**, 330–343.
29. Erslev, A. J. (1974). '*In vitro* production of erythropoietin by kidney perfused with a serum-free solution', *Blood*, **44**, 77–85.
30. Fried, W., Barone-Varelas, J., and Berman, M. (1981). 'Detection of high erythropoietin titers in renal extracts of hypoxic rats', *J. Lab. Clin. Med.*, **97**, 82–86.
31. Erslev, A. J., Caro, J., Birgegard, G., Silver, R., and Miller, O. (1980). 'The biogenesis of erythropoietin', *Exp. Hemat.*, **8**, 1–11.
32. Jelkmann, W., and Bauer, L. (1981). 'Accumulation of erythropoietin in renal cortical cells during hypoxia', *Exp. Hemat.*, **9**, 89 (abstract).
33. Erslev, A. J., Kazal, L. A., and Miller, O. (1971). 'The action and neutralization of

a renal lipid inhibitor of erythropoietin', *Proc. Soc. Exp. Biol. Med.*, **138**, 1025–1029.

34. Mitus, W. J., Toyama, K., and Braner, M. J. (1968). 'Erythrocytosis, juxtaglomerular apparatus (JGA) and erythropoietin in the course of experimental unilateral hydronephrosis in rabbits', *Ann. N.Y. Acad. Sci.*, **149**, 107–113.

35. Hebbel, R. P., Eaton, J. W., Kronenberg, R. S., Zanjani, E. D., Moore, L. G., and Berger, E. M. (1978). 'Human llamas: Adaptation to altitude in subjects with high hemoglobin oxygen affinity', *J. Clin. Invest.*, **62**, 593–600.

36. Fried, W. (1972). 'The liver as a source of extrarenal erythropoietin production', *Blood*, **40**, 671–677.

37. Gruber, D. F., Zucali, J. R., and Mirand, E. A. (1977). 'Identification of erythropoietin-producing cells in fetal mouse liver culture', *Exp. Hemat.*, **5**, 392–398.

38. Erslev, A. J., Caro, J., Kansu, E., and Silver, R. (1980). 'Renal and extrarenal erythropoietin production in anaemic rats', *Br. J. Haemat.*, **45**, 65–72.

39. Naughton, B. A., Kaplan, S. M., Roy, M., Burdowski, A. J., Gordon, A. S., and Piliero, S. J. (1977). 'Hepatic regeneration and erythropoietin production in the rat', *Science*, **196**, 301–302.

40. Fried, W., Barone, J., Schade, S., and Anagnostou, A. (1979). 'Effect of carbon tetrachloride on extrarenal erythropoietin production in rats', *J. Lab. Clin. Med.*, **93**, 700–705.

41. Anagnostou, A., Vercellotti, G., Barone, J., and Fried, W. (1976). 'Factors which affect erythropoiesis in partially nephrectomized and sham-operated rats', *Blood*, **48**, 425–433.

42. Lucarelli, G., Porcellini, A., Carnevali, C., Carmena, A., and Stohlman, F., Jr. (1968). 'Fetal and neonatal erythropoiesis', *Ann. N.Y. Acad. Sci.*, **149**, 544–559.

43. Zanjani, E. D., Peterson, E. N., Gordon, A. S., and Wasserman, L. R. (1974). 'Erythropoietin production in the fetus: Role of the kidney and maternal anemia', *J. Lab. Clin. Med.*, **83**, 281–287.

44. Radtke, H. W., Rege, A. B., LaMarche, M. B., Bartos, D., Bartos, F., Campbell, R. A., and Fisher, J. W. (1981). 'Identification of spermine as an inhibitor of erythropoiesis in patients with chronic renal failure', *J. Clin. Invest.*, **67**, 1623–1629.

45. Caro, J., Brown, S., Miller, O., Murphy, T., and Erslev, A. J. (1979). 'Erythropoietin levels in uremic nephric and anephric patients', *J. Lab. Clin. Med.*, **93**, 449–458.

46. Utiger, R. (1980). 'Decreased extrathyroidal triiodothyronine production in non-thyroidal illness. Benefit or harm?'. *Am. J. Med.*, **69**, 807–810.

47. Caro, J., Silver, R., Erslev, A. J., Miller, O. P. and Birgegard G.: Erythropoietin production in fasted rats: Effect of thyroid hormones and glucose supplementation. *J. Lab. Clin. Med.* 98:860–868, 1981.

48. Eaves, C. J., and Eaves, A. C. (1978). 'Erythropoietin dose response curves for three classes of erythroid progenitors in normal human marrow and in patients with polycythemia vera', *Blood*, **52**, 1196–1210.

49. Iscove, N. N. (1977). 'The role of erythropoietin in regulation of population size and cell cycling of early and late erythroid precursors in mouse bone marrow', *Cell Tissue Kinet.*, **10**, 323–334.

50. Glass, J., Lavidor, L. M., and Robinson, S. H. (1975). 'Use of cell separation and short-term culture techniques to study erythroid cell development', *Blood*, **46**, 705–711.

51. Papayannopoulou, T., and Finch, C. A. (1975). 'Radioiron measurements of red cell maturation', *Blood Cells,* **1**, 535–546.
52. Chamberlain, J. K., LeBlond, P. F., and Weed, R. I. (1975). 'Reduction of adventitial cell cover: An early direct effect of erythropoietin on bone marrow ultrastructure', *Blood Cells,* **1**, 655–674.
53. Chang, S. C.-S., Sikkema, D., and Goldwasser, E. (1974). 'Evidence for an erythropoietin receptor protein on rat bone marrow cells',. *Biochem. Biophys. Res. Commun.,* **57**, 399–405.
54. Roodman, G. D., Spivak, J. L., and Zanjani, E. D. (1981). 'Stimulation of erythroid colony formation *in vitro* by erythropoietin immobilized on agarose-bound lectins', *J. Lab. Clin. Med.,* **98**, 684–690.
55. Brown, J. E., and Adamson, J. W. (1977). 'Modulation of *in vitro* erythropoiesis: The influence of β-adrenergic agonists on erythroid colony formation', *J. Clin. Invest.,* **60**, 70–77.
56. Golde, D., Bersch, N., Chopra, J., and Cline, M. J. (1977). 'Thyroid hormones stimulate erythropoiesis *in vitro*', *Br. J. Haemat.,* **37**, 173–177.
57. Moriyama, Y., and Fisher, J. W. (1975). 'Effects of testosterone and erythropoietin on erythroid colony formation in human bone marrow cultures', *Blood,* **45**, 665–670.
58. Caro, J., Erslev, A. J., Silver, R., Miller, O., and Birgegard, G. (1982) 'Erythropoietin production in response to anemia or hypoxia in the newborn rat', *Blood*, (in press).

Current Concepts in Erythropoiesis
Edited by C. D. R. Dunn
© 1983 John Wiley & Sons Ltd.

CHAPTER 2

Cell amplification in erythro-poiesis: in vitro perspectives

FRANCIS C. MONETTE
Department of Biology
Boston University
Boston, U.S.A.

Contents

I. INTRODUCTION

It has only been within the last ten years or so that significant strides have been made in the analysis of red blood cell (RBC) production at the cellular level. This has largely been due to the availability of *in vitro* clonal cell assays which were pioneered by members of Axelrad's laboratory in Toronto (1–3). Much of the experimental work since that time has necessarily focused on the physiological factors and the environmental conditions controlling the growth of early erythrocytic progenitors *in vitro*. As a result, our understanding of erythrocytic regulatory mechanisms has been substantially advanced. Some groups have also endeavoured to obtain information on the cellular kinetics of early erythrocytic cell differentiation. This could only be attempted when all the major cell participants in this differentiation pathway were well-characterized. An analysis of the cellular proliferation kinetics of the morphologically non-recognizable erythron now appears feasible and this chapter will attempt to outline some of the relevant observations made in this field of study. The cellular kinetics of the morphologically-identifiable erythron have already been extensively detailed (for reviews, see references 4–7). No attempt will be made to reiterate this here except as it pertains to the non-recognizable erythron and its kinetics. Likewise, much has been learned about the kinetics of pluripotential hematopoietic stem cells, which serve as antecedents of the earliest erythrocytic progenitors. The reader is referred to more in-depth reviews on hematopoietic stem cells (6, 8–12).

II. MURINE ERYTHROPOIESIS: THE *IN VIVO* PERSPECTIVE

Of the myriad of experimental studies on erythropoiesis *in vivo*, three approaches in particular have proved particularly insightful. With the availability of cell and phase-specific radio-labeled tracers (i.e., ^{3}H-TdR, ^{55}Fe, ^{59}Fe), analyses into the proliferation kinetics of complex cell populations first became experimentally feasible. For example, the experiments of Bond *et al.* (13) and Alpen and Cranmore (14) were among the first to analyze the flow of erythrocytic cells through the morphological erythron and reveal estimates of actual cell-cycle durations. This kinetic approach was later refined by Lord (15) and Blackett and his co-workers (5). Another cell kinetics approach involved the application of erythropoietin (EPO) to animals whose endogenous hormone production had been suppressed by prior exposure to hypoxia or by hypertransfusion with homologous erythrocytes. Under these conditions, an EPO injection produces a prompt erythrocytic response, whether measured by radio-iron incorporation or enumeration of marrow RBC precursors or blood reticulocytes, which is well above the levels seen in plethoric controls. Such studies led to the notion of an EPO-responsive cell compartment which precedes the earliest morphologically-recognizable erythroblast (16, 17). These sorts of studies also led to the hypothesis that EPO might act *directly* on the hematopoietic stem cell, as this cell was thought to differentiate directly into the pronormoblast upon stimulation by EPO (18). The third experimental approach provided evidence against this latter hypothesis. In 1961, Till and McCulloch (19) developed a clonal transplantation assay which has become accepted as a quantitative measure of pluripotential hematopoietic stem cells.

The assay is based on the injection of limiting numbers of stem cells into lethally-irradiated mice. Following a suitable growth interval (i.e., 8–13 days), macroscopic nodules form on the surface of the spleen which contain at least three different hematopoietic cell lines (i.e., erythrocytic, granulocytic, and megakaryocytic). The definition of the cell which forms hematopoietic colonies is therefore an operational one, and the cell which can potentially produce a colony is referred to as the colony-forming cell, or CFC. Those CFC which actually produce nodules, are designated the colony-forming unit-spleen (or CFU-S).

The application of this assay to studies of erythropoiesis revealed that, in the short term, manipulation of the erythron had little, if any, direct effect upon the stem cell itself, and that erythrocytic differentiation can only be elicited by the action of EPO on an intermediate cell type which has become known as the EPO-responsive cell (or ERC) (20). An initial view of the structure of the erythron, based on experimental work performed *in vivo*, is shown in Figure 1. Since the mid-sixties, the model has been substantially modified to take into account a number of additional observations. The studies of Morse *et al.* (21) suggested that ERC cycled (~20% in S-phase) even in erythropoietically-suppressed rodents and the work of Lajtha *et al.* (22) implied that the cycling level of these cells was more extensive (~70%). As Kubanek *et al.* (23) point out, these two values may represent an underestimate and overestimate, respectively, of ERC cycling. In any case, the turnover of these cells is undoubtedly substantially more than that observed for pluripotential stem cells (0–20% in S-phase). Another important observation on ERC kinetics was made by Reissmann and his co-workers (24, 25), as well as others (26) who showed that EPO, in addition to stimulating ERC to differentiate into proerythroblasts, can also have an amplifying effect on the early ERC compartment. This cellular amplification results in the subsequent expansion of the ERC population. Thus, the *in vivo* role of EPO appears to be two-fold in that it augments: (1) the *differentiation* of (late) ERC, and (2) the *proliferation* of their immediate precursors. Such data fit into the ERC 'age structure' hypothesis proposed by Lajtha *et al.* (27). In their model, 'pre-ERC' were cells which, although committed to erythrocytic development, could not respond to EPO stimulation without further maturation and proliferation. Some additional work, employing a different experimental approach, measures the 'erythrocytic repopulating ability' (ERA) of marrow preparations following transfusion into irradiated mice (28–30). The discontinuity in recovery between CFU-S and ERA is usually taken as evidence for the dissimilarity between the cell-types responsible for CFU-S and ERA. It has also been shown (30) that ERA may be readily distinguished from ERC by their differences in cell kinetics. Milenkovic and Pavlovic-Kentera (30) have therefore suggested that the cell type responsible for ERA precedes ERC in differentiation, although the precise relationship of these cell-types to

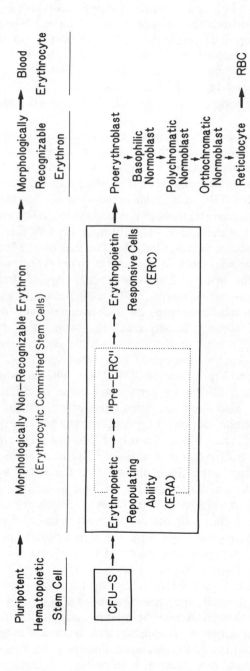

Figure 1. The cellular organization of the erythron derived from experimental work *in vivo*. See text and references 6–8, 11, 28–30 for more details

'pre-ERC' remains moot at this time. The schema in Figure 1 summarizes our present understanding of the plausible cellular make-up of the morphologically non-recognizable erythron.

A. Amplifications in erythropoiesis

By employing ^{55}Fe and following the rate at which labeled RBC enter the circulation, Tarbutt (31) estimated the cell flow into the blood of the rodent to be ~ 5.8×10^8 per day. Another estimate of daily cell production rate can be obtained by measuring the rate at which cells leave the circulation (e.g., the mean RBC lifespan). The average lifespan of blood erythrocytes in the mouse is about 35 days, thus, one can estimate a daily rate of cell loss to be ~ 4.5×10^8 (6). Since under steady-state conditions, production must balance loss, this measure of cell loss is also equivalent to the daily production rate. The two estimates of erythrocyte production rates are very similar, given the totally different experimental approaches for their measurement. One might now ask an important question. How many pluropotential stem cells are needed to maintain this daily erythrocyte production rate? or, to put it another way, how many stem cell divisions are required to produce (on the average) 5.2×10^8 erythrocytes daily? To attempt an answer to this, which would provide an estimate of the amplification potential of the stem cell, we need an estimate of the *total number* of stem cells in the mouse. Since, at present, the Till and McCulloch (19) assay provides the only reliable quantitative assay for measuring pluropotential hematopoietic stem cells, the query relates to the total number of cells which have spleen colony-forming ability (CFC). This can be approximated by first determining the number of CFU-S in a marrow cell preparation and extrapolating to the total number per tibia or femur. For C57B1/6 mice (and many other murine strains) this value ranges between 3,000 and 4,000 CFU-S per femur. However, only a small fraction of injected stem cells are actually detected by spleen colony formation. Correction for the *in vivo* efficiency of this assay (about 12%) gives a more accurate measure of the total number of femoral stem cells (i.e., $25–30 \times 10^3$). The fraction of the total marrow mass which a femur represents is about 0.05. Thus, a calculation of the total body marrow stem cell population yields a value of about $5–6 \times 10^5$ per mouse. This is similar to the 10^6 estimate calculated by Schofield and Lajtha (6) but the total body number is actually slightly more if one includes the spleen as an important extra-medullary source of stem cells (approximately 5×10^4 additional stem cells). A whole-body value of 6×10^5 will therefore be employed in all the following calculations.

Since we are trying to obtain an estimate of the amplification capacity of stem cells, we also need to approximate their daily production rate. Unfortunately, there are no direct methods for doing this, owing to our inability to identify these cells directly. Therefore, available estimates of stem cell turnover are indirect at best and subject to wide fluctuation (e.g. see Table 4). One approximation of stem cell turnover can be obtained from the proportion of cycling stem cells in normal animals. A short exposure to cytotoxic levels of ^{3}H-TdR or hydroxyurea *in vivo* will reduce the numbers of CFU-S in a cell preparation by the fraction of cells in DNA-synthesis (32). Although this fraction appears to vary according to the mouse strain employed (33) (or even the general health of the animals) and must be carefully analyzed statistically (34), a stem cell cycling level in the range 5–20% is usually observed in normal animals (an average value of 10% will be used here). A third parameter which is necessary for calculating a stem cell turnover rate is the length of the cell cycle. Since this cannot yet be determined directly, one must employ indirect estimates such as those obtained by following cell population doubling times within individual spleen colonies. Schofield and Lajtha (35) demonstrated that individual CFU-S undergo between 17 and 18 cell doublings during the first six days following cell injection into lethally-irradiated assay animals, which led them to estimate an average doubling time of about 7–8 hours. This is so short that it must be considered equivalent to the cell generation (or cycle) time (T_c). However, it must be noted that the irradiated mouse should be considered as providing an absolutely *maximal* stimulating environment for hematopoietic cell replication. Therefore, the relationship of this short stem cell cycle time to that occurring under steady-state conditions is unknown (presumably it would be much longer in normal animals). Schofield and Lajtha calculated (6) a first approximation of the total number of cycling stem cells in the normal mouse and obtained a value of 2×10^5 CFC cycling per day. Interestingly, new approaches to the kinetic analysis of hematopoietic stem cells suggest that this daily cycling value may correctly approximate the normal cycling rate of marrow stem cells. For example, two separate groups (36, 37) have employed a totally novel method of addressing the problem of stem cell turnover. They exposed murine marrow cells *in vivo* over a continuous period to the light-sensitive halogenated pyrimidine 5-bromodeoxyuridine (BRdU) which is taken up by DNA-synthesizing cells. Subsequently, the cells were exposed *in vitro* to near-UV light which resulted in the elimination of only those cells containing the substituted base. Extrapolation to controls over a given exposure period allows an estimate of the average stem cell entry rate into DNA synthesis. Both groups observed that *most* (i.e. 90–95%) of the marrow stem cells turnover within an approximate two-day (37) to more than six-day (36) period, strongly suggesting a kinetically active cell compartment in normal animals. For example, from the work of Hagan and MacVittie (37), it is possible to estimate a daily turnover of approximately 37% of the marrow stem cell pool. Assuming a constant rate of cell-cycle progression throughout the day (which was, in fact, suggested by both BrdU studies), this means that on the average 2.2×10^5 CFC (i.e. $0.37 \times 6 \times 10^5$) are available for use each day. This value is not unlike previous estimates of stem cell turnover rates (6).

However, on the average only half of these cells would be available for differentiation into blood cells since Vogel *et al.* (38) and others have shown that normally at least half (actually about 0.6) of the stem cells produced in the mouse are retained within the stem cell compartments. This is essential for the maintenance of the steady state. One must note though, that this fraction is usually obtained under experimental conditions and may not actually apply to the situation in normal marrow except as a crude mathematical approximation (39). When this correction for the actual number of stem cells available for differentiation is made an over-all value of 1.1×10^5 stem cells per day is obtained (i.e. $2.2 \times 10^5 \times 0.5$).

The end result of these mathematical 'games' is an approximation of the amplification which stem cells undergo during their differentiation into blood cells in the marrow. If 1.1×10^5 stem cells are available for differentiation daily and half of these enter the erythrocytic pathway, then 5.5×10^4 stem cells produce, on the average, 5.2×10^8 erythrocytes daily. This results in an over-all amplification factor of 9,455 which extrapolates to about 13 cell division cycles. Schofield and Lajtha (6) calculated a very similar value.

Now we must ask where these amplification divisions are located in the pathway of erythrocytic differentiation between the stem cell and the last dividing erythroblast. Experiments *in vivo* provide a partial answer. In their analysis of cell population kinetics of recognizable erythrocytic cells, Tarbutt and Blackett (5) compared the results obtained in rats employing ^{3}H-TdR autoradiography and ^{55}Fe labeling and autoradiography. Their best-fit estimates produced the data summarized in Table 1. The total number of mitoses observed within the recognizable erythron was 6.6. Lord (8) effectively argues that this estimate depends somewhat on short-term measures and is consequently biased in favor of the more rapidly cycling cells in the population. Therefore, one should probably consider these values as maximal estimates. In fact, the work of Covelli *et al.* (40), which employed corrections for ^{55}Fe labeling curves, suggested a proerythroblast cell-cycle time of 24.8 hours and an average number of only 1.5 cell cycles within this single morphologically-re-cognizable cellular compartment. Earlier estimates emphasized the variability of the cell-cycle number in the recognizable erythron (14, 41) ranging between three and five cell divisions in total. Obviously, then, a unanimity of opinions does not exist on the total number of cell divisions within the recognizable erythron. The range of suggested values (three to six divisions) may also reflect a variety of physiological states. An average value of four cell divisions within the recognizable erythron shall be assumed for the subsequent calculations of total erythrocytic amplification. In this context, it is noteworthy that Bessis *et al.* (42) demonstrated an average of four mitotic events when erythrocytic marrow cells were followed directly *in vitro*.

We are now faced with the following situation with regard to amplification within the erythron;

Table 1. Kinetic parameters of morphologically-recognizable erythrocytic cells in the rat*

Measured parameter	Pro-erythroblast	Basophilic normoblast	Polychromatic normoblast	All erythroid
Hourly birth rate (as fraction of total cells)	0.07	0.06	0.05	0.053
Average number of cell cycles	2.9	2.1	1.6	6.6
Transit time (hours)	28	23	18	69
Average cell-cycle time (T_c) (hours)	—	9.9	11.0	—

* Adapted from references (5) and (8).

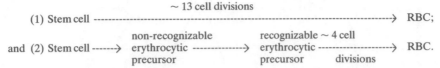

Thus, we must try to account for the cellular basis for the approximately nine remaining cell divisions in the erythrocytic pathway. This has proved all but impossible to approach experimentally *in vivo* although gallant attempts have been made. Presumably, the residual nine cell divisions are a property of the cellular compartments responsible for EPO responsiveness and ERA (Figure 1) but any further analysis in the intact animal is not feasible without specific cell assays (6, 8, 43). Since the cells which respond to EPO by producing hemoglobin-synthesizing cells are detected only subsequent to the synthesis of hemoglobin and thus following a long time delay, they cannot be measured directly *in vivo* with present experimental techniques. Although this fact has been one of the major drawbacks in further kinetic investigations of erythropoiesis under *in vivo* conditions, it has also served as a major impetus for the development of specific erythrocytic cell assays. These have all evolved within the last decade and are all based on the clonal growth of primitive erythrocytic progenitors *in vitro*.

III. MURINE ERYTHROPOIESIS: THE *IN VITRO* PERSPECTIVE

The development of clonal cell assays for discrete stages of mammalian erythrocytic cell differentiation rapidly followed the initial reports of the successful growth of early erythrocytic progenitors in semi-solid cultures (2, 3). The following is a brief over-view of our present knowledge of erythropoiesis based on these clonal cell assays. [The reader is referred to Chapters 1, 4, and 7 for a more-detailed review (see also 43, 44).] The early reports from the Toronto group (2, 45) established the *in vitro* assay for mature-type cellular units with colony-forming ability (termed; CFU-E). These colony-forming cells rapidly develop into hemoglobin-synthesizing cells in the presence of exogenous EPO. Cormack (46) showed with reverse microcinematography that CFU-E divided once or twice before commencing hemoglobin synthesis and assuming the morphological appearance of typical erythroblasts. Later (3) Axelrad's group described a second erythrocytic cell type which formed large, diffuse colonies in culture but required high concentrations of EPO and longer (i.e., 7+ days) incubation periods for their full manifestation *in vitro*. These have been commonly referred to as erythrocytic 'burst-forming units' (BFU-E) and are usually designated according to the length of their *in vitro* growth period, i.e., day 7 BFU-E, day 10 BFU-E, etc. Since then, a cellular differentiation stage intermediate between BFU-E and CFU-E has been described *in vitro* (47; day 3–4 BFU-E),

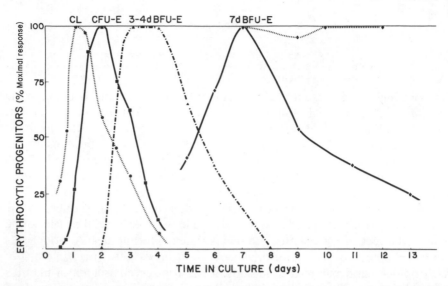

Figure 2. *In vitro* growth curves of four classes of erythrocytic progenitors. Data obtained from the following: reference 62 (clusters and CFU-E); 47 (day 3–4 BFU-E); 47 and 84 (day 7+ BFU-E). Day 3–4 BFU-E are termed as such since they maintain similar levels *in vitro* on either day. Two colony responses for day 7 BFU-E are shown. Solid line, growth in plasma clot without exogenous BPA (84); dotted line, the cumulative colony growth in methylcellulose cultures in the presence or absence of BPA (47). Growth of CFU-mix or 'macrobursts' is not shown

as well as one which probably precedes day 7 BFU-E (48, referred to as 'macrobursts') and another which follows CFU-E in differentiation (49, erythrocytic-clusters). Thus, it is now readily apparent that erythropoiesis in the mouse as well as in man (50) is characterized by a spectrum of cellular subtypes which demonstrate tremendous heterogeneity not only in their time of appearance *in vitro* (Figure 2), but also in their EPO requirements and over-all colony size. These and other properties have helped re-shape our thinking of the cellular make-up of the non-recognizable erythron, and more importantly, have allowed us to address experimental questions which were not possible just a few years ago. Table 2 summarizes some of the more important biological properties of primitive erythrocytic precursors for which specific clonal cell assays are available. Some salient properties will be discussed briefly below.

A. Late (mature) erythrocytic colony-forming cells

The cells responsible for the formation of small erythrocytic colonies (i.e., CFU-E) have a limited capacity for proliferation as evidenced by the range of cell numbers found in these colonies (eight to about 64 per colony) and from the fact that further incubation beyond the two-day optimum does not result in an increase in the average colony size. CFU-E average between twelve and 17 cells per colony (2) and thus undergo 3.5–4.0 cell divisions during their 48-hour culture period. In both plasma and methylcellulose culture systems, murine marrow CFU-E attain maximal efficiency between 400–500 per 10^5 nucleated cells at EPO concentrations ranging from 0.05 units/ml (44) to about 0.25 units/ml. Guilbert and Iscove (51) showed that the serum requirement of CFU-E could be reduced 100-fold with the addition of albumin, transferrin, selenium, and phospholipid. Under such conditions, and with the addition of inhibitor-free EPO preparations as well as growth-promoting thiols at very low concentrations ($< 5 \times 10^{-4}$ M) (52), the frequency of CFU-E can be increased to $\sim 600/10^5$ (53). The clonal origin of CFU-E has been demonstrated by time-lapse microcinematography in the mouse (46) and by isoenzyme markers in man (54). Gregory and her co-workers (55, 56) have shown both the lack of correlation between CFU-S and CFU-E within individual spleen colonies and the close correlation between CFU-E and morphologically recognizable erythrocytic precursors, thus placing CFU-E near the terminal stages of differentiation of the non-recognizable erythron. However, it is clear from the work of Cormack (46) and others (49, 57) that CFU-E are removed from proerythroblasts by one or more cell divisions and cannot, therefore be considered identical to these cells.

In sharp contrast to earlier stages of progenitor cell differentiation, the population size of CFU-E is largely regulated by EPO. Hypertransfusion-induced plethora, which profoundly lowers plasma EPO levels, reduces the size of the marrow CFU-E compartment by $\sim 70\%$ but leaves unchanged the *in vitro* EPO requirements of the remaining 30% CFU-E fraction (58). Likewise, administration of partially 'purified' EPO preparations or the induction of an anemic state in intact mice greatly augments marrow (and splenic) CFU-E levels (55, 59, 60). The requirement of CFU-E for exogenous EPO *in vitro* appears absolute since few colonies form in its absence and colony numbers are diminished greatly when EPO is withheld for even brief periods (61). Although EPO appears to regulate the population size of CFU-E, it does not seem essential for maintaining the CFU-E cycling rate *in vivo* since nearly the same proportion of CFU-E is cycling in normal, regenerating, and plethoric marrow preparations (59). Nor does EPO usually affect the over-all size of CFU-E colonies *in vitro* (62) although it may under some specific growth conditions (63). Since the fraction of CFU-E in S-phase of the cell cycle can be shown by both ^{3}H-TdR (59, 60) and hydroxyurea 'suicide' (62) to be very high (70–75%), a high cycling rate for these cells is also inferred. Cormack (46) showed that first-to-third generation cells derived from CFU-E had an average T_c ranging from 7.6 hours to 11 hours. In another study, Wagemaker and Visser (64) observed the rate of increase in modal cell volumes following hydroxyurea administration and calculated a CFU-E cell-cycle duration of

Table 2. Physical and biological characteristics of primitive murine marrow erythrocytic progenitor cells detected by clonal cell assays

Characteristic	Pluripotential stem cell	Burst-forming cells			Colony-forming cell	Cluster-forming cell
		Macro	Primitive (Early)	Mature (Late)		
Abbreviation	CFU-S	Macro-burst	Day 7+ BFU-E	Day 3–4 BFU-E	CFU-E	Cluster-forming cell
Assay interval	9–11 days (*in vivo*)	9–14 days (*in vitro*)	7–14 days (*in vitro*)	3–4 days (*in vitro*)	2 days (*in vitro*)	1 day (*in vitro*)
Scoring criteria	Macroscopic Surface Colony	Macroscopic Red Colony	50–200 cells	3+ colony clusters	8+ cells	2–7 cells
Incidence (No/10^5 nucleated cells)	20–40	5–10	up to 100–125	50–80	400–600	$12–16 \times 10^2$
Proliferative capacity (No. cells/colony)	$0.2–16 \times 10^6$	$0.3–12 \times 10^5$	5×10^1– 10^4–10^5	24–150	8–64	2–7
% In S-phase	5–20%	?	15–25	50–65	70–77	75–85
Average number cell divisions per colony	20 (if 10^6 cells)	18 (2×10^5)	9 (5×10^2)	5–6	3.5–4	2

Cell size:						
A) modal velocity sedimentation (in mm/hr)	4.0	?	4.0	4.4	6.4–7.4	5.9
B) Modal cell diameter in G_1 (in μm)	7.0	—	7.0	7.6	10–13	N.D.
Buoyant density (g/cm^3)	1.070	?	1.070	N.D.	1.077	?
Erythropoietin sensitivity* (units/ml)	? none	0.5 (+)	0.5 (+)	0.05–0.4 (++)	0.04 (+++)	0.01 (++++)
Requirement for burst-promoting activity (BPA)	– – – –	(++++)	(++)	(±)	(±)	(±)

* Defined as the amount of the hormone needed to obtain 50% of the maximal response under optimal *in vitro* conditions. Observed variations are also due to the differences between plasma clot and methylcellulose assay systems.

N.D., Not determined.

about seven hours. The rapid turnover of CFU-E is therefore strongly supported by these studies. The heterogeneity of CFU-E has long been implied, not only from the wide variation in cell number per colony (2) but also by the width of EPO dose/response curves (52, 65). The reasons for this heterogeneity are not fully explained, but may be due in part to prior EPO exposure *in vivo* as well as to a limited coupling of cell-cycle position to EPO sensitivity (58). Interestingly, Kennedy *et al*. (66) postulate the existence of a minor CFU-E subpopulation which requires only a very short exposure to EPO for full colony expression. That CFU-E are not identical with proerythroblasts was first indicated by the work of Cormack (46) and more recently by work from my laboratory (49, 57, 67). Since the criteria for scoring CFU-E arbitrarily sets a threshold at eight or more cells per colony, we attempted to characterize erythrocytic clusters containing fewer than eight cells. Two important observations were made. First, clusters attained optimal numbers after only a 24-hr incubation period and their marrow frequency was found to be three-times as great as CFU-E (i.e., 1200 per 10^5 *vs* 400 per 10^5). This suggested to us the possibility that erythrocytic cluster-forming cells were further along the erythrocytic differentiation pathway than CFU-E; a conclusion which was more directly demonstrated in subsequent experiments (57). Secondly, cluster-forming cells are characterized by an EPO sensitivity which is at least four-fold greater than that of CFU-E. Thus, these cells can be considered as progeny of CFU-E although perhaps intermediate with proerythroblasts, since the latter have a greater marrow frequency and show different kinetic patterns following manipulations of the erythron (57).

The late stages of erythrocytic progenitor cell differentiation can therefore be envisioned as a cellular continuum characterized by increasing sensitivity to EPO (*in vitro* and *in vivo*), a decreasing proliferative capacity (although a high proliferative rate), and a fairly high frequency in normal marrow.

B. Early (primitive) erythrocytic colony-forming cells

The growth of primitive BFU-E *in vitro* has proved to be more demanding than CFU-E owing largely to their specific growth requirements which only recently have been systematically explored. Although Axelrad *et al*. (3) first reported the high EPO requirements of these cells *in vitro*, it was only later appreciated that it was a factor(s) within the crude EPO preparation, and not the EPO itself, that was responsible for the early growth of BFU-E *in vitro*. This factor(s) has become known as 'burst-promoting (or enhancing) activity (or factor)' (thus, BPA or BEF). Two critical observations, one *in vivo* the other *in vitro*, demonstrated the relative EPO-independence of BFU-E. Both Iscove (59) and Hara and Ogawa (60) reported that marrow BFU-E do not decline in plethoric mice, thus establishing their EPO-independence *in vivo*. Iscove (61) likewise showed that BFU-E could be maintained *in vitro* and continue to produce nucleated cell progeny in the absence of exogenous EPO. Presumably, EPO is needed only for the terminal stages of BFU-E differentiation which lead to the induction of hemoglobin synthesis (61). Nevertheless, the Naples group (68, 69) has shown that early fluctuations in BFU-E pool size do occur after erythrocyte transfusion or the administration of a 'purified' EPO preparation, this effect probably being mediated via BFU-E cycling. In contrast to the relative EPO-independence of BFU-E *in vitro*, Iscove (61) also showed an $\sim 80\%$ reduction in BFU-E growth when cells were deprived of BPA for two or more days, thus suggesting the *in vitro* requirement of these cells for this factor(s). This might explain why burst growth is so critically dependent on the serum used for culture, BPA-poor sera yielding low BFU-E growth. Serum does not appear to be the only source of BPA since Aye (70) demonstrated that conditioned medium derived from human peripheral blood leukocytes could enhance marrow burst growth. Other sources of BPA include lectin-stimulated spleen cell conditioned medium (71) and 1500 R-irradiated marrow cell feeder layers (72, 73). The physiological nature of this material is suggested from its presence in the sera of anemic mice (72) and humans with bone marrow aplasia (74), and its relative specificity for earlier burst forms than the mature bursts, CFU-E or non-erythrocytic cells (61, 75, 76). In the presence of BPA, BFU-E growth *in vitro* increases over a wide EPO dose range, and some groups report a reduction in the amount of EPO required for full maturation *in vitro* (61, 73, 74). In fact, in the presence of BPA, Wagemaker (77) observed that BFU-E levels plateaued at about 1 unit EPO/ml and the cell dose/response curve extrapolated to the origin (73), two findings which have yet to be seen by others (75). These data seem to imply that the number of BFU-E detected in culture as well as their sensitivity to EPO is directly related to the BPA concentration. The active component in BPA preparations appears to be a glycoprotein with a molecular weight in the 24,000–35,000 D range (61, 75). Wagemaker (75) has been successful in purifying BPA 600-fold with gel filtration on Sephadex G-150. While further characterization and purification of BPA will be necessary to establish its full chemical identity, some preliminary work on the cell types which produce this factor has already been accomplished. Wagemaker (77) showed that BPA was associated with a non-dividing population of murine bone marrow cells with a fairly homogeneous buoyant density of 1.083 g/cm^3 which was quite distinct from BFU-E. This group has also produced evidence that the BPA-associated (producing?) cell may have phagocytic properties (78). BPA would therefore appear to be a necessary factor for the growth of primitive erythrocytic precursors *in vitro*. Whether or not BFU-E actually express EPO receptors is not yet known but it is clear that they can produce progeny that do, so that an early increase in EPO receptors may represent one of the first discernable steps in erythropoietic cell differentiation (44). (See Chapters 3, 4, and 14 for further discussion regarding the properties of BPA).

Given the optimal growth conditions for BFU-E as defined above, it should be possible to learn something about the growth kinetics of these cells. Iscove and Sieber (52) suggested that BFU-E colonies may contain from 50 cells to 10^4 cells, but it is now clear that under certain conditions, burst-like colonies appear in culture containing 10^6 cells or more (79). These colonies, which can achieve macroscopic proportions, have been called 'uncommitted' or 'macroscopic' bursts (48) and evidence has been presented for their pluripotentiality. Other groups have also detailed similar mixed colonies *in vitro* (71, 80, 81). The existence of mixed colonies raises several important questions regarding the nature of the cells giving rise to such colonies. First, are the colonies clonal in origin? Second, what factors underlie colony heterogeneity and can they be controlled so as to give reproducible assay results? Although large burst colonies are very diffuse in appearance and often contain two or more differentiated cell types (although most are predominantly erythrocytic), their clonal origin has been demonstrated by several groups. Johnson and Metcalf (71) showed with single-cell transfer experiments that fetal liver BFU-E are derived from a single cell. The following year Strome *et al.* (82) confirmed the clonal nature of marrow-derived BFU-E by evaluating individual bursts for the presence of the Y-chromosome in cultures seeded with mixtures of male and female cells. Lastly, Hara and Noguchi (83) have recently performed single-cell transfer experiments of separated murine marrow cells in which they were also able to demonstrate the clonal origin of mixed colonies. Regarding the heterogeneity of bursts, most groups describe similar *in vitro* requirements for their growth: a source of BPA, EPO (usually at concentrations of 1 or more units/ml), and long culture intervals (7–14 days). Mixed burst formation usually requires the longer time intervals, and the growth of 'macrobursts' appears to require nearly two full weeks (76). Thus, clonal cell assays now appear available for the *in vitro* growth of all stages of erythrocytic differentiation.

Most workers report that a minimum of seven days in culture is required for optimal burst growth (Figure 2). However, under some culture conditions this growth peak is followed by an abrupt decline (84) as in the assay of other erythrocytic progenitors, whereas in other culture systems, most notably methylcellulose, BFU-E tend to be maintained following day 7 or only show a modest decline in number (47) (Figure 2). In our hands (84), day 7 BFU-E do not increase in size with further culturing as some have reported (63) and the colonies tend to be predominantly erythrocytic in their make-up. Colonies of this sort are usually scored by applying a low threshold of > 50 cells per colony, although some groups score > 200 cells. The upper range in cell number may average in the order of 10^3 cells although colonies of 10^4 or more have been scored. An average of ~ 500 cells/colony would appear typical for day 7 bursts, so these colony-forming cells probably undergo at least nine cell divisions during the seven-day culture period. The growth potential of day

7 BFU-E is therefore considerably more than what is observed for CFU-E colonies (Table 2). However, the proliferative capacity of cells responsible for large, mixed colonies or 'macrobursts' far outstrip that of day 7 BFU-E. For example, Humphries *et al*. (76) have shown upper size limits of 1.2×10^6 cells per colony for 10–14 day 'macrobursts'. Assuming an average colony size of 2×10^5 cells, this would amount to ~ 18 cell divisions. Thus, the separation in proliferative capacity between day 7 BFU-E and 'macrobursts' appears to be greater than between day 7 BFU-E and CFU-E. Bursts must therefore be considered very heterogeneous with regard to their proliferative capacity *in vitro*. This heterogeneity may suggest that additional steps in cell differentiation occur between 'macrobursts' and day 7 BFU-E. One such category of events is undoubtedly the restriction in cellular differentiation, i.e., commitment to erythropoiesis. The frequency of primitive bursts in murine marrow is variable, owing to the variability in culture conditions. However, an incidence of up to 100 (day 10) BFU-E per 10^5 cells has been reported when irradiated feeder cells are employed as the BPA source (73) although the usually observed range is ~ 35–$55/10^5$ marrow cells. Recently, we have also shown that modulation of the culture environment can raise the efficiency of (day 7) BFU-E to about $100/10^5$ cells (84). In contrast to day 7 BFU-E, 'macrobursts' are thus far characterized by a rather low plating efficiency of about 5–$10/10^5$ in spite of the fact that marrow subpopulations are preselected for growth in flask cultures and the 'macrobursts' are grown in the presence of lectin-stimulated cell conditioned media plus irradiated marrow feeder cells (79). The turnover of erythrocytic bursts has been measured by standard 'suicide' experiments by short exposures to cytotoxic doses of ^{3}H-TdR or hydroxyurea. Although early reports employing *in vitro* ^{3}H-TdR suicide indicated that about 30–40% of normal marrow BFU-E were in S-phase (59, 60, 85), the work of Suzuki and Axelrad (86) suggests that this moderate rate of BFU-E cycling might apply only to certain murine strains and that a quiescent (86) or a low cycling state (i.e., 15–20%) might apply to other murine strains (73, 87, 88). It is therefore not surprising that a profound stimulation of the hematopoietic system will produce an increase (albeit often transient) in the proportion of BFU-E in cycle. For example, although neither Iscove (59) nor Hara and Ogawa (60) observed any substantial change in BFU-E cycling following the induction of acute anemia, Adamson *et al*. (85), in contrast, saw a 75% increase in the BFU-E cycling level following an acute bleeding and we (89) have observed a nearly three-fold cycling increase ($20 \rightarrow 60\%$) in BDF_1 mice treated with phenylhydrazine. However, the increase in cycling is transient, occurring only on certain days following the erythropoietic stimulus. Likewise, BFU-E can be shown to be maximally cycling in regenerating marrow (59, 87). Peschle *et al*. (90) have pointed out the transient nature of the BFU-E cycling patterns following erythrocytic perturbations and suggest that BFU-E cycling is correlated with their over-all pool size. If this is indeed the case, the

mechanism controlling BFU-E proliferation must itself be finely tuned to account for such abrupt changes in cell cycling.

The length of time needed to fully express erythrocytic bursts *in vitro*, their extensive proliferative capacity, and their ability to modulate their cycling suggests a close relationship with the most primitive hematopoietic cell progenitors. When one compares the numbers of CFU-S and BFU-E within a single spleen colony, a correlation is obtained between these two cell types which is as good as a comparison between CFU-S/CFU-S (56). These results therefore confirm the notion that BFU-E are closely related to pluripotential stem cells. Large macroscopic bursts and colonies which contain two or more cell types may indeed prove to be identical with spleen colony-forming cells as some authors have argued. Recent evidence for this possibility has come from the Vancouver group (79), who demonstrated that 'macrobursts' fulfill two important stem cell properties: first, and most important, macroscopic bursts are capable of self-renewal, i.e., the replating of primary colonies will produce (about 30% of the time) large, secondary colonies which themselves resemble macroscopic bursts. This is in marked contrast to all other erythrocytic colonies. Secondly, macroscopic bursts contain cells capable of spleen colony-formation (i.e., CFU-S). These studies therefore provide strong support for the likelihood that the culture of macroscopic bursts will provide an *in vitro* assay for pluripotential stem cells which are at a similar (or identical) state of differentiation as spleen colony-forming cells.

In 1976 Gregory (47) described an *in vitro* class of erythrocytic progenitor cells which appeared intermediate between CFU-E and the large, diffuse bursts which had been previously described. She referred to these as day 3 BFU-E thus reflecting their optimal growth period *in vitro*, and presented several lines of data for considering these cells as a distinct stage in erythrocytic differentiation. In addition to their intermediate growth kinetics in culture, day 3 BFU-E fell between CFU-E and day 8 BFU-E in EPO sensitivity, and perhaps more convincingly, Gregory showed that the correlation between CFU-S and day 3 BFU-E in spleen colonies was substantially less than observed for CFU-S and day 8 BFU-E. Lastly, an intermediate cell-cycling level for day 3 BFU-E has also been reported (73, 87, 88). However, the physiological significance of these erythrocytic progenitors is still to be fully appreciated. Since CFU-E are reduced by about 70% in plethoric animals it has often been suggested that EPO-responsive cells must therefore precede CFU-E in differentiation. Although day 3 BFU-E were initially thought to be independent of EPO *in vivo* (88), subsequent studies have shown a 40–50% reduction in plethoric animals (57, 85, 87). Thus, the population sizes of CFU-E, and to some degree day 3 BFU-E, are EPO-dependent. In regenerating marrow, however, the increase in both day 3 BFU-E and CFU-E occurs independently of EPO. Seidel (91) and Wagemaker (92) showed that following drug-induced marrow cell depletion, the pattern of erythrocytic

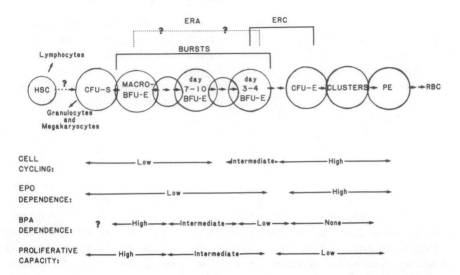

Figure 3. The cellular organization of the erythron as derived from *in vitro* clonal cell assays. See text for a fuller explanation. Abbreviations: HSC, the hematopoietic stem cell; PE, proerythroblast; ERA, erythrocytic repopulating ability; ERC, erythropoietin-responsive cell; EPO, erythropoietin; BPA, burst-promoting activity

progenitor cell recoveries was similar in both normal and plethoric animals. These results have been confirmed in my laboratory (87) and raise the possibility that EPO may more specifically affect the fate of erythrocytic progenitors (i.e. differentiation into the next cellular stage) including survival, rather than regulate the proliferation of these cells. In other words, controlling cellular differentiation and not proliferation may be the primary role of this hormone (44). An over-all view of the cellular stages of murine erythropoiesis and their regulation is schematized in Figure 3.

IV. CELL PROLIFERATION KINETICS OF ERYTHROCYTIC PROGENITORS

With the possible exception of CFU-E no direct cell kinetic analyses of erythrocytic progenitors have been attempted. Although the concentrations of both early and late progenitors can be increased somewhat by selective or separative techniques (64, 79), none of these cells has been isolated in sufficient quantities to permit detailed kinetic analyses. It is unlikely that this will be accomplished until specific preparative techniques are developed for each cell subtype. In the meantime numerous indirect techniques are available (46, 64) which can be coupled to quantitative and qualitative data (see below) to obtain at least a general idea of their proliferation kinetics both *in vivo* and *in vitro*. One important prerequisite must be met, however, before an analysis of this sort is feasible: *in vitro* cell assays should be standardized so as to consistently yield maximal plating efficiencies, otherwise gross underestimates of cell amplification will be obtained. This is a difficult undertaking since the 'true' plating efficiency of erythrocytic progenitors is not really known. For the present, the lower limits of their 'true' incidence may be approximated by the upper limits observed *in vitro*. For the purposes of this analysis, the incidence given in Table 2 will be assumed in each case. However, the reader should keep in mind that the actual incidence of these erythrocytic progenitors may exceed the values given. Figure 4a summarizes the absolute frequency of each erythrocytic progenitor in the tibia of the adult mouse. The numbers of both morphologically recognizable erythrocytic cells as well as non-recognizable progenitors assayed *in vitro* are shown. In addition, the total tibial stem cell pool was estimated by correcting the tibial CFU-S number for splenic seeding. Thus, each cellular compartment should be directly comparable in quantitative terms. Table 3a compares the marrow frequencies observed between successive cell compartments. These ratios therefore serve as a crude approximation of the total cellular amplification occurring between each compartment. This, of course, assumes a pipeline arrangement throughout the non-recognizable erythron, which may not be entirely correct. The most noticeable finding is the observation that in both normal marrow and spleen, the greatest cell amplification occurs between day 3–4 BFU-E and CFU-E cell compartments. Interestingly, the amplification between day 3–4 BFU-E and CFU-E is nearly 70% greater in the spleen (Table 3b) than in the marrow (twelve-fold vs. 7.1-fold, respectively). Secondly, the ratio between CFU-S and all bursts is < 1. This might be easily explained by the difference in efficiencies between *in vivo* and *in vitro* assays. Alternatively, the greater total marrow CFU-S number may reflect the pluripotentiality of these cells, i.e., the need for additional differentiation into the non-erythrocytic cell compart-

---

Figure 4. (a) Total marrow erythrocytic progenitors in normal (light part of histogram) and anemic (dark portion) mice. Data adapted, in part, from references. 59, 60, 79, 85, 89 and 90. Stem cell (CFU-S) levels were corrected for a splenic seeding efficiency of 0.12 in both normal and anemic animals since the cycling level in both organs was similar (i.e., range: 10–25% in S-phase). Anemia was induced either by an acute bleeding or by the injection of phenylhydrazine on three successive days. Abbreviations as given for Table 2; Macro, macroburst of Humphries *et al.* (79); Cl, cluster-forming cells; PE, proerythroblast; TRCP, total morphologically-recognizable erythrocytic precursors, including PE. Data from anemic animals were obtained at the maximal cellular response interval, usually between days 3 and 5 following bleeding or phenylhydrazine. The numbers in parenthesis refer to the average cycling level obtained with either ^{3}H-TdR or hydroxyurea suicide in at least two separate experiments. Arrows indicate possible underestimates of day 7 BFU-E. The proerythroblast level in anemic spleen is only an estimate. (b) Total splenic erythrocytic progenitors in normal (dark part of histogram) and anemic (light portion) mice.

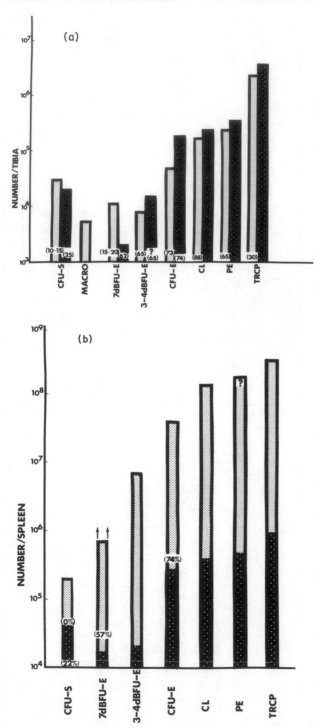

Table 3. Comparison of the total inter-compartmental amplification of erythrocytic progenitors in normal vs. anemic animals*

	Progeny/progenitor ratio in:			Ratio	
	Normal	Anemic	% Change	Anemic/Normal	
(a) Bone marrow					
Day 7 BFU-E/CFU-S;	< 1.0	< 1.0	0	< 1.0	
Day 3–4 BFU-E/Day 7 BFU-E:	< 1.0	7.5	> +750%	1.3	
CFU-E/Day 3–4 BFU-E:	7.1	13.3	+187%	25.0	
Cluster/CFU-E:	2.7	2.1	(−22%)	7.3	
Proerythroblast/Cluster:	1.3	2.0	+154%	22	
(b) Spleen					
Day 7 BFU-E/CFU-S:	< 1.0	3.5	> +350%	15.9	
Day 3–4 BFU-E/Day 7 BFU-E:	~ 1.0	8.6	+860%	300	
CFU-E/Day 3–4 BFU-E:	12.0	7.2	(−40%)	2000	
Cluster/CFU-E:	1.6	3.6	+225%	533	

* Data from Figure 4.

ments. In any case, both marrow and spleen (Figure 4b) display proportionately similar levels for all categories of erythrocytic bursts, thus making the numerical transition to CFU-E very conspicuous. The average S-phase distribution for each cell type is also given in Figure 4. Day 3–4 BFU-E show a substantially greater cycling level than do day 7 BFU-E (65% *vs* 20%). Taken together, these data therefore suggest that the average age of day 3–4 BFU-E is much less than day 7 BFU-E in normal bone marrow. Figure 4 also shows the level of erythrocytic progenitors in marrow and spleen following the induction of acute anemia by both bleeding and the administration of phenylhydrazine. These results were gleaned from the available literature (59, 60) as well as from recent work in my laboratory (89). Clearly, the amplifying role of the murine spleen in erythropoiesis is reaffirmed (93) by these findings. By comparing the ratio of the cell progeny in anemic animals to the baseline level of their progenitors in normal mice, it is possible to obtain a measure of the total amplification that has occurred between successive compartments as a consequence of the anemia (Table 3). Again, the greatest amplification of cells is found between day 3–4 BFU-E and CFU-E (a 2000-fold increase in the spleen would suggest about eleven extra cell divisions). In contrast to the situation observed in normal spleen, an amplification of all cell compartments is observed in the spleens of anemic animals. The situation in the marrow of anemic mice is somewhat different, however. Anemia appears to mainly increase the day 7 BFU-E → day 3–4 BFU-E → CFU-E amplifications. As a consequence of the anemia, it appears that only the day 7 BFU-E significantly augment their cycling levels (from a value of ∼ 20% in normals to levels of ∼ 60% in anemic animals (Figure 4a). Although this result is inconsistent with some findings (59, 60), it does reflect what we (89) and others (85, 90) have consistently obtained for anemia-induced changes in day 7–10 BFU-E cycling. Since Hara and Ogawa (60, 94) observed a substantial increase in the number of day 9–10 BFU-E being transported by the blood following the induction of anemia by both phenylhydrazine and bleeding, it is very likely that substantial BFU-E migration from marrow to spleen is occurring in addition to the marrow emigration of CFU-S (95). Thus, the total amplification of marrow erythrocytic progenitors is muted relative to that of the spleen as a consequence of the marrow loss of early progenitors with high proliferative potential. These data seem to suggest that amplification in erythropoiesis is actually a property of the cellular stages of erythrocytic differentiation and not just the more mature ones (42). In normal animals, steady-state erythropoiesis is maintained by a minimal amplification of cellular stages preceding day 3–4 BFU-E whereas under conditions of greatly increased demand for erythrocytes the increase in amplification stretches further and further back toward the most primitive hematopoietic elements. Since, under the anemic conditions described, the spleen assumes the principal erythropoietic role, the increase in cell amplification may be considerable as evidenced by the eleven extra cell divisions occurring between day 3–4 BFU-E → CFU-E alone. In fact, one can calculate an approximate total of 32 'extra' cell divisions occurring in the spleen of anemic animals from CFU-S → clusters (discounting migration) when compared to normal spleen (Table 3). Erythrocytic amplification, then, must be considered a flexible variable which is subject to regulation and a property of all erythrocytic progenitors. Obviously, a detailed dissection of the regulatory mechanisms governing these amplifications is sorely needed.

Another kinetic measure which is applicable to erythrocytic progenitors grown *in vitro* is an estimation of their proliferative ability from colony size distributions. One point worth emphasizing, however, is the fact that these data reflect over all *in vitro* growth conditions so the relationship to the theoretical value *in vivo* is unknown. Table 4 summarizes average colony size distributions obtained from a number of reports in the literature. From these values, one may extrapolate to the average number of cell divisions over the duration of the assay. The cell division estimates can then be expressed as the daily frequency. All progenitor cell-types exhibit an average of about two daily cell divisions independently of their state of differentiation. This also includes CFU-S which are assayed *in vivo*, even when spleen colonies of various sizes are analyzed. An estimate of the average duration of the cell cycle (T_c) is easily calculated and reveals estimates ranging from ten to 18 hours, with a definite tendency to cluster around a value of 12–13 hours. Of course, it must be realized that these estimates are, at best, a first approximation of progenitor cycling rates and that the 'true' cycling level may be considerably greater (i.e., shorter T_c), especially if 'ineffective' cell production is a significant factor in the production of these colonies. However, a noticeable lack of cellular debris, even in seven-day colonies, may argue against ineffective cell production being a significant liability in these estimates. In addition, a recent study (96) has shown that in day 3–4 marrow cell cultures, RBC destruction may be well within tolerable limits. Also shown in Table 4 are average T_c values for CFU-E and CFU-S which have been previously measured directly (CFU-E) or estimated from *in vivo* colony growth patterns (CFU-S). The agreement between estimated and measured T_c for CFU-E is quite good. In contrast, the variation in measured T_c values for CFU-S (range: 8.6–40 hr) suggests that the *in vivo* measures are subject to too many variables to be considered even as a first approximation. These results suggest a fairly constant minimum proliferation rate of about two daily cell divisions (giving an average cycle duration of ~ 12–13 hr) when erythrocytic progenitors are assayed *in vitro* under 'standard' conditions. Unfortunately, sizing data are lacking for colonies obtained under stimulated conditions. It would certainly be of interest to see whether an increase in the erythrocytic cycling rate occurs in severe anemia, for example.

The length of time it takes to express colony formation *in vitro* (Figure 2)

Table 4. Average cell-cycle number and duration of primitive marrow progenitors

Cell type	Average no. cells/colony	Total no. cell divisions	No. cell divisions per day	Average T_c (hr.)	
				Estimated*	Measured†
Cluster-forming cells	4	2.0	2.0	12.0	N.D.
CFU-E	14	3.75	1.9	12.6	7.0 (64)
					11.0 (46)
Day 3–4 BFU-E	48	5.5	1.8	13.3	N.D.
Day 7 BFU-E	500‡	9.0	1.3	18.5	N.D.
	1000	10.0	1.43	16.8	
	10,000§	13.4	1.9	12.6	
Macrobursts$ (day 9)	2×10^5	17.5	1.9	12.6	N.D.
CFU-S (day 9)	5×10^5	19.0	2.1	11.4	24.5 (97)
	1×10^6	20.0	2.2	10.9	36.0 (35)
					8.6 (39)
	16×10^6 (day 10)	24	2.4	10.0	8.0 (33)
					40.0 (98)

* Obtained from these data.
† Obtained from the reference given in parentheses.
‡ Marginal growth conditions, no exogenous BPA.
§ With the addition of exogenous BPA.
$ From reference number 79.
N.D., Not determined.

Table 5. Average time in culture for the initiation and full expression of colony-forming capacity*

Colony type	Time (hr) for colony:		
	Initiation†	Full expression‡	Ratio
Cluster-forming cell	~ 18	~ 36	0.5
CFU-E	~ 30	~ 48	0.6
Day 3–4 BFU-E	~ 60	~ 72	0.8
Day 7 BFU-E	~ 128	~ 90	1.4

* Estimates obtained from *in vitro* growth curve data (Figure 2).
† Defined as the length of time from plating to obtain 50% of the maximal colony response.
‡ Defined as the interval between the mid-points of the ascending and descending portions of the growth curve (Figure 2).

has been taken as a barometer of the state of differentiation of erythrocytic progenitors *in vivo* (47). The longer the time interval needed to observe the formation of colonies, the more primitive the progenitor. Not surprisingly, this relationship also appears to hold true for the length of time *in vitro* needed to obtain full colony expression. This is shown in Table 5 where a comparison is made between the length of time needed to initiate colony formation and the length of time needed to obtain full expression of the colony type once colony formation is initiated. The estimates derive from the *in vitro* growth curves (Figure 2) and are obtained by mid-point approximations. One will note that the colony 'initiation' and 'expression' intervals are not equivalent, and that the 'initiation' of colony formation takes proportionately longer than does colony 'expression' as one compares mature and primitive progenitors. On the average it took twice as long to initiate colony formation as it did to obtain full colony expression (110 hr *vs* 54 hr, respectively). This may suggest that 'initiation' of colony formation *in vitro* involves a number of events which must be completed before colony formation can proceed. Since these data appear independent of colony size, cell division would not appear to be a major factor in the initiation of colonies *in vitro*. If this is indeed true, then estimated day 7 BFU-E cell cycle times (Table 4) will be overestimated by the length of the 'initiation' period. Presumably, then, other 'conditioning' events occur during 'initiation' to permit colony formation.

Another view of the kinetics of primitive erythrocytic progenitors can be obtained from an analysis of their population doubling times (i.e. T_2). Table 6 compares marrow T_2 estimates obtained *in vivo* following a variety of hematopoietic perturbations to growth curve doubling times observed *in vitro*. With the exception of two reports (91, 92), the *in vivo* doubling times for all the erythrocytic progenitors show remarkably little variation around an

Table 6. Measured doubling times of primitive erythrocytic progenitors in murine bone marrow*

	Doubling time (hr)	
Progenitor	*in vivo*†	*in vitro*‡
Cluster-forming cell	12 (87) §	6 (67)
CFU-E	16 (68)	
	16 (62)	6–7 (67)
	~ 20 (94)	> 10 (2)
	< 4 (91, 92)	
Day 3–4 BFU-E	14 (87)	
	< 4 (91, 92)	~ 9 (47)
Day 7 BFU-E	15 (92)	
	16 (87)	~ 24 (47)
		18 (73)
		7.3 (84)
CFU-S	16 (92)	—
	~ 31 (99)	

* Since considerable marrow → spleen migration probably occurs in many states of perturbed hematopoiesis, estimates of T_2 in the spleen will underestimate the true value and therefore are not considered here.
† Estimated from marrow growth curves following a variety of perturbations *in vivo*.
‡ Estimated from growth curves *in vitro* under 'optimal' growth conditions.
§ Numbers in parenthesis refer to the reference from which the data were obtained.

average of ~ 15–16 hr. This is only slightly longer (~ 3 hr) than the cell-cycle durations obtained from the data on colony size distributions (Table 4) and might suggest that cell proliferation *in situ* is partly responsible for the increase in the number of progenitor cells following various perturbations. The fact that the average T_2 is ~ 3 hr longer than the average T_c could be taken as circumstantial evidence for cell loss, presumably through differentiation into succeeding cell compartments. The two exceptions noted in T_2 estimates (91, 92) employed a single experimental protocol of drug-induced marrow aplasia. In this case, the rate of increase in both marrow CFU-E (91, 92) and day 3–4 BFU-E (91) was < 4 hr. Since both protocols evaluated marrow progenitors, it is unlikely that immigration from other hematopoietic sources played a significant role in augmenting the cellular doubling time. Influx from precursor cell compartments was therefore most likely a major contributing factor to the short T_2 estimates. Alternatively, the short doubling times could have been due to the release of synchronized cells by the cycle-active drug employed in these studies. In contrast to the growth of cell progenitors *in vivo* the progenitor doubling times following cell plating *in vitro* averaged only ~ 8+ hr (Table 6). It should be noted, however, that these *in vitro* intervals are most likely a measure of the rate of cellular expression rather than a measure of their proliferation *per se*. As such, the relationship to specific cell-cycle parameters is rather moot. As was previously noted for measures of CFU-S T_c (Table 4), T_2 measures for these cells usually exhibit wide fluctuations (Table 6). The variations in T_2 measures for day 7–10 BFU-E may also reflect the variety of culture conditions under which these cells are grown in addition to the heterogeneity which exists in this category of cellular progenitors. Taken together, the observations on cell doubling times would tend to argue against such measures being an accurate estimate of any single cell kinetic parameter. More likely, *in vivo* T_2 estimates represent the net contribution of cell proliferation, migration and fluxes through contiguous cellular compartments.

V. ERYTHROPOIESIS: CELLULAR KINETICS *IN VITRO*

In the absence of available measures for directly estimating the proliferation rate of primitive erythrocytic progenitors, we are forced to derive proliferation estimates from very indirect measures. Those available include colony size distributions, progenitor ratios in marrow and spleen in normal and stimulated animals, as well as those gleaned from cellular growth patterns *in vitro* and *in vivo*. Analysis of such data permits the following major generalizations regarding the proliferation kinetics of primitive erythrocytic progenitors.

First, under normal steady-state conditions, erythrocytic progenitor cell amplification in marrow and spleen is primarily a property of mature burst-forming cells (i.e., day 3–4 BFU-E) whereas, under stimulated conditions (i.e., anemia) the substantial increase in erythrocytic cell production is largely a consequence of amplifications within earlier, more primitive cellular compartments. These observations strongly imply that the amplifying capacity of erythrocytic stem cells is subject to very precise regulation.

A second conclusion pertains to the average cell-cycle times derived from colony sizing data. These T_c estimates exhibit remarkable similarity for all progenitor cell stages, suggesting that under optimal *in vitro* growth conditions, the average turnover at the cellular level is about the same throughout the erythron (i.e., ~ 12–13 hr). This cell-cycle interval is similar to that of CFU-S and their progeny which grow within individual spleen colonies (Table 4). Thus, both *in vivo* and *in vitro* colony sizing data yield similar cell-cycle values. One must note, however, that cell-cycle data obtained by analyzing cell populations reflect the kinetics of the entire population and not individual cells within the colony. Such data are also biased in favor of the largest subpopulations within the colony, which in this case, are the more mature erythrocytic progenitors. In addition to estimating the duration of T_c, it is also possible to obtain an estimate of the total amplification capabilities of the erythron, which, in the above analysis amounts to a minimum of 17–18 total cell

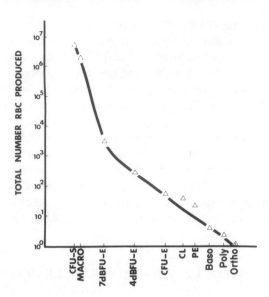

Figure 5. The net effect of a single, extra cell division on the total marrow production of blood erythrocytes. An increase by a factor of two over the average number of cell divisions given in Table 2 was assumed in this calculation. Abbreviations, as for Figure 4. Baso, basophilic normoblast; Poly, poly-chromatophilic normoblast; Ortho, orthochromatic normoblast

divisions. It becomes quite clear that an 'extra' cell division at the earliest stages of erythrocytic differentiation greatly enhances the over-all output of the erythron. Figure 5 illustrates the net effect of an extra cell division at the level of a single erythrocytic progenitor cell. The proliferation of erythrocytic progenitors *in vitro* would therefore seem to suggest that the total amplifying capability of the non-recognizable erythron is considerably more than what has been previously thought, particularly if one sums the capacity within each compartment of the erythron. A capability of ~ 20 cell divisions from stem cell→ RBC (Table 4) would appear to far exceed the 13 or so divisions needed for full erythrocyte production in normal animals. In fact, since the data in Table 4 indicate that the cell which forms a day 7 BFU-E colony has the capability of undergoing a total of ~ 9–13+ cell divisions, it would appear that this cell type has the capacity for maintaining normal erythrocytic amplification. However, the daily number of cell divisions within a seven-day colony is only about two (Table 4) (or perhaps a maximum of three to four if one corrects for the five-day lag phase needed for the 'initiation' of day 7 BFU-E colonies, Table 5). If one then sums the total number of daily cell divisions occurring from day 7 BFU-E → clusters, a total of about eight (or nine plus) is obtained, which, added to the two daily cell divisions occurring within the recognizable erythron yields a daily figure of about ten (or eleven or more) cell divisions within the day 7 BFU-E $\rightarrow$ RBC sequence. At least two more cell divisions can also be assumed to originate from the stem cell compartment itself. Since the assays for 'macrobursts' and CFU-S may actually overlap, the about two plus cell divisions which these two cell types collectively represent (Table 4) would provide the twelve (or 13) needed to account for the daily production of 5.2×10^8 RBC (see Figure 6). Lastly, under stimulated conditions, the increased cell amplification within the non-recognizable erythron is reflected by the greatly augmented rate of RBC production, which, in anemic animals, may be the consequence of 25 or more 'extra' cell divisions within these same cellular compartments. Thus, *in vitro* assays appear to provide cell kinetic measurements which are generally consistent with those obtained from other techniques (i.e., RBC lifespan, spleen colony formation, etc.) which depend on entirely different physiologic variables.

VI. EPILOGUE: WHAT HAVE WE LEARNED?

The techniques for the growth of erythrocytic progenitor cells *in vitro* are still rapidly developing and undoubtedly will continue to increase in sophistication and precision in the very near future. However, a picture of erythropoiesis is emerging which permits one to identify and analyze kinetically some of the major cellular stages of erythrocytic development prior to hemoglobinization. In so far as the proliferative capacity of cells residing within the non-recognizable erythron is concerned, it is quite clear that these cells are characterized by a significant, but variable, capacity for cell amplification, and that this capacity is expressed to some extent *in vitro*. Whether or not the **full** proliferative capacity of these cells is expressed *in vitro* is still unclear. The lag time between plating and full colony expression *in vitro* as well as the great variability in cellular growth patterns *in vitro* would tend to suggest that colony-forming cells do not always proliferate at their maximum in culture. This, of course, could be due to a number of reasons, most notably to suboptimal growth conditions, the absence or suboptimal concentrations of the required growth factor(s), and the like. However, the greatest variability in the proliferation of colony-forming cells *in vitro* appears localized precisely within the erythron where one might expect the greatest amplification capacity to reside: at the level of the most primitive erythrocytic progenitors (Figure 6). It is therefore tempting to suggest the possibility that amplification within the erythron is a controlled variable which exhibits great variance at the cellular level of commitment to erythropoiesis. One of the most important tasks in the near future will be to detail the mechanisms which regulate erythrocytic amplification at early stages of cellular development.

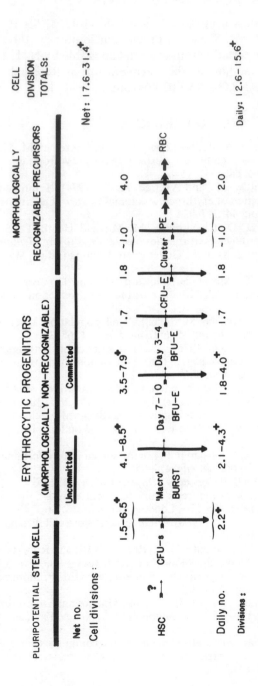

Figure 6. Amplification divisions in normal murine marrow erythrocytic progenitors. The cell division number is expressed in two ways. (1) as the *net* number between successive cell stages, and (2) as the average daily number for each cell stage. Data from Table 4. The net number of cluster cell divisions was assumed to be 1.0 because of the overlap with proerythroblasts (PE). Likewise, the number of stem cell divisions was assumed to overlap with 'macrobursts'. The maximum number of daily cell divisions for day 7 BFU-E was assumed to equal 3.5 by correcting for the five-day time lag in the initiation of colony formation (Table 5)

VII. ACKNOWLEDGMENTS

The author wishes to express his gratitude to Ms S. Holden, Mr R. Ziegelstein, Mr P. Faletra, and Dr E. Weiner for their contributions to this chapter. The laboratory research reported herein was made possible by N. I. H. grant No. AMDD-17735. The author is the recipient of a Research Career Development Award (No. 1-KO4-AM00200) from the N. I. H.

VIII. REFERENCES

1. Stephenson, J. R., Axelrad, A. A., McLeod, D. L., and Shreeve, M. M. (1971). 'Induction of colonies of hemoglobin-synthesizing cells by erythropoietin *in vitro*', *Proc. Nat. Acad. Sci. USA*, **68**, 1542–1546.
2. McLeod, D. L., Shreeve, M. M., and Axelrad, A. A. (1974). 'Improved plasma culture system for production of erythrocytic colonies *in vitro*: Quantitative assay method for CFU-E', *Blood*, **44**, 517–534.
3. Axelrad, A. A., McLeod, D. L., Shreeve, M. M., and Heath, D. S. (1973). 'Properties of cells that produce erythrocytic colonies *in vitro*', in *Hemopoiesis in Culture*, (Ed. W. A. Robinson), U.S. Government Printing Office, Washington, D.C., pp. 226–234.
4. Stohlman, F. Jr., Ebbe, S., Morse, B., Howard, D., and Donovan, J. (1968). 'Regulation of erythropoiesis. XX. Kinetics of red cell production', *Ann. N.Y. Acad. Sci.*, **149**, 156–172.
5. Tarbutt, R. G., and Blackett, N. M. (1968). 'Cell population kinetics of the recognizable erythroid cells in the rat,' *Cell Tissue Kinet.*, **1**, 65–80.
6. Schofield, R., and Lajtha, L. G. (1976). 'Cellular kinetics of erythropoiesis', in *Congenital Disorders of Erythropoiesis*, Ciba Foundation Symposium 37 (New Series), Elsevier Excerpta Medica, N.Y., pp. 3–24.
7. Izak, G. (1977). 'Erythroid cell differentiation and maturation', in *Progress in Hematology*, (Ed. E. B. Brown), Grune and Stratton, N.Y., vol. 10, pp. 1–41.
8. Lord, B. I. (1979). 'Kinetics of the recognizable erythrocyte precursor cells', in *Clinics in Haematology*, W. B. Saunders Co. Ltd., London, vol. 8 (no. 2), pp. 335–350.
9. Schofield, R. (1978). 'The relationship between the spleen colony-forming cell and the haemopoietic stem cell', *Blood Cells*, **4**, 7–25.
10. Lajtha, L. G. (1979). 'Stem Cell Concepts', *Differentiation*, **14**, 23–34.
11. Lord, B. I. (1979). 'Proliferation regulators in haemopoiesis', in *Clinics in Haematology*, W. B. Saunders Co. Ltd, London, vol. 8 (no. 2), pp. 435–451.
12. Till, J. E., and McCulloch, E. A. (1980). 'Hemopoietic stem cell differentiation', *Biochim. Biophys. Acta*, **605**, 431–459.
13. Bond, V. P., Fliedner, T. M., Cronkite, E. P., Rubini, J. R., and Robertson, J. D. (1959). 'Cell turnover in blood and blood forming tissues studied with tritiated thymidine,' in *The Kinetics of Cellular Proliferation*, (Ed. F. Stohlman, Jr.), Grune and Stratton, N.Y., pp. 188–200.
14. Alpen, E. L., and Cranmore, D. (1959). 'Cellular kinetics and iron utilization in bone marrow as observed by Fe[59] radioautography,' *Ann. N.Y. Acad. Sci.*, **77**, 753–765.
15. Lord, B. I. (1965). 'Cellular proliferation in normal and continuously irradiated rat bone marrow studied by repeated labelling with tritiated thymidine', *Brit. J. Haemat.*, **11**, 130–143.

16. Jacobson, L. O., Goldwasser, E., Plzak, L. F., and Gurney, C. W. (1957). 'Studies on erythropoiesis. IV. Reticulocyte response of hypophysectomized and polycythemic rodents to erythropoietin'. *Proc. Soc. Exp. Biol. Med.*, **94**, 243–246.

17. Erslev, A. J. (1964). 'Erythropoietin *in vitro*. II. Effect on "stem cells" ', *Blood*, **24**, 331–342.

18. Alpen, E. L., and Cranmore, D. (1959). 'Observations on the regulation of erythropoiesis and on cellular dynamics by Fe^{59} autoradiography', in *Kinetics of Cellular Proliferation*, (Ed. F. Stohlman, Jr.), Grune and Stratton, N.Y., pp. 290–300.

19. Till, J. E., and McCulloch, E. A. (1961). 'A direct measurement of the radiation sensitivity of normal mouse bone marrow cells', *Rad. Res.*, **14**, 213–222.

20. Bruce, W. R., and McCulloch, E. A. (1964). 'The effect of erythropoietic stimulation on the haemopoietic colony-forming cells of mice', *Blood*, **23**, 216–232.

21. Morse, B. S., Rencricca, N. J., and Stohlman, F. Jr., (1970). 'Relationship of erythropoietin effectiveness to the generative cycle of erythroid precursor cell', *Blood*, **35**, 761–774.

22. Lajtha, L. G., Pozzi, L. V., Schofield, R., and Fox, M. (1969). 'Kinetics of haemopoietic stem cells', *Cell Tissue Kinet.*, **2**, 39–49.

23. Kubanek, B., Bock, O., Heit, W., Bock, E., and Harriss, E. B. (1973). 'Size and proliferation of stem cell compartments in mice after depression of erythropoiesis', in *Haemopoietic Stem Cells*, Ciba Foundation Symposium 13 (New series), Elsevier, Excerpta Medica, North Holland, Amsterdam, pp. 243–262.

24. Reissmann, K. R., and Samorapoompichit, S. (1970). 'Effect of erythropoietin on proliferation of erythroid stem cells in the absence of transplantable colony-forming units,' *Blood*, **36**, 287–296.

25. Reissmann, K. R., and Udupa K. B. (1972). 'Effect of erythropoietin on proliferation of erythropoietin-responsive cells', *Cell Tissue. Kinet.*, **5**, 481–489.

26. Fogh, J. (1970). 'Studies on the mechanism of the increased dose–response of erythropoietin after stimulation with erythropoietin', *Blood*, **35**, 476–492.

27. Lajtha, L. G., Gilbert, C. W., and Guzman, E. E. (1971). 'Kinetics of haemopoietic colony growth', *Brit. J. Haemat.*, **20**, 343–354.

28. Twentyman, P. R., and Blackett, N. M. (1970). 'Action of cytotoxic agents on erythroid system of the mouse', *J. Nat. Cancer Inst.*, **44**, 117–123.

29. Millar, J. L., Constable, T. B., and Blackett, N. M. (1974). 'Delayed response to erythropoietin in polycythemic animals treated with cytotoxic agents', *Cell Tissue Kinet.*, **7**, 363–370.

30. Milenkovic, P., and Pavlovic-Kentera, V. (1980). 'Regeneration of erythroid committed precursor cells in polycythaemic mice treated with cyclophosphamide', *Exp. Hemat.*, **8**, 44–51.

31. Tarbutt, R. G. (1967). 'A study of erythropoiesis in the rat', *Exp. Cell Res.*, **48**, 473–483.

32. Becker, A. J., McCulloch, E. A., Siminovitch, L., and Till, J. E. (1965). 'The effect of differing demands for blood cell production on DNA synthesis by hemopoietic colony forming cells of mice', *Blood*, **26**, 296–308.

33. Vassort, F., Winterholer, M., Frindel, E., and Tubiana, M. (1973). 'Kinetic parameters of bone marrow stem cells using *in vivo* suicide by tritiated thymidine or by hydroxyurea', *Blood*, **41**, 789–796.

34. Quesenberry, P. J., and Stanley, K. (1980). 'A statistical analysis of murine stem cell suicide techniques', *Blood*, **56**, 1000–1005.

35. Schofield, R., and Lajtha, L. G. (1969). 'Graft size considerations in the kinetics of spleen colony development', *Cell Tissue Kinet.,* **2**, 147–155.
36. Patt, H. M., Maloney, M. A., and Lamela, R. A. (1980). 'Hematopoietic stem cell proliferative behavior as revealed by bromodeoxyuridine labeling', *Exp. Hemat.,* **8**, 1075–1079.
37. Hagan, M. P., and MacVittie, T. J. (1981). 'CFU-S kinetics observed *in vivo* by bromodeoxyuridine and near-UV light treatment', *Exp. Hemat.,* **9**, 123–128.
38. Vogel, H., Niewisch, H., and Matioli, G. (1968). 'The self renewal probability of hemopoietic stem cells', *J. Cell. Physiol.,* **72**, 221–229.
39. Schofield, R., Lord, B. I., Kyffin, S., and Gilbert, C. W. (1980). 'Self-maintenance capacity of CFU-S', *J. Cell. Physiol.,* **103**, 355–362.
40. Covelli, V., Briganti, G., and Silini, G. (1972). 'An analysis of bone marrow erythropoiesis in the mouse', *Cell Tissue Kinet.,* **5**, 41–51.
41. Stohlman, F. Jr., (1970). 'Regulation of red cell production', in *Formation and Destruction of Blood Cells*, (Eds. T. J. Greenwalt and G. A. Jamieson) J.B.Lippincott Co., Philadelphia, pp. 65–84.
42. Bessis, M., Mize, C., and Prenant, M. (1978). 'Erythropoiesis: Comparison of *in vivo* and *in vitro* amplification', *Blood Cells,* **4**, 155–174.
43. Testa, N. G. (1979). 'Erythroid progenitor cells: Their relevance for the study of haematological disease', in *Clinics in Haematology*, W. B. Saunders Co. Ltd, London, vol. 8, (no. 2), pp. 311–333.
44. Eaves, C. J., Humphries, R. K., and Eaves, A. C. (1979). '*In vitro* characterization of erythroid precursor cells and the erythropoietic differentiation process', in *Cellular and Molecular Regulation of Hemoglobin Switching*, (Eds. G. Stamatoyannopoulos and A. W. Nienhuis), Grune and Stratton, N.Y., pp. 251–273.
45. Heath, D. S., Axelrad, A. A., McLeod, D. L., and Shreeve, M. M. (1976). 'Separation of the erythropoietin-responsive progenitors BFU-E and CFU-E in mouse bone marrow by unit gravity sedimentation', *Blood,* **47**, 777–792.
46. Cormack, D. (1976). 'Time-lapse characterization of erythrocytic colony-forming cells in plasma cultures', *Exp. Hemat.,* **4**, 319–327.
47. Gregory, C. J. (1976). 'Erythropoietin sensitivity as a differentiation marker in the hemopoietic system: Studies of three erythropoietic colony responses in culture', *J. Cell. Physiol.,* **89**, 289–302.
48. Humphries, R. K., Eaves, A. C., and Eaves, C. J. (1979). 'Characterization of a primitive erythropoietic progenitor found in mouse marrow before and after several weeks in culture', *Blood,* **53**, 746–763.
49. Ouellette, P. L., and Monette, F. C. (1980). 'Erythroid progenitors forming clusters *in vitro* demonstrate high erythropoietin sensitivity,' *J. Cell. Physiol.,* **105**, 181–184.
50. Gregory, C. J., and Eaves, A. C. (1977). 'Human marrow cells capable of erythropoietic differentiation *in vitro*: Definition of three erythroid colony responses', *Blood,* **49**, 855–864.
51. Guilbert, L. J., and Iscove, N. N. (1976). 'Partial replacement of serum by selenite, transferrin, albumin and lecithin in haemopoietic cell cultures', *Nature,* **263**, 594–595.
52. Iscove, N. N., and Sieber, F. (1975). 'Erythroid progenitors in mouse bone marrow detected by macroscopic colony formation in culture', *Exp. Hemat.,* **3**, 32–43.
53. Iscove, N. N. (1978). 'Regulation of proliferation and maturation at early and late stages of erythroid differentiation', in *Cell Differentiation and Neoplasia*, (Ed. G. F. Saunders), Raven Press, N.Y., pp. 195–209.
54. Prchal, J. F., Adamson, J. W., Steinmann, L., and Fialkow, P. J. (1976). 'Human erythroid colony formation *in vitro*: Evidence for clonal origin', *J. Cell. Physiol.,* **89**, 489–492.

55. Gregory, C. J., McCulloch, E. A., and Till, J. E. (1973). 'Erythropoietic progenitors capable of colony formation in culture: State of differentiation', *J. Cell. Physiol.*, **81**, 411–420.
56. Gregory, C. J., and Henkelman, R. M. (1977). 'Relationships between early hemopoietic progenitor cells determined by correlation analysis of their numbers in individual spleen colonies,' in *Experimental Hematology Today*, (Eds. S. J. Baum and G. D. Ledney), Springer-Verlag, N.Y., pp. 93–101.
57. Monette, F. C., Weiner, E. J., and Faletra, P. P. (1981). 'The state of differentiation of erythroid cells forming clusters *in vitro*', *Exp. Hemat.*, **9**, 711–715.
58. Monette, F. C., Ouellette, P. L., Thorson, J. A., Hausdorff, W., Weiner, E. J., and Jarris, R. F., Jr. (1980). 'The *in vitro* erythropoietin sensitivity of late erythroid progenitors subjected to opposing physiologic demands', *Exp. Hemat.*, **8**, 947–953.
59. Iscove, N. N. (1977). 'The role of erythropoietin in regulation of population size and cell cycling of early and late erythroid precursors in mouse bone marrow', *Cell Tissue Kinet.*, **10**, 323–334.
60. Hara, H., and Ogawa, M. (1977). 'Erythropoietic precursors in mice under erythropoietic stimulation and suppression', *Exp. Hemat.*, **5**, 141–148.
61. Iscove, N. N. (1978). 'Erythropoietin-independent stimulation of early erythropoiesis in adult marrow cultures by conditioned media from lectin-stimulated mouse spleen cells,' in *Hematopoietic Cell Differentiation*, ICN-UCLA Symposia on Molecular and Cellular Biology, (Eds. D. W. Golde, M. J. Cline, D. Metcalf, and C. F. Fox), Academic Press, N.Y., vol. X, pp. 37–52.
62. Monette, F. C., Kent, R. B., Weiner, E. J., Jarris, R. F., Jr. Ouellette, P. L., Thorson, J. A., and Zelick, R. D. (1980). 'Cell-cycle properties and proliferation kinetics of late erythroid progenitors in murine bone marrow', *Exp. Hemat.*, **8**, 484–493.
63. Gerard, E., Carsten, A. L., and Cronkite, E. P. (1978). 'The proliferative potential of plasma clot erythroid colony-forming cells in diffusion chambers', *Blood Cells*, **4**, 105–128.
64. Wagemaker, G., and Visser, T. P. (1981). 'Analysis of the cell cycle of late erythroid progenitor cells by sedimentation at unit gravity', *Stem Cells*, **1**, 5–15.
65. Gregory, C. J., Tepperman, A. D., McCulloch, E. A., and Till, J. E. (1974). 'Erythropoietic progenitors capable of colony formation in culture: Response of normal and genetically anemic W/W^v mice to manipulations of the erythron', *J. Cell. Physiol.*, **84**, 1–12.
66. Kennedy, W. L., Alpen, E. L., and Garcia, J. F. (1980). 'Regulation of red blood cell production by erythropoietin: Normal mouse marrow *in vitro*,' *Exp. Hemat.*, **8**, 1114–1122.
67. Monette, F. C., Ouellette, P. L., and Faletra, P. P., (1981). 'Characterization of murine erythroid progenitors with high erythropoietin sensitivity *in vitro*', *Exp. Hemat.*, **9**, 249–256.
68. Peschle, C., Magli, M. C., Cillo, C., Lettieri, F., Pizzella, F., Migliaccio, G., and Mastroberardino, G. (1978). 'Erythroid stem cell kinetics: Experimental and clinical aspects', *Blood Cells*, **4**, 233–252.
69. Peschle, C., Cillo, C., Rappaport, I. A., Magli, M. C., Migliaccio, G., Pizzella, F., and Mastroberardino, G. (1979). 'Early fluctuations of BFU-E pool size after transfusion or erythropoietin treatment', *Exp. Hemat.*, **7**, 87–93.
70. Aye, M. T. (1977). 'Erythroid colony formation in cultures of human marrow: effect of leukocyte conditioned medium', *J. Cell. Physiol.*, **91**, 69–78.
71. Johnson, G. R., and Metcalf, D. (1977). 'Pure and mixed erythroid colony formation *in vitro* stimulated by spleen conditioned medium with no detectable erythropoietin', *Proc. Natl. Acad. Sci. USA.*, **74**, 3879–3882.

72. Wagemaker, G. (1978). 'Cellular and soluble factors influencing the differentia-
    tion of primitive erythroid progenitor cells (BFU-E) *in vitro*', in *In Vitro Aspects of
    Erythropoiesis*, (Eds., M. J. Murphy, Jr., C. Peschle, A. S. Gordon, and
    E. Mirand), Springer-Verlag, N.Y., pp. 44–57.
73. Wagemaker, G., Peters, M. F., and Bol, S. J. L. (1979). 'Induction of
    erythropoietin responsiveness *in vitro* by a distinct population of bone marrow
    cells', *Cell Tissue Kinet.*, **12**, 521–537.
74. Nissen, C., Iscove, N. N., and Speck, B. (1979). 'High burst-promoting activity
    (BPA) in serum of patients with acquired aplastic anemia', in *Experimental
    Hematology Today* (Eds., S. J. Baum and G. D. Ledney), Springer-Verlag, N.Y.,
    pp. 79–87.
75. Wagemaker, G. (1980). 'Early erythropoietin-independent stage of *in vitro*
    erythropoiesis: Relevance to stem cell differentiation', in *Experimental Hematol-
    ogy Today*, 1980, (Eds. S. J. Baum, G. D. Ledney, and D. van Bekkum),
    S. Karger, Basel, pp. 47–60.
76. Humphries, R. K., Eaves, A. C., and Eaves, C. J. (1979). 'Characterization of a
    primitive erythropoietic progenitor found in mouse marrow before and after
    several weeks in culture', *Blood*, **53**, 746–763.
77. Wagemaker, G. (1978). 'Induction of erythropoietin responsiveness *in vitro*', in
    Hematopoietic Cell Differentiation, (Eds., D. W. Golde, M. J. Cline, D. Metcalf,
    and C. F. Fox), Academic Press, N.Y., pp. 109–118.
78. Ploemacher, R. E., van Soest, P. L., Wagemaker, G., and van't Hull, E. (1979).
    'Particle-induced erythropoietin-independent effects on erythroid precursor cells
    in murine bone marrow', *Cell Tissue Kinet.*, **12**, 539–550.
79. Humphries, R. K., Eaves, A. C., and Eaves, C. J. (1981). 'Self-renewal of
    hemopoietic stem cells during mixed colony formation *in vitro*', *Proc. Natl. Acad.
    Sci. USA*, **78**, 3629–3633.
80. Hara, H., and Ogawa, M. (1978). 'Murine hemopoietic colonies in culture
    containing normoblasts, macrophages, and megakaryocytes', *Am. J. Hemat.*, **4**,
    23–34.
81. Fauser, A. A., and Messner, H. A. (1979). 'Identification of megakaryocytes,
    macrophages and eosinophils in colonies of human bone marrow containing
    neutrophilic granulocytes and erythroblasts', *Blood*, **53**, 1023–1027.
82. Strome, J. E., McLeod, D. L., and Shreeve, M. M. (1978). 'Evidence for the
    clonal nature of erythropoietic bursts: Application of an *in situ* method for
    demonstrating centromeric heterochromatin in plasma cultures', *Exp. Hemat.*, **6**,
    461–467.
83. Hara, H. and Noguchi, K. (1981). 'Clonal nature of pluripotent hemopoietic
    precursors *in vitro* (CFU-Mix)', *Stem Cells*, **1**, 53–60.
84. Holden, S. A., and Monette, F. C. 'The effect of hemin on primitive erythroid
    precursors', (submitted).
85. Adamson, J. W., Torok-Storb, B., and Lin, N. (1978). 'Analysis of erythropoiesis
    by erythroid colony formation in culture', *Blood Cells*, **4**, 89–103.
86. Suzuki, S., and Axelrad, A. A. (1980). 'Fv-2 locus controls the proportion of
    erythropoietic progenitor cells (BFU-E) synthesizing DNA in normal mice', *Cell*,
    19, 225–236.
87. Weiner, E. J. (1981). '*Proliferation kinetics of primitive murine marrow erythro-
    poietic progenitors: A comparison of erythropoietin responsiveness assayed in vivo
    and in vitro*,' Ph.D. thesis, Boston University, Boston, MA.
88. Gregory, C. J., and Eaves, A. C. (1978). 'Three stages of erythropoietic progenitor
    cell differentiation distinguished by a number of physical and biologic properties',
    Blood, **51**, 527–537.

89. Faletra, P. P., and Monette, F. C. 'Cell proliferation kinetics of erythroid progenitors in anemic mice', (submitted).
90. Peschle, C., Cillo, C., Migliaccio, G., and Lettieri, F. (1980). 'Fluctuations of BFUe and CFUe cycling after erythroid perturbations: Correlation with variations of pool size', *Exp. Hemat.*, **8**, 96–102.
91. Seidel, H. J., and Opitz, U. (1979). 'Erythroid stem cell regeneration in normal and plethoric mice treated with hydroxyurea', *Exp. Hemat.*, **7**, 500–508.
92. Wagemaker, G., and Visser, T. P. (1980). 'Erythropoietin-independent regeneration of erythroid progenitor cells following multiple injections of hydroxyurea', *Cell Tissue Kinet.*, **13**, 505–517.
93. Schooley, J. C. (1970). 'The significance of the spleen in recruitment of erythropoietin-sensitive cells', in *Hemopoietic Cellular Proliferation*, (Ed., F. Stohlman, Jr.), Grune and Stratton, N.Y., pp. 171–179.
94. Hara, H., and Ogawa, M. (1976). 'Erythropoietic precursors in mice with phenylhydrazine-induced anemia', *Am. J. Hemat.*, **1**, 453–458.
95. Rencricca, N. J., Rizzoli, V., Howard, D., Duffy, P., and Stohlman, Jr., F. 'Stem cell migration and proliferation during severe anemia', *Blood*, **36**, 764–771.
96. Samson, D., Tikerpae, J., and Crowne, H. (1981). 'A simple *in vitro* method for the assessment of ineffective erythropoiesis', *Blood*, **58**, 782–787.
97. Wu, A. M. (1981). 'A method for measuring the generation time and length of DNA synthesizing phase of clonogenic cells in a heterogenous population', *Cell Tissue Kinet.*, **14**, 39–52.
98. Blackett, N. M. (1976). 'Cell cycle characteristics of haemopoietic stem cells', in *Stem Cells of Renewing Cell Populations*, (Eds., A. B. Cairnie, P. K. Lala, and D. G. Osmond), Academic Press, N.Y., pp. 157–164.
99. Millar, J. L., Blackett, N. M., and Hudspith, B. N. (1978). 'Enhanced post-irradiation recovery of the haemopoietic system in animals pretreated with a variety of cytotoxic agents', *Cell Tissue Kinet.*, **11**, 543–553.

Current Concepts in Erythropoiesis
Edited by C. D. R. Dunn
© 1983 United States Government

CHAPTER 3

Involvement of cells of the immune system in regulation of erythropoiesis

JOAN WRIGHT GOODMAN
Biology and Medicine Division
University of California
Berkeley

and

DIANA R. GOODMAN
Department of Philosophy
University of California
Berkeley

The last ten years has seen a burgeoning of interest in cells of the immune system that appear to affect blood formation either in a direct regulatory sense, i.e., helper or suppressor activity at the progenitor level; or in a secondary way, e.g., by increased demand placed on precursors through depletion of mature, circulating elements. Malfunction of the immune system might thus be seen to underlie such hematologic disorders as aplastic anemia as well as autoimmune hemolytic anemia and all forms of myelogenous malignancy. Many of the experimental studies in this area involve erythro-poiesis specifically; it is to this aspect of blood formation and the level of direct regulation that this chapter will be addressed. Expansion of interest in cellular regulatory mechanisms in the seventies was accompanied by and to some extent dependent on a resurgence of interest in the thymus and in thymus-dependent (or T) lymphocytes following the important finding in 1966 (1,2) that two kinds of lymphocytes were required for some immune functions. The subsequent virtual explosion in cellular immunology expanded the consideration of cellular regulation of biologic functions and developed a variety of *in vitro* experimental methods to explore control mechanisms.

That the thymus might be involved in erythropoiesis was not exactly a new concept clinically. Existence of the organ in the thoracic cavity of man had been known for centuries (e.g., 3) before speculation as to its function began to be made. William Hewson (4) in the mid-eighteenth century promulgated an interesting theory linking erythropoiesis with the thymus, which he considered an appendage to the lymphatic 'glands'. Although credited with the first good description of a lymphocyte (5), he believed the white cells in lymphatic fluid were the 'central particles' around which would be formed red vesicles yielding red blood cells (or 'particles') (4, p. 274). Hewson's theory did not of course survive subsequent scientific advances, but similar conjectures about the function of the thymus persisted. A 1919 review of nineteenth and early twentieth century investigations of the effects of thymus extirpation in animals of various species cites a number of researchers who speculated that the thymus plays some essential role in blood formation (6). Only at the beginning of this century, with the demonstration by Pfeiffer and Marx (cited in 5), that lymph nodes, bone marrow, and spleen are involved in antibody production, was any appreciation gained of the central role played by lymphatic tissue in resistance to infection or in immune processes as we think of them today. Yet another 50 years passed before cellular immunology began really to flower. As late as 1956 in a cytology and pathology text (7) could be found such statements as, under the heading 'Lymphocyte': 'These cells represent an unsolved problem. In spite of numerous investigations, the fate and functions of the lymphocytes of the blood and lymphoid tissue are mainly unknown ...' (p. 52); and, under the heading 'Functions of the lymphocyte': 'Little can be said on this subject. A vague and indefinite connection exists between the accumulations of lymphocytes in inflammatory processes and defence mechanisms, but there is no knowledge of the actual part played by these cells ...' (p. 53). During that 50 years, however, clinical data provided good circumstantial evidence that blood formation was in some way linked to the thymus, since tumors of that organ in man were observed to be associated with abnormalities of the hematopoietic system. Among thymoma patients studied in this regard, hematologic disorders were found in some cases before, in others at the same time a tumor was diagnosed. In many other instances, however, the finding of a tumor preceded that of the blood dyscrasia (8). This association of thymic abnormality with hematopoietic disorder was described in the literature as early as 1928 (9), but more than 80% of those cases listed in a discussion by

Fisher in 1964 (8) had been reported in the ten years immediately preceding his compilation. Among 39 patients he reviewed, there were 27 cases of 'pure' red cell agenesis, two of anemia and thrombocytopenia, one of anemia and neutropenia, and eight of pancytopenia. Remission or significant hematologic improvement was seen in more than half the patients whose thymomas were removed and who survived the post-operative period, a development strengthening the possible link between the thymus and hematopoiesis.

In response to the suggestive clinical observations that were appearing occasionally in the literature, laboratory experiments were devised to explore the relationship of the thymus to erythropoiesis. Unsuccessful attempts were made to find a humoral suppressor of erythropoiesis in anemic patients with a thymoma by injecting rats with the patient's serum (10,11) or with saline extracts from tumors (8). Using mouse tissues, Auerbach (12) found that thymus fragments cultured *in vitro* with embryonic spleen fragments had a beneficial effect on the subsequent growth of all elements of the splenic tissue. This effect was confirmed *in vivo* by Metcalf (13), who found a 67% greater mass in splenic fragments implanted subcutaneously with thymus than in splenic fragments implanted alone. This increased mass represented all splenic components and, as Metcalf pointed out, was in agreement with the converse finding of decreased splenic size of both follicles and red pulp after thymectomy in adult mice (14). That the thymus may be involved in control of red blood cell (RBC) formation was further indicated by (a) the anemia subsequent to neonatal thymectomy of mice (13), and (b) maturation arrest of erythrocytic cells in the neonatally thymectomized opossum (15). Results of studies on congenitally athymic (nude) and asplenic-athymic (lasat) mice revealed abnormalities in bone marrow cellularity (16,17) and in kinetics of RBC formation (18). Despite these irregularities in marrow erythropoiesis, normal hemoglobin, reticulocyte, and RBC values have been recorded in the peripheral blood of these animals, a result not predictable from the anemia of neonatally thymectomized mice.

More recent experimental data have shown a positive or augmentative effect of normal lymphocytes on hematopoiesis. These studies have made use of radiation chimeras (19,20), neonatally thymectomized mice, and congenitally athymic (nude) mice (21), and they have shown that thymic and lymph node lymphocytes affect not only erythrocytic elements but also other hemato-poietic cell lines (22). In these latter papers, Zipori and Trainin suggested that thymic humoral factor played a major role in hematopoiesis. In contrast, Goodman *et al.* (23,24) held that thymocytes or thymus-dependent cells were of primary importance, thymic hormone being essential secondarily to promote normal development of T-cells from progenitors (25). Although some experimentalists have interpreted their data in terms of a cell–cell interaction, implying a requirement of contact (23,26,27), it is doubtful, definitive evidence being absent, that any would argue strongly against the interactions being mediated by one or more of the ever increasing numbers of known lymphokines (e.g., see 28).

In 1977 Wiktor-Jedrzejczak et al (29) reported that a Thy-1-bearing cell in bone marrow was necessary for curing the anemia of W/W^v mice. Sharkis (30), extending these studies in vivo with histologic examination of recipients' spleens, concluded that removal of thymocytes resulted in a greater percentage of granulocytic colonies in either W/W^v or irradiated $+/+$ mice and that administration of $+/+$, but now W/W^v, thymocytes along with the θ-poor marrow restored the erythrocytic:granulocytic (E:G) ratio of spleen colonies to that seen initially. This finding is in direct conflict with data of others showing that inclusion of thymic or lymph node lymphocytes in parental bone marrow transplants into F_1 hybrid mice ($P \rightarrow F_1$) results in increased numbers of granulocytic colonies (31). In addition, removal of θ-bearing cells from marrow transplanted isogenically to five kinds of standard laboratory mice results in a decrease in granulocytic colonies and thereby an increase in the E:G ratio (32). Marrow from thymectomized mice, presumably devoid of T-cells, on transplantation also gave rise to low numbers of granulocytic colonies in the experiments of Petrov et al (33) and in those of Burek et al (34) further underlining conflicts in the published data. An explanation of the apparent contradiction may lie in the nature of the W/W^v defect. One could speculate, for example, that abnormal suppression is exerted on the pluripotential stem cell (CFU-S) and even on the differentiating, more mature cell lines in these unusual mice. Administration of thymocytes, by furnishing cells to restore balance between help and suppression, brings the E:G ratio back to that of the normal mouse. Extending his study to the putatively normal $+/+$ mouse (30), Sharkis and co-workers found that addition of $+/+$ thymocytes augmented $+/+$ marrow growth in these irradiated mice as well. As previously stated (22), we were unable to confirm this result in normal mice of other strains.

The interest in hematopoietic regulation stimulated by the report of involvement of a θ-bearing cell in blood formation led to further investigations in which recently developed in vitro methods were brought to bear. Sharkis et al (35) added thymocytes to cultures of W/W^v and $+/+$ bone marrow (BM) and found augmentation of the late erythrocytic progenitors (CFU-E) at a $+/+$ thymocyte: W/W^v BM cell ratio of 20 and inhibition at a ratio of 0.02. This dual role (augmentative and inhibitory) for thymocytes seemed to hold also for B10, CBA and C57BL/6 mice for both CFU-E and the early erythrocytic progenitors (BFU-E). It is curious that Sawada and Adler (36), using W/W^v mice from the same supplier could not confirm Sharkis' findings of; (a) considerable augmentation of CFU-E by $+/+$ thymocytes and (b) a difference between the effects of $+/+$ and W/W^v thymocytes on erythropoiesis in vitro.

We have repeated some of these experiments using two of the same strains used by Sharkis et al, CBA and C57BL/6, in addition to B6D2F$_1$'s, with the results shown in Table 1. At first glance (experiments A–C) it appears that we

Table 1. Effect of thymocytes on CFU-E

Experiment (Donor strain)	T-cells	BM Concentration plated 10^{-5}	T:BM	CFU-E/10^5BM
A (B6D2F$_1$)	−	2.5	—	154 ± 11
	+	2.5	20	†214 ± 12
	+	2.5	0.02	155 ± 13
B (B6D2F$_1$)	−	2.5	—	133 ± 12
	+	2.5	20	†273 ± 26
	+	2.5	0.02	125 ± 10
C (B6D2F$_1$)	−	2.0	—	116 ± 12
	+	2.0	20	†309 ± 26
	+	2.0	0.02	206 ± 20
D (B6D2F$_1$)	−	2.0	—	1205 ± 18
	+	2.0	20	*
E (CBA)	−	0.4	—	427 ± 55
	+	0.4	20	†712 ± 47
	+	0.4	0.02	548 ± 50
	−	2.0	—	1155 ± 28
	+	2.0	20	1245 ± 43
	+	2.0	0.02	1135 ± 35
F (C57BL/6)	−	0.4	—	256 ± 21
	+	0.4	20	†377 ± 28
	+	0.4	0.02	310 ± 26
	−	2.0	—	856 ± 26
	+	2.0	20	815 ± 18
	+	2.0	0.02	†768 ± 24

* Unable to count colonies as too many clumps of cells obscured field
† Significantly different from marrow-only group at $p < 0.05$

confirmed the data of Sharkis *et al* as far as the positive effect was concerned; but the first three experiments, our earliest attempts at growing CFU-E, yielded very low numbers, only 1/5–1/10 the number we now get routinely when we plate cells under carefully controlled conditions at comparable concentrations (i.e. 2–5×10^5/ml). In experiments D, E, and F, for example, we counted respectively, 1205, 1155, and 856 CFU-E/10^5 cells plated, and were unable to record any augmentation. When a marrow concentration low enough to yield a submaximal number of CFU-E was plated, in experiments E and F, thymocytes at 20:1 (T:BM) produced significant augmentation not revealed by the same cell preparations at the same ratio when plated at a marrow concentration five-fold greater. In only one case (experiment F) was an inhibitory effect seen in our experiments at very low T:BM ratios, while in another instance (experiment C) a significant augmentation was recorded. Zanjani (37) in two separate experiments using C57BL mice could show no augmentation of CFU-E by thymocytes at a T:BM ratio of 20:1, when cells were cultured under optimal conditions yielding 800–1200 colonies/10^5 cells plated; nor was there any evidence of inhibition or suppression at low T:BM ratios. Other investigators have also reported augmentation and at least a suggestion of suppression (36), but they, like Sharkis et al (35), were recording relatively low CFU-E yields. It is extremely difficult to compare other investigators' data that are derived from a technique that appears to be so variable from one laboratory to another. One might conclude from the CFU-E data cited and presented in Table 1 that only when the system is working suboptimally or submaximally, as is the case also in vivo with P → F_1 transplantation, can thymocytes be shown to augment. Nathan et al (38) have recently come to similar conclusions based on results of in vitro cultures of human cells.

There are many additional suggestions in the literature that thymocytes or Thy-1-bearing cells have a regulatory function in hematopoiesis in general, some of them in conflict with each other. For instance, the inhibitory effect of rabbit anti-mouse brain serum (RAMBS) on CFU-S content of mouse marrow has been reported to be the result of removal of Thy-1-bearing cells, for addition of thymocytes to such treated suspensions led to expression of at least some of the 'lost' stem cells (39–41). However, using antibody similarly raised, but probably differently absorbed, others have not been able to 'rescue' such cells (24). One is at a loss to explain the positive findings with RAMBS in view of the inability of anti Thy-1 serum to affect CFU-S content in other experiments (22,42). Interestingly, Tyan (42) found that although marrow from young adult mice was insensitive to anti Thy-1.2 and specific anti-helper (Ly 1.2) or anti-suppressor (Ly 2.2) activity, that from older mice showed clear evidence of regulatory T-cells.

The BFU-E, early progenitors that are relatively insensitive to homeostatic control by erythropoietin (EPO) (43–45), may be more subject than are CFU-E to regulation by other cells or their products. The requirement for burst-promoting activity (BPA) to achieve growth of BFU-E in vitro is itself evidence for such regulation, as BPA is produced by actively dividing cells (44,46–49). At least one investigator has linked BPA production to a cell line with T-cell characteristics (50).

As early as the mid-seventies Cerny and his colleagues (51,52) studied changes in marrow stem cells that were caused by activated lymphocyte products. They showed that marrow cells cultured for short periods in the presence of PHA-conditioned medium were more actively dividing, as judged by [^{3}H]thymidine uptake, and expressed more CFU-S when injected into irradiated recipient mice, than did controls cultured without the factor, which they called SAF (stem cell-activating factor). Additional data suggesting a dependent relationship of hematopoietic progenitors on factors resulting from immunologic stimuli come from data of Frindel *et al* (53) and Lepault *et al* (54), who showed that stimulation of mice by T-dependent antigens caused cycling of previously quiescent CFU-S; and of Burstein *et al* (55), who noted changes in BFU-E following administration of rabbit anti-platelet serum, which they believed constituted an immune stimulation.

In vitro studies along similar lines have added weight to the notion that erythropoiesis, and probably hematopoiesis in general, can be regulated by cells of the immune system. For example, Torok-Storb and her associates (56) found that lymphocytes from sensitized dogs suppressed erythrocytic colony growth *in vitro*; Banisadre *et al* (57) found that mitogen-activated T-lymphocytes suppressed human BFU-E; and a similar *in vitro* suppression of erythropoiesis, but mediated by bone marrow adherent cells, has been reported by Zanjani *et al* (58) for some patients with fungal infections. Those individuals whose marrow produced normal erythrocytic colony (EC) numbers showed a decrease in performance when macrophages were removed, but those whose EC were abnormally low when grown from whole marrow showed much better growth in the absence of adherent cells. *In vitro* testing of nonadherent cells from a patient who had developed pancytopenia showed strong inhibition of autologous but not allogenic CFU-E (59). Such genetic restriction has not been a common feature of recent reports of regulatory interactions in blood formation.

Despite continuing research effort in the late 1970s and early 1980s, controversy as to the role of T-lymphocytes in RBC formation persists. Nathan (48) attributed to T-cells an obligatory role in human BFU-E growth, and recently Haq *et al* (60), using the monoclonal antibodies OKT-3, -4, and -8 to eliminate all or specific subpopulations of T-cells, came to the same conclusion. The latter group of workers, however, found that the absolute requirement for T-cells was non-specific and that T_H (helper) and T_S (suppressor) cells had no differential effects. This conclusion contrasts with the interpretation Torok-Storb and her colleagues had given to their data (61,62), which were obtained from cells similarly separated by reaction with the specific antisera 7.2, which recognizes human Ia and therefore probably reacts with BFU-E themselves (63); 7.28, which recognizes a lympho-hematopoietic differentiation antigen present on most T-cells; and 9.3, which recognizes an antigen on a subset of T-cells larger than but including that identified by OKT-4. Torok-Storb's data are illustrated in Figures 1 and 2. The explanation of the apparent conflict might be found in considerations of the particular subsets of cells recognized by the different antibodies used by the various groups. It is quite possible that the helpers and suppressors for this particular committed progenitor are not recognized by OKT-4 and -8.

The collected abstracts from the 1979 annual meeting of the American Society of Hematology contains a report (64) that T-cells were found to augment human peripheral blood (PB) mononuclear cell-derived BFU-E but

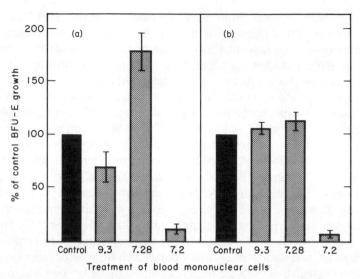

Figure 1. The effect of antibody (9.3, 7.28, or 7.2) and complement treatment on BFU-E growth from either unfractionated peripheral blood mononuclear cells (A) or from T-cell-depleted mononuclear cells (B). The data are shown as percentage of BFU-E growth from control cells treated with complement only. Each bar represents the mean ±S.E. of normalized data from 4–6 experiments. Control BFU-E growth in different experiments ranged from 15 ± 1.7 to 59 ± 2.5/10⁵ cells. Reproduced by permission from 'Regulation of *in vitro* erythropoiesis by normal T-cells: evidence for two T-cell subsets with opposing function. B. Torok-Storb, P. J. Martin, and J. A. Hansen, *Blood*, **58**, 171–174, 1981

not those developing from BM precursors. The rather unorthodox interpretation was put forth '... that PB BFU-E utilize T-cell help for erythroid colony expression, but the *mature BM BFU-E, which are derived from them and multiply to dominate the marrow* (our italics) no longer require T-cell help to interact with EPO and form colonies ...'. From the data of Micklem *et al* (65,66) and Rosendaal *et al* (67), we are accustomed to think of circulating stem cells as 'second class', or at least already started toward terminal differentiation, destined never to return to marrow. On the other hand, we consider those in marrow less mature, and capable of self-renewal as well as differentiation. It is consequently a somewhat unusual proposal that committed progenitors, such as BFU-E, leave the marrow in a relatively immature state to circulate peripherally, then return to marrow to mature before going on to further differentiation. No compelling evidence is known to us that would substantiate this point of view. If such a progression to maturation were to occur, from blood to marrow, these data might be interpreted as evidence for the disappearance of a receptor or differentiation antigen recognized by T-cells, as progenitors become relatively more mature — an interesting possibility. Inexplicably, other investigators on the basis of negative data from

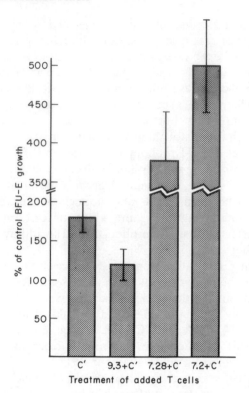

Figure 2. The effect of antibody (9.3, 7.28, or 7.2) and complement treatment on the ability of T-cells to stimulate BFU-E growth is shown as percentage of control BFU-E growth. Each bar represents the mean ± s.e. of data from five experiments. Control BFU-E were grown without T-cells. The number of BFU-E grown in control groups from five separate experiments ranged from 9.3 ± 1.9 to 56 ± 4.2/10^5 non-T PBM. Reproduced by permission from 'Regulation of *in vitro* erythropoiesis by normal T-cells: evidence for two T-cell subsets with opposing function'. B. Torok-Storb, P. J. Martin, and J. A. Hansen, *Blood*, **58**, 171–174, 1981

human *in vitro* colony studies, have concluded that T-lymphocytes play no role at all in erythropoiesis. Finlay (68), for example, could find no effect on human PB BFU-E when T-cells were depleted by monoclonal antibodies. The negative conclusion reached by Nomdedeu *et al* (69,70) was derived from cultures of isolated populations of PB null cells in the presence or absence of isolated PB T-cells. One might question the absolute depletion in the first instance (68): possibly a few undetected helper cells remained. In the second instance (69,70), one can only speculate that here too the isolated populations were not so pure as assumed. Failure of isolated T-cells to modify growth of null cells might represent an artifactual balance between helpers and suppressors that results from particular separation procedures. It should be emphasized that these speculations are not suggested by any flaws perceived in experimental design or execution of the work cited, but were instead motivated by the need to reconcile the vastly different conclusions in current literature.

Three years after Nathan's original paper (48), an absolute requirement of human BFU-E for T-cells was similarly reported by Reid et al (71), who found that monocytes (adherent cells) could also promote expression of BFU-E from peripheral blood null cells but were less effective than T-lymphocytes. Monocytes, although stimulatory at low numbers (up to 4×10^5), did not show increasing effects, as did T-lymphocytes, on either BFU-E number or size when greater cell doses were used. When both cell types were cocultured with BFU-E, a greater response was seen than with either alone, suggesting a positive interaction between T-cells and monocytes. Zuckerman (72,73) on the other hand, employing the same kinds of cell populations, found monocytes more effective than T-lymphocytes and no additive effect of the two populations together.

Despite the strong implication from the evidence cited above that a T-cell is able to augment or 'help' erythropoiesis in vitro, some doubt has been cast on the helper cell's identity by the work of Kanamaru et al (74). They found that thymocytes markedly augmented BFU-E (fourfold) from marrow of specific pathogen free (SPF) CBA and C57BL/6 mice but found a much less impressive (1.5-fold) effect on marrow from conventional mice. Irradiated spleen and marrow cells also could augment BFU-E, but frozen-thawed cells from spleen, marrow, or thymus lost their activity. The lack of effectiveness of non-viable cells in vitro was later confirmed by Sawada and Adler (75). The fact that anti-θ serum and complement pretreatment of BFU-E-containing marrow had no effect on erythropoiesis in vitro was taken by Kanamaru et al as evidence that the helper cell in their system, also shown to be cortisone resistant, was not T-dependent.

Mangan and Desforges (76) also examined effects of T-cells and monocytes on BFU-E and concluded that proliferation of these early committed erythrocytic progenitors was directly proportional to the T-cell concentration but, as Rinehart et al (77) had reported earlier, inversely proportional to the monocyte concentration in culture. In the work of Mangan and Desforges, monocytes, separated from PB mononuclear (PBM) cells by adherence to plastic, were harvested by gentle scraping, and they were judged at least 95% pure by criteria of morphologic appearance, non-specific naphthylacetate-esterase staining, and phagocytosis of latex particles (0.8 μm). These investigators found BPA in supernatant fluids from mixed lymphocyte cultures and conversely found burst inhibitory activity in supernatant fluids from 48hr cultures of monocytes. It is difficult to reconcile these data with the findings of Lipton et al (78) who were using comparable monocyte percentages in analogous studies but could find no effects. The latter group believed the discrepant results might be explained by differences in separated populations,

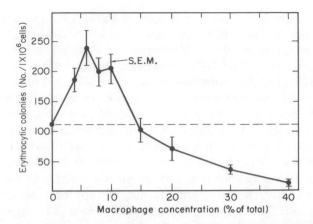

Figure 3. Effect of human bone marrow macrophages on erythrocytic colony formation by normal peripheral blood BFU-E. Bone marrow macrophages derived from liquid culture, when added to peripheral blood mononuclear cells and assayed for BFU-E in the plasma clot system, cause stimulation of the BFU-E at low concentrations and inhibition at high concentrations. Reproduced by permission from 'Regulation of colony formation by bone marrow macrophages' L. I. Gordon, W. J. Miller, R. F. Branda, E. D. Zanjani, and H. S. Jacob. *Blood,* **55**, 1047–1050, 1980

and to substantiate this suggestion they cited a review of separation techniques (79) that points out errors inherent in each method. Alternatively, it was suggested that the explanation might be found in differences in EPO preparations used by the two groups with the possibility that endotoxin contamination of EPO gave rise to erroneously interpreted enhancement of erythropoiesis. Gordon *et al* (80), on the other hand, by varying macrophage percentages in human PBM cell cultures, found enhancement of BFU-E below 4% and inhibition above 15%. Figure 3 illustrates the bimodal effect of bone marrow macrophages on BFU-E grown from PBM cells by these investigators. Their data are compatible with those of Murphy and Urabe (81) resulting from cultures of BDF_1 mouse BM in the presence of macrophages. They found increasing enhancement of erythrocytic colony growth as the percentage of peritoneal macrophages in cultures was increased from 2.5 to 10.

Some of the most intriguing recent data on the relationship of erythropoiesis to cells of the immune system come from human hematologic disorders, in particular from aplastic anemias. These bring us back to the early clinical indications, mentioned above, of a connection *via* the thymus. Mathé and his collaborators (82) using antilymphocyte globulin (ALG) to condition patients for marrow transplantation from HLA-non-identical donors, found a beneficial effect on some of the patients with severe aplastic anemia irrespective of the outcome of the bone marrow graft. Speck *et al* (83) relate the historically interesting circumstances leading to the deductions from Mathé's cases that;

'(a) it was unlikely that spontaneous recovery accounted for all improvements; and (b) a complete take of donor marrow could not be demonstrated in any of the patients who recovered (a few patients had a partial and temporary take [split chimaerism])'. They (83) presented data concerning 29 patients treated with ALG either alone or together with allogenic marrow, and they recorded hematologic improvement in twelve of them over a four-and-a-half year period. Since there were no permanent bone marrow 'takes', the amelioration could not be ascribed to transplanted cells. Instead, they concluded their data were consistent with the disease's having its basis in an autoimmune block of residual stem cell development. Not disparate from this interpretation is the recovery from aplastic anemia reported by Thomas and his group (84) of a patient following conditioning therapy for transplanted marrow that was rejected. The following year, Sensenbrenner (85) reported a similar case in which the patient's marrow cells taken before any therapy was initiated were studied after culture in diffusion chambers placed in cyclophosphamide (CY)-conditioned mice for up to twelve days. The patient's cells in chambers, presumably isolated from suppressive influences, behaved like normal marrow cells similarly cultured. There have been other clinical reports (e.g., 86,87) linking marrow aplasia with immunologic suppression, many of them cited by Shadduck et al (88) and Zanjani et al (27). A recent study by Shadduck et al (89) of twelve aplastic anemia patients treated with antithymocyte globulin (ATG) suggests that administration of such serum is indeed useful as a treatment in cases where transplantation is contraindicated.

These clinical reports are supplemented by in vitro studies showing that a certain percentage of patients suffering from aplastic anemia or the closely related congenital hypoplastic anemia harbor in their peripheral blood, lymphocytes capable of suppressing erythrocytic colony growth (90–94). In some cases, T-cell depletion from autologous cultures of cells from anemic patients was shown to enhance an otherwise depressed rate of colony growth; re-introduction of T-cells into cultures restored suppression in some but not all of these cases (93,94). It is well known that aplastic anemia has no single etiology, and the complex results of the in vitro studies reflect this. It is hoped that increasingly precise in vitro tests will make it possible to identify those anemic patients whose disease has an immune etiology and, by identifying the immune cell subsets that are active in the disease, make it possible to predict a patient's response to therapy. Mangan et al (95), addressing this issue with regard to three of their patients, have found the correlation between in vitro culture data and clinical results of therapy to be imperfect at present, but nonetheless worth considering. Shadduck (96) has suggested refinement of the culture systems to be used in clinical studies.

Further progress toward defining the mechanisms of immune-mediated aplastic anemias has come from very interesting recent studies of the pure red cell aplasia (PRCA) associated with chronic lymphocytic leukemia (CLL).

Over half of all CLL patients are anemic (97). This condition was originally thought to result from disease-related overcrowding of the marrow or from nutritional deficiency, but that view has not been substantiated. Instead, recent work indicates a likelihood that CLL-associated PRCA is immune-mediated, implicating specific abnormalities in T-cell subpopulations. Hoffman *et al* (98) in 1978 reported a case of relatively rare T-cell CLL in which the patient's peripheral blood T-cells were found to suppress normal erythrocytic colony growth. The following year, Chiorazzi *et al* (99) reported that CLL-PRCA patients exhibited an abnormally low proportion of circulating T_μ (helper) cells; and in a related study, Kay *et al* (100) demonstrated a significant increase in numbers of T_γ (suppressor) cells in similar patients. This was followed by a report by Linch *et al* of a case of aplastic anemia associated with abnormally elevated T_γ, and by a series of investigations by Mangan and co-workers (101–103) ultimately linking a disproportionately large T_γ population in CLL-PRCA patients to their abnormal suppression of erythropoiesis. Increasingly it appears that those cells (T_γ's and T_μ's) which are considered suppressors and helpers in immune functions are suppressors and helpers in erythropoiesis as well.

The question of how T-lymphocytes and monocytes exert the effects reported in the literature remains open. Although many titles include the words 'cellular interaction', thus implying need for contact between two viable cells, there is a dearth of definitive data to substantiate the necessity for membrane communication. There are, on the other hand, many solid data indicating that humoral substances with effects measurable in *in vitro* systems, such as CFU-E and BFU-E colony growth, are produced by activated T-cells and by rapidly dividing, sometimes including malignant, cells of other types (see, e.g., 104–106, and many other works cited above). Yet it is unlikely that all the cellular effects on erythropoiesis that have been reported are explicable simply in terms of BPA production or of the various other products of activated macrophages and T-lymphocytes, respectively (28). For example, the evidence of Kanamaru *et al* (74) from studies of mouse BFU-E strongly indicate a cellular rather than a humoral effect inasmuch as heavily irradiated, but not frozen-thawed, spleen, or bone marrow cells increased colony yield, whereas conditioned medium from thymus cultures or from pokeweed mitogen stimulated spleen cells did not. Perhaps one of the most convincing arguments in favor of close cell contact can be based on our knowledge of nurse cells first described by Bessis in 1958 (107) around which normoblasts are arrayed in the marrow and with which each is in physical touch. These reticular elements, which are reasonably believed to play an essential role in erythropoiesis, undoubtedly have as their counterparts in the long term Dexter marrow culture system (108) the fat-containing, adherent cells on which hematopoietic progenitors depend for maintenance and with which according to Bentley (109) they are physically in close association. Particularly compelling, with regard to the need for cell–cell interaction are the phase contrast time lapse observations of Boll and Domeyer showing the hematopoietic progenitor cells touched by locomotive lymphocytes are triggered into mitosis (110,111). In all probability there are at least several ways in which T-lymphocytes and monocytes can effect their modifications of erythropoiesis; the evidence on hand does not permit exclusion of either cell–cell contact or a purely humoral mode. The basic importance of stromal cells in the process of hematopoietic differentia-tion was made obvious again in the work of Wolf and Trentin (112,113) and more recently of Chertkov (114) and Werts (115) and their respective associates. Whether histiocytic/reticular/stromal cells are properly part of the immune system is debatable. Surely they can be considered if not ancestors at least relatives.

It would be nice to conclude that there are definite, invariant effects of lymphocytes and macrophages, each cell type defined by specific surface markers or distinctive functional characteristics, on individual maturational steps in erythropoiesis. Unfortunately, the data in the literature do not permit so clear a picture to emerge. Definite, repeatable (within a given research group) regulatory effects can be seen in laboratory animal experiments and *in vitro* using cells cultured from patients with hematologic disturbances. Furthermore, successful treatment of such patients by protocols that suppress T-lymphocyte activity strongly suggest involvement of the immune system in the etiology of the disorder and by inference in normal blood formation. However, 'suggestion' and 'inference' do not provide enough substance for strong conclusions. The disagreements about whether or not T-cells are required for EC growth and whether or not monocytes play a major role will have to be resolved. But more than that, it needs to be established that *in vitro* systems, as wonderful as they are for producing, under controlled conditions, myriad colonies to count, truly reflect normal physiology; that hematologic disorders give valid clues as to regular order; even that *in vivo* studies of suboptimal growth, allowing experimental modulation of hematopoiesis, truly tell us what goes on in a properly functioning intact organism.

ACKNOWLEDGMENTS

The authors' work referred to in this paper was supported by the Office of Health and Environmental Research of the U.S. Department of Energy under Contract No. DE-AC03-76SF00098 with the University of California, and by NIH Grant AM28430–01.

REFERENCES

1. Claman, H. N., Chaperon, E. A., and Triplett, R. F. (1966). 'Immunocompet-ence of transferred thymus-marrow cell combinations', *J. Immunol.*, **97**, 828–832.

2. Claman, H. N., Chaperon, E. A., and Triplett, R. F. (1966). 'Thymus-marrow cell combinations. Synergism in antibody production', *Proc. Soc. Exp. Biol. Med.*, **122**, 1167–1171.
3. Berengario da Carpi, J. (1523). *A Short Introduction to Anatomy (Isagogae Breves)*, University of Chicago Press, Chicago, 1959.
4. Gulliver, G. (1846). *The Works of William Hewson, F.R.S.*, Syndenham Society, London.
5. Kay, N. E., Ackerman, S. K., and Douglas, S. D. (1979). 'Anatomy of the immune system', in *Seminars in Hematology*, (Eds. P. A. Miescher and E. R. Jaffe), vol. 16, no. 4, pp. 252–282. Grune and Stratton, New York.
6. Park, E. A., and McClure, R. D. (1919). 'The results of thymus extirpation in the dog, with a review of the experimental literature on thymus extirpation', *Am. J. Dis. Child.*, **18**, 317–524.
7. Marshall, A. H. E. (1956). *An Outline of the Cytology and Pathology of the Reticular Tissue*, Oliver and Boyd, London.
8. Fisher, E. R. (1964). 'Pathology of the thymus and its relation to human disease', in *The Thymus in Immunobiology*, (Eds. R. A. Good and A. E. Gabrielson), Hoeber-Harper, New York, pp. 676–726.
9. Matras, A., and Priesel, A. (1928). 'Uber einige gewachse des Thymus', *Beitr. Path. Anat.*, **80**, 270–306.
10. Jacobs, E. M., Hutter, R. V., Pool, J. L., and Ley, A. B. (1959). 'Benign thymoma and selective erythroid aplasia of the bone marrow', *Cancer*, **12**, 47–57.
11. Parry, E. H. O., Kilpatrick, G. S., and Hardisty, R. M. (1959). 'Red-cell aplasia and benign thymoma. Studies on a case responding to prednisone', *Brit. Med. J.*, **1**, 1154–1156.
12. Auerbach, R. (1963). 'Developmental studies of mouse thymus and spleen', *J. Nat. Canc. Inst. Monogr.*, **11**, 23–33.
13. Metcalf, D. (1964). 'Functional interactions between the thymus and other organs', in *The Thymus*, (Eds. V. Defendi and D. Metcalf), The Wistar Institute Symposium Monograph No. 2., The Wistar Press, Philadelphia. pp. 53–73.
14. Metcalf, D. (1960). 'The effect of thymectomy on the lymphoid tissues of the mouse', *Brit. J. Haemat.*, **6**, 324–333.
15. Miller, J. F. A. P., Block, M., Rowlands, D. J., Jr., and Kind, P. (1965). 'Effect of thymectomy on hematopoietic organs of the opossum "embryo" ', *Proc. Soc. Exp. Biol. Med.*, **118**, 916–921.
16. Bamberger, E., Machado, E. A., and Lozzio, B. B. (1977). 'Hematopoiesis in hereditarily athymic mice', *Lab. Animal Sci.*, **27**, 43–49.
17. Aggio, M. C., and Lozzio, B. B. (1979). 'Hematopoiesis of hereditarily asplenic-athymic (Lasat) mice', *Exp. Hemat.*, **7**, 197–205.
18. Harris, G., and Wickramasinghe, S. N. (1979). 'Effect of T-lymphocytes on normal haemopoiesis: studies in congenitally athymic nude mice', *Blut*, **39**, 191–199.
19. Goodman, J. W., and Shinpock, S. G. (1968). 'Influence of thymus cells on erythropoiesis of parental marrow in irradiated hybrid mice', *Proc. Soc. Exp. Biol. Med.*, **129**, 417–422.
20. Lord, B. I., and Schofield, R. (1973). 'The influence of thymus cells in hemopoiesis: stimulation of hemopoietic stem cells in a syngeneic, *in vivo*, situation', *Blood*, **42**, 395–404.
21. Zipori, D., and Trainin, N. (1973). 'Defective capacity of bone marrow from nude mice to restore lethally irradiated recipients', *Blood*, **42**, 671–678.
22. Zipori, D., and Trainin, N. (1975). 'Impaired radioprotective capacity and reduced proliferative rate of bone marrow from neonatally thymectomized mice', *Exp. Hemat.*, **3**, 1–11.

23. Goodman, J. W., and Grubbs, C. G. (1970). 'The relationship of the thymus to erythropoiesis', in *Hemopoietic Cellular Proliferation*, (Ed. F. Stohlman, Jr.) pp. 26–35. Grune and Stratton, Inc., New York.

24. Goodman, J. W., Chervenak, R. P., and Shinpock, S. G. (1980). 'Thymic regulation of stem cell division', in *Experimental Hematology Today, 1980*, (Eds. S. J. Baum, G. D. Ledney, and D. W. Van Bekkum), S. Karger, Basel, pp. 119–123.

25. Komuro, K., and Boyse, E. A. (1973). 'Induction of T lymphocytes from precursor cells *in vitro* by a product of the thymus', *J. Exp. Med.,* **138**, 479–482.

26. McCulloch, E. A. and Till, J. E. (1970). 'Cellular interactions in the control of hemopoiesis', in *Hemopoietic Cellular Proliferation*, (Ed. F. Stohlman, Jr.), Grune and Stratton, New York, pp. 15–25.

27. Zanjani, E. D., and Kaplan, M. E. (1979). 'Cell–cell interaction in erythropoiesis', in *Progress in Hematology*, Grune and Stratton, New York, vol. XI, pp. 173–191.

28. Cohen, S., Pick, E., and Oppenheim, J. J. eds. (1979). *Biology of the Lymphokines*, Academic Press, new York.

29. Wiktor-Jedrzejczak, W., Sharkis, S., Ahmed, A., and Sell, K. W. (1977). 'Theta-sensitive cell and erythropoiesis: Identification of a defect in W/W^v anemic mice', *Science*, **196**, 313–315.

30. Sharkis, S. J., Wiktor-Jedrzejczak, W., Ahmed, A., Santos, G. W., McKee, A., and Sell, K. W. (1978). 'Anti-theta-sensitive regulatory cell (TSRC) and hematopoiesis: regulation of differentiation of transplanted stem cells in W/W^v anemic and normal mice', *Blood,* **52**, 802–817.

31. Basford, N. L., and Goodman, J. W. (1974). 'Effects of lymphocytes from the thymus and lymph nodes on differentiation of hemopoietic spleen colonies in irradiated mice', *J. Cell Physiol.,* **84**, 37–48.

32. Goodman, J. W. and Shinpock, S. G. (1980). 'Interaction between T lymphocytes and hemopoietic stem cells. A critical mini-review', in *Biology of Bone Marrow Transplantation*, ICN-UCLA Symposia on Molecular and Cellular Biology, (Eds. R. P. Gale and C. F. Fox), Academic Press, New York, vol. XVII, pp. 461–476.

33. Petrov, R. V., Khaitov, R. M., Aleinikova, N. V., and Gulak, L. V. (1977). 'Factors controlling stem cell recirculation. III. Effect of the thymus on the migration and differentiation of hemopoietic stem cells', *Blood,* **49**, 865–872.

34. Burek, V., Plavljanic, D. J., Slamberger, S., and Vitale, B. (1977). 'Studies on the mechanism of allogenic disease in mice. I. The influence of bone marrow T lymphocytes on the differentiation and proliferation of hemopoietic stem cells', *Exp. Hemat.,* **5**, 465–479.

35. Sharkis, S. J., Spivak, J. L., Ahmed, A., Misiti, J., Stuart, R. K., Wiktor-Jedrzejczak, W., Sell, K. W., and Sensenbrenner, L. L. (1980). 'Regulation of hematopoiesis: helper and suppressor influences of the thymus', *Blood,* **55**, 524–527.

36. Sawada, U., and Adler, S. S. (1980). '*In vitro* hemopoiesis of W/W^v and +/+ marrow cells cultured alone and with thymocytes', *Exp. Hemat.,* **8**, 702–708.

37. Zanjani, E. D. (1982). Personal communication.

38. Nathan, D. G. (1981). 'Monoclonal antibody assessments of T cell interaction in erythropoietin studies', *Int. J. Immunopharmacol.,* **3**, 233–247.

39. Poverenny, A. M., Semina, O. V., Semenets, T. N., and Yarilin, A. A. (1980). 'Probable mechanism of spleen colony formation suppression with rabbit antimouse brain antiserum', *Exp. Hemat.,* **8**, 1216–1221.

40. Monette, F. C., and Wassef, W. Y. (1981). 'Thymocyte involvement in spleen colony formation by subpopulations of hematopoietic stem cells', *Exp. Hemat.,* **9**, 1011–1019.

41. Testa, N. G., Schofield, R., and Eliason, J. F. (1980). 'Enhancement of spleen colony formation by live syngeneic thymus cells: Effects on subpopulations of CFU-S', in *Experimental Hematology Today*, (Eds. S. J. Baum, D. Ledney, and D. W. van Bekkum) S. Karger, Basel. pp. 103–108.

42. Tyan, M. L. (1980). 'Marrow colony forming units: age-related changes in responses to anti-θ-sensitive helper/suppressor stimuli', *Proc. Soc. Exp. Biol. Med.,* **165**, 354–360.

43. Iscove, N. N., and Guilbert, L. J. (1978). 'Erythropoietin-independence of early erythropoiesis and a two regulator model of proliferative control in the hemopoietic system', in *In Vitro Aspects of Erythropoiesis*, (Ed. M. J. Murphy, Jr.), Springer-Verlag, New York, pp. 3–7.

44. Aye, M. J. (1976). 'Erythroid colony formation in cultures of human marrow: effect of leukocyte conditioned medium', *J. Cell. Physiol.,* **91**, 69–78.

45. Wagemaker, G. (1978). 'Cellular and soluble factors influencing the differentiation of primitive erythroid progenitor cells (BFU-E) *in vitro*', in *In Vitro Aspects of Erythropoiesis*, (Ed. M. J. Murphy, Jr.), Springer-Verlag, New York, pp. 44–57.

46. Gregory, C. J., and Eaves, A. C. (1977). 'Human marrow cells capable of erythropoietic differentiation *in vitro*: definition of three erythroid colony responses', *Blood,* **49**, 855–864.

47. Johnson, G. R., and Metcalf, D. (1977). 'Erythropoietin-independent erythroid colony formation *in vitro* by fetal mouse cells,' *Exp. Hemat.,* **5 (Supp 2)**, 75.

48. Nathan, D. G., Chess, L., Hillman, D. G., Clark, B., Breard, J., Merler, E., and Housman, D. E. (1978). 'Human erythroid burst forming unit (BFU-E): T cell requirement for proliferation *in vitro*', *J. Exp. Med.,* **147**, 324–339.

49. Porter, P. N., Ogawa, M., and Leary, A. G. (1980). 'Enhancement of the growth of human early erythroid progenitors by bone marrow conditioned media', *Exp. Hemat.,* **8**, 83–88.

50. Hamburger, A. W. (1980). 'Enhancement of human erythroid progenitor cell growth by media conditioned by a human T-lymphocyte line', *Blood,* **56**, 633–639.

51. Cerny, J. (1974). 'Stimulation of bone marrow hemopoietic stem cells by a factor from activated T cells', *Nature,* **249**, 63–66.

52. Cerny, J., Waner, E. B., and Rubin, A. S. (1975). 'T cell products activating stem cells: further studies on the origin and action of the factor(s)', *J. Immunol.,* **115**, 513–518.

53. Frindel E., Leuchars, E., and Davies, A. J. S. (1976). 'Thymus dependency of bone marrow stem cell proliferation in response to certain antigens', *Exp. Hemat.,* **4**, 275–284.

54. Lepault, F., Dardenne, M., and Frindel, E. (1979). 'Restoration by serum thymic factor of colony-forming unit (CFU-S) entry into DNA synthesis in thymecto-mized mice after T-dependent antigen treatment', *Eur. J. Immunol.,* **9**, 661–664.

55. Burstein, S. A., Erb, S. K., Adamson, J. W., and Harker, L. A. (1981). 'Immunologic stimulation of early murine hematopoiesis and its abrogation by cyclosporin A (cyA)', *Blood,* **58 (Suppl 1)**, 93a.

56. Torok-Storb, B. J., Storb, R., Graham, T. C., Prentice, R. L., Weiden, P. L., and Adamson, J. W. (1978). 'Erythropoiesis *in vitro*: Effect of normal versus "transfusion-sensitized" mononuclear cells', *Blood,* **52**, 706–718.

57. Banisadre, M., Ash, R. C., Ascensao, J. L., Kay, N. E., and Zanjani, E. D. (1981). 'Suppression of erythropoiesis by mitogen-activated T lymphocytes *in vitro*', in *Experimental Hematology Today*, (Eds. S. J. Baum, G. D. Ledney, and

A. Kahn), S. Karger, Basel, pp. 151–159.
58. Zanjani, E. D., McGlave, P. B., Davies, S. F., Banisadre, M., Kaplan, M. E., and Sarosi, G. A. (1982). '*In vitro* suppression of erythropoiesis by bone marrow adherent cells from some patients with fungal infection', *Brit. J. Haemat.*, **50**, 479–490.
59. Roodman, G. D., Ascensao, J. L., Banisadre, M., Bloom, P. M., and Zanjani, E. D. (1980). 'Autoimmune pancytopenia. Lymphocyte inhibition of autologous but not allogenic bone marrow growth *in vitro*', *Am. J. Med.*, **69**, 325–328.
60. Haq, A. U., Rinehart, J. J., and Balcerzak, S. P. (1981). 'T-cell subset effects on blood erythroid burst forming units', *Blood*, **58 (Suppl. 1)**, 97a.
61. Torok-Storb, B., Martin, P. J., and Hansen, J. A. (1981). 'Regulation of *in vitro* erythropoiesis by normal T cells: evidence for two T-cell subsets with opposing function', *Blood*, **58**, 171–174.
62. Torok-Storb, B., Martin, P. J., and Hansen, J. A. (1981). 'Cellular interactions in the regulation of *in vitro* erythropoiesis', in *Hemoglobins in Development and Differentiation*, (Eds. G. Stamatoyannopoulos and A. W. Nienhuis) Alan R. Liss, Inc., New York, pp. 137–143.
63. Winchester, R. J., Meyers, P. A., Broxmeyer, H. E., Wang, C. Y., Moore, M. A. S., and Kunkel, H. G. (1978). 'Inhibition of human erythropoietic colony formation in culture by treatment with Ia antisera', *J. Exp. Med.*, **148**, 613–618.
64. Lipton, J., Breard, J., Kudisch, M., Jackson, P., Schlossman, S., and Nathan, D. G. (1979). 'Mature bone marrow erythroid burst forming units (BFU-E) do not require T cell help', *Blood*, **54**, **(Suppl. 1)**, 140a.
65. Micklem, H. S., Ogden, D. A., Evans, E. P., Ford, C. E., and Gray, J. G. (1975). 'Compartments and cell flows within the mouse haemopoietic system II. Estimated rates of interchange', *Cell Tissue Kinet.*, **8**, 233–248.
66. Micklem, H. S., Anderson, N., and Ross, E. (1975). 'Limited potential of circulating haemopoietic stem cells', *Nature*, **256**, 41–43.
67. Rosendaal, M., Hodgson, G. S., and Bradley, T. R. (1979). 'Organization of haemopoietic stem cells: the generation-age hypothesis', *Cell Tissue Kinet.*, **12**, 17–29.
68. Finlay, J. L., Link, M. P., Shatsky, M. G., and Gladen, B. E. (1981). 'Influence of T-lymphocyte depletion by monoclonal antibodies on human peripheral blood erythroid colony (BFU-E) growth', *Blood*, **58 (Suppl. 1)**, 96a.
69. Nomdedeu, B., Gormus, B. J., Rinehart, J. J., Kaplan, M. E., and Zanjani, E. D. (1978). 'Are T-lymphocytes required for growth and differentiation of human erythroid burst-forming units (BFU-E) *in vitro*?' *Blood*, **52 (Suppl. 1)**, 213.
70. Nomdedeu, B., Gormus, B. J., Banisadre, M., Rinehart, J. J., Kaplan, M. E., and Zanjani, E. D. (1980). 'Human peripheral blood erythroid burst forming unit (BFU$_e$): evidence against T-lymphocyte requirement for proliferation *in vitro*', *Exp. Hemat.*, **8**, 845–852.
71. Reid, C. D. L., Baptista, L. C., and Chanarin, I. (1981). 'Erythroid colony growth *in vitro* from human peripheral blood null cells: evidence for regulation by T-lymphocyts and monocytes', *Brit. J. Hemat.*, **48**, 155–164.
72. Zuckerman, K. S. (1980). 'Stimulation of human BFU$_e$ by products of human monocytes and lymphocytes', *Exp. Hemat.*, **8**, 924–932.
73. Zuckerman, K. S. (1981). 'Human erythroid burst-forming units. Growth *in vitro* is dependent on monocytes, but not T lymphocytes', *J. Clin. Invest.*, **67**, 702–709.
74. Kanamaru, A., Durban, E., Gallagher, M. T., Miller, S. C., and Trentin, J. J. (1980). 'Augmentation of erythroid burst formation by the addition of thymocytes and other myelo-lymphoid cells', *J. Cell. Physiol.*, **104**, 187–197.

75. Sawada, U., and Adler, S. S. (1981). '*In vitro* interactions between thymocytes and hemopoietic precursor cells', *Blut*, **42**, 1–12.
76. Mangan, K. F., and Desforges, J. F. (1980). 'The role of T lymphocytes and monocytes in the regulation of human erythropoietic peripheral blood burst forming units', *Exp. Hemat.*, **8**, 717–727.
77. Rinehart, J. J., Zanjani, E. D., Nomdedeu, B., Gormus, B. J., and Kaplan, M. E. (1978). 'Cell–cell interaction in erythropoiesis. Role of human monocytes', *J. Clin. Invest.*, **62**, 979–986.
78. Lipton, J. M., Link, N. A., Breard, J., Jackson, P. L., Clarke, B. J., and Nathan, D. G. (1980). 'Monocytes do not inhibit peripheral blood erythroid burst forming unit colony formation', *J. Clin. Invest.*, **65**, 219–223.
79. Blaese, R. M., Lawrence, E. C., and Poplack, D. G. (1977). 'A critique of techniques of macrophage-monocyte depletion in studies of human peripheral blood mononuclear leukocyte (MNL) function', in *Regulatory Mechanisms in Lymphocyte Activation*, (Ed. D. O. Lucas) Academic Press, New York, pp. 579–582.
80. Gordon, L. I., Miller, W. J., Branda, R. F., Zanjani, E. D., and Jacob, H. S. (1980). 'Regulation of erythroid colony formation by bone marrow macrophages', *Blood*, **55**, 1047–1050.
81. Murphy, M. J., and Urabe, A. (1978). 'Modulatory effects of macrophages on erythropoiesis', in *In Vitro Aspects of Erythropoiesis* (Ed. M. J. Murphy Jr.), Springer-Verlag, New York, pp. 189–191.
82. Mathé, G., Amiel, J. L., Schwarzenberg, L., Choay, J., Trolard, P., Schneider, M., Hayat, M., Schlumberger, J. R., and Jasmin, C. L. (1970). 'Bone marrow graft in man after conditioning by antilymphocytic serum', *Brit. Med. J.*, **ii**, 131–136.
83. Speck, B., Gluckman, E., Haak, H. L., and Van Rood, J. J. (1977). 'Treatment of aplastic anemia by antilymphocyte globulin with and without allogeneic bone marrow infusions, *Lancet*, **ii**, 1145–1148.
84. Thomas, E. D., Storb, R., Giblett, E. R., Longpre, B., Weiden, P. L., Fefer, A., Witherspoon, R., Clift, R. A., and Buckner, C. D. (1976). 'Recovery from aplastic anemia following attempted marrow transplantation', *Exp. Hemat.*, **4**, 97–102.
85. Sensenbrenner, L. L., Steele, A. A., and Santos, G. W. (1977). 'Recovery of hematologic competence without engraftment following attempted bone marrow transplantation for aplastic anemia: Report of a case with diffusion chamber studies', *Exp. Hemat.*, **5**, 51–58.
86. Baran, D. T., Griner, P. F., and Klemperer, M. R. (1976). 'Recovery from aplastic anemia after treatment with cyclophosphamide', *New Engl. J. Med.*, **295**, 1522–1523.
87. Ascensao, J., Kagan, W., Moore, M. Pahwa, R., Hansen, J., and Good, R. (1976). 'Aplastic anaemia: evidence for an immunological mechanism', *Lancet*, **i**, 669–671.
88. Shadduck, R. K., Winkelstein, A., Zeigler, Z., Lichter, J., Goldstein, M., Michaels, M., and Rabin, B. (1979). 'Aplastic anemia following infectious mononucleosis: possible immune etiology', *Exp. Hemat.*, **7**, 264–271.
89. Shadduck, R. K., Winkelstein, A., Zeigler, Z., and Mangan, K. F., (1982). 'Response to antithymocyte globulin (ATG) in severe aplastic anemia', *Clin. Res.*, (in press).
90. Hoffman, R., Zanjani, E. D., Vila, J., Zalusky, R., Lutton, J. D., and Wasserman, L. R. (1976). 'Diamond–Blackfan syndrome: lymphocyte-mediated suppression of erythropoiesis', *Science*, **193**, 899–900.

91. Hoffman, R., Zanjani, E. D., Lutton, J. D., Zalusky, R., and Wasserman, L. R. (1977). 'Suppression of erythroid colony formation of lymphocytes from patients with aplastic anemia', *N. Eng. J. Med.*, **296**, 10–13.

92. Takaku, F., Suda, T., Mizoguchi, H., Miura, Y., Uchino, H., Nagai, K., Kariyone, S., Shibata, A., Akabane, T., Nouma, T., and Maekawa, T. (1980). 'The effect of peripheral blood mononuclear cells from aplastic anemia patients on granulocyte-macrophage and erythroid colony formation in samples from normal human bone marrow *in vitro* — A co-operative work', *Blood*, **55**, 937–943.

93. Linch, D. C., Cawley, J. C., MacDonald, S. M., Masters, G., Roberts, B. E., Antonis, A. H., Waters, A. K., Sieff, C., and Lydyard, P. M. (1981). 'Acquired pure red cell aplasia associated with an increase of T cells bearing receptors for the Fc of IgG', *Acta Haemat.*, **65**, 270–274.

94. Torok-Storb, B. J., Sieff, C., Storb, R., Adamson, J., and Thomas, E. D. (1980). '*In vitro* tests for distinguishing possible immune mediated aplastic anemia from transfusion induced sensitization', *Blood*, **55**, 211–215.

95. Mangan, K. F., Shadduck, R. K., and Winkelstein, A. (1982). 'Plasmapheresis and antithymocyte globulin treatment of chronic refractory pure red cell aplasia: correlation of clinical results with *in vitro* erythroid culture studies', *Clin. Res.*, (in press).

96. Shadduck, R. K. (1982). '*In vitro* colony studies may not predict response to antithymocyte globulin in severe aplastic anemia', *Clin. Res.*, (in press).

97. Wintrobe, M. M., Lee, G. R., Boggs, D. R., Bithell, T. C., Athens, J. W., and Foerster, J. (1974). *Clinical Hematology*, Lea and Febiger, Philadelphia.

98. Hoffman, R., Kopel, S., Hsu, S. D., Dainiak, N., and Zanjani, E. D. (1978). 'T cell chronic lymphocytic leukemia. Presence in bone marrow and peripheral blood of cells that suppress erythropoiesis *in vitro*', *Blood*, **52**, 255–260.

99. Chiorazzi, N., Fu, S. M., Montazeri, G., Kunkel, H. G., Rai, K., and Gee, T. (1979). 'T cell helper defect in patients with chronic lymphocytic leukemia', *J. Immunol.*, **122**, 1087–1090.

100. Kay, N. E., Johnson, J. D., Stanek, R., and Douglas, S. D. (1979). 'T cell subpopulations in chronic lymphocytic leukemia. Abnormalities in distribution and *in vitro* receptor maturation', *Blood*, **54**, 540–544.

101. Mangan, K. F., Chikkappa, G., Scharfman, W. B., Desforges, J. F. (1981). 'Evidence for reduced erythroid burst (BFU_e) promoting function of T lymphocytes in the pure red cell aplasia of chronic lymphocytic leukemia', *Exp. Hemat.*, **9**, 489–498.

102. Mangan, K. F., Chikkappa, G., Bieler, L. Z., and Scharfman, W. B. (1981). 'The role of T lymphocytes bearing Fc receptors for IgM or IgG in the pathogenesis of pure red cell aplasia in a patient with chronic lymphocytic leukemia', in *Experimental Hematology Today* (Eds. S. J. Baum, G. D. Ledney, and A. Khan) S. Karger, Basel, pp. 161–168.

103. Mangan, K. F., Chikkappa, G., and Farley, P. C. (1981). 'T Gamma ($T_γ$) cells suppress erythropoiesis in B cell chronic lymphocytic leukemia', *Blood*, **58**, (**Suppl. 1**), 98a.

104. Tsang, R. W., and Aye, M. T. (1979). 'Evidence for proliferation of erythroid progenitor cells in the absence of added erythropoietin', *Exp. Hemat.*, **7**, 383–388.

105. Golde, D. W., Quan, S. G., and Cline, M. J. (1978). 'Human T lymphocyte cell line producing colony-stimulating activity', *Blood*, **52**, 1068–1072.

106. Ascensao, J. L., Kay, N. E., Earenfight-Engler, T., Koren, H. S., and Zanjani, E. D. (1981). 'Production of erythroid potentiating factor(s) by a human monocytic cell line', *Blood*, **57**, 170–173.

107. Bessis, M. (1958). 'L'ilot erythroblastique, unite fonctionelle de la moelle osseuse', *Rev. Hemat.*, **13**, 8–11.
108. Dexter, T. M., and Lajtha, L. G. (1974). 'Proliferation of haemopoietic stem cells *in vitro*', *Brit. J. Haemat.*, **28**, 525–530.
109. Bentley, S. A. (1981). 'Close range cell:cell interaction required for stem cell maintenance in continuous bone marrow culture', *Exp. Hemat.*, **9**, 308–312.
110. Boll, I. J. M., and Domeyer, C. (1981). 'Cell–cell interaction between lymphocytes and hematopoietic progenitor cells inducing mitosis. Time lapse phase contrast observations with 16 mm film.' *Exp. Hematol.*, **9 (Suppl. 9)**, 147.
111. Boll, I. J. M., and Domeyer, C. (1982). 'Lymphocytes as inducers of mitosis of human morphologically identifiable progenitor cells. Phase contrast observations.' *Exp. Hemat.*, **10**, 326–331.
112. Wolf, N. S., and Trentin, J. J. (1968). 'Hemopoietic colony studies V. Effect of hemopoietic organ stroma on differentiation of pluripotent stem cells', *J. Exp. Med.*, **127**, 205–215.
113. Trentin, J. J. (1970). 'Influence of hematopoietic organ stroma (hematopoietic inductive microenvironments) on stem cell differentiation', in *Regulation of Hematopoiesis*, (Ed. A. S. Gordon), Appleton-Century-Crofts, New York, vol. I, pp. 161–186.
114. Chertkov, J. L., Gurevitch, O. A., and Udalov, G. A. (1980). 'Role of bone marrow stroma in hemopoietic stem cell regulation', *Exp. Hemat.*, **8**, 770–778.
115. Werts, E. D., DeGowin, R. L., Knapp, S. K., and Gibson, D. P. (1980). 'Characterization of marrow stromal (fibroblastoid) cells and their association with erythropoiesis', *Exp. Hemat.*, **8**, 423–433.

Current Concepts in Erythropoiesis
Edited by C. D. R. Dunn
© 1983 John Wiley & Sons Ltd.

CHAPTER 4

Erythroid burst-promoting activity (BPA)

PAMELA N. PORTER and MAKIO OGAWA
Department of Medicine, Medical University of South Carolina and VA Medical Center, Charleston

Contents

I. INTRODUCTION

The initial step in the production of mature blood cells is the commitment of pluripotential hematopoietic precursors to a particular path of differentiation.

The precise mechanism of commitment has been a key question in hemato-poiesis research. Two models have been proposed for the commitment process. According to the first, commitment would occur in a stochastic manner (1,2). According to the second model, commitment would be regulated by the local microenvironment (3,4), either by direct cell–cell interactions or by factors produced by cells in the hematopoietic environment. Regardless of the model, commitment is thought to be irreversible and the replication of stem cells appears to be associated with commitment in a manner which insures that the pluripotential cell compartment is not depleted. In order to distinguish between these two models, investigators have searched for humoral factors and types of cells which are involved in the commitment of pluripotential stem cells to erythropoiesis and for cell types and/or factors which promote the early stages of erythrocytic differentiation.

Initially, the question arose as to whether or not erythropoietin (EPO) which is known to be required for the maturation of red blood cell (RBC) precursors (see 5, for a review), regulates the rate of commitment to erythropoiesis. *In vivo* studies on the mechanism of action of EPO showed that it has no effect on pluripotential hematopoietic progenitors (6). The alternative possibility is that EPO regulates the rate at which committed erythrocytic progenitors become erythroblasts. Support for the latter possibility came from studies in which RBC production was manipulated by injection of EPO into hypertransfused mice. Committed erythrocytic progenitors are depleted in hypertransfused mice. Proerythroblasts appeared 24 hr after EPO injection and erythroblasts and reticulocytes were seen 72 hr following EPO injection (7,8). The cell responding to EPO is operationally termed the erythropoietin responsive cell (ERC). During accelerated erythropoiesis, such as that induced by hypoxia or bleeding, a greater number of ERC are forced into differentiation. In order to sustain the EPO responsive population, the greater cell outflow must be balanced either by increased inflow from earlier cell compartments or by increased self-replication of ERC. When busulfan was used to deplete stem cells (9,10), injections of EPO restored the ERC population in proportion to the dose of EPO but had no effect on the pluripotential stem cells. Without EPO, no ERC were detectable for twelve days following busulfan treatment. These results were interpreted to mean that in addition to its role in transforming immediate precursors into proerythroblasts, EPO stimulates the proliferation of committed erythrocytic progenitors.

The development of clonal cell culture techniques has allowed further investigation of the nature of the ERC and the control of different stages of erythropoiesis. Stephenson *et al* (11) first documented that erythrocytic progenitor cells can be detected in culture by their ability to form clones of hemoglobin (Hb) containing cells. Subsequent studies have shown that different types of clones appear sequentially as a function of incubation time. The clonal precursors have been rather arbitrarily divided into three categories

(12–14). The most mature progenitor cells (CFU-E) form small colonies containing eight to thirty-two cells after a short culture period (two days for mice and four to seven days for human cells). Intermediate precursors form larger colonies at later times (three days for mice and seven to nine days for human). Early (primitive) erythrocytic progenitors (BFU-E) form macroscopic colonies or bursts containing as many as 10^4 cells after longer culture periods (nine days for mice and 14–21 days for human cells). BFU-E and CFU-E can also be distinguished by differences in sedimentation velocity (14), sensitivity to tritiated thymidine (15, 16) and by their EPO requirement (17, 18).

Using clonal cell culture techniques, it became possible to examine the effect of EPO and other humoral agents on erythrocytic progenitors at different stages of differentiation. The number of CFU-E is reduced but not eliminated in the marrow of plethoric mice (13). Stimulation of erythropoiesis by phenylhydrazine or bleeding increased the marrow content of CFU-E and stimulated the migration of BFU-E from the marrow to the spleen (15, 19), and EPO injection increased CFU-E numbers but not BFU-E numbers in the marrow (15). Neither the induction of anemia nor polycythemia changed the proliferative state of the progenitors. Approximately 35% of the BFU-E and 75% of the CFU-E from both anemic and plethoric mice were sensitive to a short incubation with [^{3}H]-thymidine (15, 16). When hematopoietic regeneration was induced by cytosine arabinoside or hydroxyurea, a similar rebound of CFU-E was seen whether or not mice were hypertransfused (20,22).

Test of the hypothesis that commitment is governed by competition between EPO and granulocytic colony stimulating factor (CSF) for the same stem cell population has resulted in conflicting conclusions. At high cell density, Van Zant and Goldwasser (23) found that high levels of EPO suppressed granulocyte-macrophage colonies, and that increasing amounts of CSF caused a decrease in stimulated Hb synthesis. The cell densities required for these effects were so high that the possibilities of overlapping colonies and depletion of the media have to be considered. In contrast, Metcalf and Johnson (24) found that excess amounts of EPO did not reduce the number of non-erythrocytic colonies and that excess CSF did not reduce the number of erythrocytic colonies.

It may be concluded from cell culture studies that unlike the production of CFU-E, which increases at high EPO levels (25), the earliest steps in erythrocytic differentiation are relatively independent of EPO levels. For this reason, investigators have searched for factors other than EPO which influence the early stages of erythropoiesis. A number of cell types and their products have been found to increase the growth of erythrocytic bursts in culture. Axelrad et al (26) first reported that pokeweed mitogen (PWM) stimulated-spleen cell conditioned media (SCM) enhanced the survival of BFU-E during preincubation in the absence of EPO and reduced the EPO requirement of BFU-E. Furthermore, larger bursts were seen in cultures containing PWM–SCM and EPO than in those containing only EPO. Aye (27) reported that erythrocytic colony formation by non-adherent human bone marrow cells is enhanced by the addition of leucocyte conditioned medium (LCM). At that same time, Johnson and Metcalf (28) reported that PWM–SCM enhanced the growth of pure and mixed erythrocytic colonies. Wagemaker (29) found that the addition of irradiated bone marrow cells increased the number of mouse bursts when cells were plated at low density. The cells with burst feeder activity could be distinguished from BFU-E by density centrifugation. Subsequently, Porter et al. (30) found that human bone marrow conditioned media (BMCM) was a good source of human BPA.

II. DEFINITION OF BPA

As a working definition, we have chosen to define BPA as any growth factor which stimulates the production of erythrocytic bursts in culture. We have chosen to exclude from the discussion factors which are known not to be specific for hematopoietic cells. Factors such as growth hormone, insulin, and transferrin were not included since they have been shown to promote the growth of non-hematopoietic cells in culture (31). Analysis of the specificity of factors presumed to be BPA will be a critical aspect of their characterization. After determining that a factor is specific for hematopoietic cells, the next step will be to determine whether or not it is specific for erythrocytic versus granulocytic cells, and finally, the determination of its specificity for early *versus* late erythrocytic progenitors. As BPA studies progress, factors may be found in each of these categories. For example, Aye et al (32) described a lipoprotein fraction which supported the growth of both BFU-E and CFU-C.

III. TYPES OF CELLS PRODUCING BPA

Evidence has accumulated that both T-lymphocytes and monocytes produce BPA. Rinehart et al (33) reported that peripheral blood monocytes inhibited BFU-E growth when unfractionated mononuclear cells were cultured at high density. Subsequent work from their laboratory, however, demonstrated dual effects of macrophages on erythropoiesis in culture; 1–10% monocytes stimulated, but more than 15% were inhibitory (34). Kurland et al (35) also demonstrated an effect of macrophages. The addition of increasing numbers of mouse peritoneal macrophages to agar underlayers resulted in three to five times as many bursts as seen with EPO alone. In contrast, Nathan et al (36) found that T-cells and T-cell conditioned media increased burst formation by the null cell fraction. These studies were carried out at a cell density of 5×10^6 cells/ml without removal of monocytes. Therefore, both inhibition and stimulation from monocytes may have been present. In a later study, treatment of peripheral blood mononuclear cells with complement and a monoclonal cytotoxic antibody prepared against circulating T-cells reduced burst formation (37). In diffusion chambers, erythrocytic colony formation was enhanced by treatment of mouse bone marrow cells with phytohemagglutinin (PHA) prior to culture (38). PHA did not augment erythrocytic colony formation when bone marrow was depleted of Thy-1-bearing cells. BPA as well as CSF was released during secondary immune responses by mouse spleen cells in culture (39). Activity was released when helper T-cells were cultured with specific antigens. This release depended upon interaction with accessory cells present in the spleen or peritoneal cavity. Specific pathogen-free CBA and C57BL/6 mice had low numbers of bursts which could be increased by co-culture with thymocytes (40). Clinically, however, T-lymphocytes do not seem to be essential for erythropoiesis. Anemia is not seen in patients with DiGeorge syndrome nor is it a cardinal feature of severe combined immune deficiency. Therefore, it is unlikely that T-cells are the sole source of any essential erythropoietic factor.

Zuckerman (41,42) examined the production of BPA by human monocytes and lymphocytes in detail. His arguments for a predominant role for monocytes are the following: (a) the reduction of BFU-E after depletion of monocytes alone; (b) the relatively large number of T-lymphocytes that are required for an effect [2×10^5 T-cells vs 10^4 monocytes]; (c) the complete return to expected numbers of BFU-E to cell suspensions depleted of both monocytes and T-lymphocytes by the addition of small numbers of monocytes; and (d) higher BPA in monocyte CM than in T-lymphocyte CM. Reid et al (43) also found that either T-lymphocytes or monocytes induce the growth of BFU-E and that co-culture of null cells with both T-cells and monocytes gave a greater response than either did alone.

Further evidence that BPA is produced by lymphocytes and monocytes--macrophages comes from studies of established cell lines. Golde et al (44) found that the human T-lymphoblast cell line, Mo, produces BPA as well as CSF (45). This cell line was obtained from a patient with a T-cell variant of hairy-cell leukemia. Mo cells have the following characteristics: (a) lymphoblastic morphology; (b) formation of rosettes with sheep red blood cells; (c) sensitivity to anti-thymocyte globulin; (d) inability to synthesize immunoglobulin; and (e) absence of Epstein–Barr antigens. Another T-lymphocyte cell line, ATCC.CCL 119 (CCRF–CEM) derived from a patient with T-cell acute lymphocytic leukemia, also produces BPA (46). The mouse macrophage cell line, WEHI-3 (47), and two human monocyte cell lines, GCT (48), and U-937 (49), have also been reported to produce BPA. U-937 was derived from a pleural effusion of a patient with histiocytic lymphoma, and these cells have macrophage characteristics (50).

Monocytes and T-lymphocytes may not be the only sources of BPA. Recently, Meytes et al (51) found that BPA is produced by phytohemagglutinin stimulated, radio-resistant, peripheral blood mononuclear cells which originated in a non-adherent, non-rosetting (T-cell depleted) cell population. Marrow stromal cells also appear to produce BPA (52). DeGowin and Gibson (53) confirmed the enhancement of the growth of erythrocytic colonies by small numbers of marrow stromal cells and found that indomethacin suppressed this enhancement. They postulated that E-type prostaglandins may mediate the effects of marrow stromal cells on erythrocytic development.

IV. BPA ASSAY

A major problem in comparing the BPA in various sources is the lack of a standard assay. A recurrent problem has been the control of endogenous levels of BPA since many of the commonly used tissue culture reagents (particularly fetal calf serum, human plasma and crude EPO) probably contain BPA. Johnson and Metcalf (28) used fetal mouse liver cells in semi-solid agar containing human plasma and found that lectin-stimulated SCM supported the formation of pure and mixed erythrocytic colonies in the absence of EPO. Iscove (54) assayed the BPA in mouse SCM in methylcellulose cultures of mouse bone marrow cells containing reduced serum concentrations. Ultimately, the use of serum-free defined media should alleviate these problems. Iscove *et al* (55) have successfully cultured mouse CFU-E in a defined serum-free culture system supplemented with bovine serum albumin, transferrin, Fe^{2+}, selenium, cholesterol, and lecithin. The culture of BFU-E in the complete absence of serum, however, has proven to be more difficult. Belger *et al* (56) have had some success, but at a substantially reduced plating efficiency. Another problem is that the BPA and EPO preparations commonly used are crude extracts and often contain more than one hematopoietic factor. The development of a standardized, quantitative assay for BPA is complicated by the fact that EPO and BPA may act synergistically (26, 30, 54). Varying levels of burst feeder activity make it difficult to compare the responses of cells from different sources. The ideal culture system for the assay of BPA would be a serum-free culture system which uses a cell fraction from which burst feeder activity had been removed, while maintaining good recovery of BFU-E.

V. TARGETS OF BPA

Early committed erythrocytic precursors are generally thought to be the primary target cell for BPA. Initially, Gregory and Eaves (12) found the effect of LCM to be restricted to large bursts. The BPA in lectin-stimulated mouse CM promotes the growth of mouse BFU-E but not CFU-E (54), and reduces the requirement of BFU-E for fetal calf serum and EPO. Similar results were obtained by Porter *et al* (30) using human BMCM as a source of BPA and also by Humphries *et al* (57) using PWM-SCM. Many of the large, day 14 BFU-E analyzed by Humphries *et al* revealed a mixed cellular composition. These results are consistent with earlier observations by Johnson and Metcalf (28) that one-third to one-half of the day 7 erythrocytic colonies seen in cultures of mouse fetal liver cells contained non-erythrocytic cells.

Somewhat different results have been observed by others. Human macrophage CM increased the numbers of both erythrocytic colonies (day 7) and erythrocytic bursts (day 14) (34). Similar results were observed for CM from the monocyte cell line U-937 (49). Feeder layers of peritoneal macrophages increased the plating efficiency of murine CFU-E and BFU-E equally (35). Although such cells are assumed not to release EPO, this possibility is probably worthy of reinvestigation, since an erythrocytic stimulating factor was detected in the supernatant when fetal liver, adult bone marrow or spleen macrophages were incubated with silica (58). Evidence that suggests that this factor may be EPO includes its activity in the polycythemic mouse EPO assay, its sensitivity to anti-EPO and its ability to support the growth of fetal liver CFU-E (59). Golde *et al* (44) also found that CM from their lymphoblast cell line promoted the growth of human CFU-E (day 7–8) and BFU-E (day 14), and for this reason, they have chosen to call their factor ESA (erythrocytic stimulating activity) instead of BPA. Because their ESA is not specific for BFU-E, they have suggested that this may reflect a difference between human and mouse erythrocytic factors. However, Porter *et al* (30) have found that the BPA in human BMCM promotes the growth of BFU-E but not CFU-E. This apparent difference may be due to differences in precursor classification. Different classes of erythrocytic cells are well-defined for mouse marrow cells (17): CFU-E mature on day 2, mature BFU-E on day 3 and BFU-E on day 7. However, more variability exists in the classification of human cells. Human CFU-E have been scored as early as days 4–5 (14) or as late as days 7–8 (12). In studies of BPA specificity, Golde *et al* (44) scored human CFU-E on days 7–8; whereas Porter *et al* (30) scored human CFU-E on day 5.

Confusion as to the target cell for BPA may also be the result of the use of rather ill-defined culture systems. Generally, endogenous levels of BPA have not been well controlled. Non-hematopoietic cells within the cultured population may provide an appreciable amount of burst feeder activity. Although it is now generally accepted that sensitivity to EPO parallels the maturity of erythrocytic progenitors (29), the relative sensitivity to other erythropoietic factors remains to be established. In this regard, it is conceivable that the apparent differences in the target cell are quantitative rather than qualitative. Both BFU-E and CFU-E could be sensitive to BPA with BFU-E being more sensitive than CFU-E. Another possibility is that ESA, which acts on both CFU-E and BFU-E, is a different factor from BPA, which is specific for BFU-E.

VI. EFFECTS OF BPA

In studying the response of BFU-E to BPA under different culture conditions, Iscove (54) found that his partially-purified mouse spleen BPA reduced the serum and EPO requirement of mouse BFU-E but had no effect on the plating efficiency of CFU-E. He carried out delayed addition studies to determine if BPA and EPO acted simultaneously or sequentially. In cultures containing BPA, BFU-E were indifferent to the absence of EPO for up to seven days. Four days following the addition of EPO, large bursts were seen, which suggests that the role of EPO was to allow hemoglobinization of the later maturational stages. If, however, the addition of BPA was delayed for one day, there was a 75% reduction in the number of bursts which subsequently developed. Thus, BPA is required for the functional survival of BFU-E and it seems to act earlier in the maturational sequence than EPO. Wagemaker *et al* (60) have argued that the absence of erythrocytic bursts at low cell concentrations implies that BFU-E are not able to directly respond to EPO but are dependent on an accessory activity designated as burst feeder activity. This activity is specific for BFU-E. They also confirmed the observation (54) that increasing the BPA concentration decreases the requirement of BFU-E for EPO. Similar responses of human BFU-E to BPA have been reported by Porter *et al* (30) in that the BPA in BMCM reduces the serum and EPO requirements of BFU-E, and BMCM protects against the effect of the delayed addition of EPO for up to four days after the initiation of the cultures.

Another aspect of the characterization of BPA is its effect on burst size. In their initial report, Axelrad *et al* (26) noted that bursts were larger when SCM was included in the medium. Eliason *et al* (61) studied hemoglobin (Hb) synthesis by erythrocytic colonies and bursts. Plots of burst number *versus* number of cells plated were compared to plots of Hb synthesis *versus* the number of cells plated. The slope of the Hb synthesis curve was greater than that of the burst number curve. In contrast, essentially parallel curves were seen for CFU-E. These results indicate enhanced Hb synthesis at high cell densities and are consistent with the presence of burst feeder activity at high cell density (19). Porter *et al* (30, 62) reported that addition of BMCM results in a larger increase in the incorporation of ^{59}Fe into heme than in burst number. The question of the effect of BPA on Hb synthesis was investigated in detail by Ogawa *et al* (63). They found that when burst feeder activity was reduced by adherence and by lowering the serum concentration, a much larger effect of crude BPA was seen on Hb synthesis (700% of control values) than on burst number (160% of control values). Similar results were seen for human and rabbit cells. Rabbit bone marrow cells, which form particularly large bursts, were cultured in the presence and absence of BMCM, and the size and Hb synthesis of individual bursts measured. Cumulative, relative frequency distributions showed a shift in the size of the bursts in cultures containing BMCM. A similar shift was seen for Hb synthesis in individual bursts. Since BPA increases both the number of erythrocytic bursts in culture and the size of these bursts, we have postulated that BPA has dual functions: (a) the recruitment of BFU-E into proliferation in culture; and (b) the enhancement of cell division during the early phase of burst formation.

BPA has also been shown to influence the type of Hb synthesized by culture cells. Initially, Kidoguchi *et al* (64) showed that the relative rate of fetal hemoglobin (HbF) biosynthesis in culture depended upon the concentration of EPO. However, since crude preparations of EPO were used, the observed effects may have been due to factors other than EPO in these preparations. The observation by Fauser and Messner (65) that the addition of PHA–LCM increased the number of HbF-containing erythrocytic bursts gave support for this idea. Therefore, we reinvestigated the effects of preparations of EPO, varying in purity, and BPA on HbF biosynthesis. Using pure EPO, there was no dose-response relationship between EPO concentration and HbF biosynthesis. Two different sources of BPA, BMCM and T-lymphocyte cell line (Mo) CM increased the ratio of HbF/(HbF + HbA) (66). While we have no insight into the mechanism of BPA augmentation of HbF biosynthesis, these preliminary studies with BPA suggest that it may be possible to manipulate HbF synthesis in culture to some extent. In this regard, it is of interest that high levels of BPA have been found in the sera of patients with aplastic anemia (67, 68) and significantly high levels of HbF have been detected in patients with various hematological disorders associated with severe anemia, including recipients of bone marrow transplants (69).

VII. PURIFICATION OF BPA

Purification of BPA from different sources has been initiated in several laboratories, but is far from complete for any source of BPA. The first material used for purification was lectin-stimulated mouse SCM — a particularly rich source of many hematopoietic factors. Iscove (54) subjected concanavalin A stimulated SCM to two purification steps. First, concentrated SCM was applied to a concanavalin A Sepharose column, and BPA was eluted with α-methylglucoside. The active fraction was then gel filtered on Sephadex G-150. The apparent molecular weight of this BPA was estimated to be 35,000D. Enrichment, but not complete purification, of BPA was obtained. Burgess *et al* (70) have also attempted to separate the different hematopoietic factors present in SCM. The factors were bound to concanavalin A Sepharose and were eluted with α-methyl-D-glucopyranoside. All colony stimulating factors showed the same apparent molecular weight by gel filtration on Sephadex G-150. However, charge differences were detected by isoelectric focusing. Granulocyte CSF had a pI of 4.8; eosinophil CSF had a pI of 5.8. Erythrocyte and megakaryocyte CSFs were detected between 4.6 and 7.1. Thus far, they have not been able to completely separate BPA from CSF. Using CM from a T-lymphoblast cell line, Mo, as a source of starting material, Golde *et al* (44) have partially purified human BPA. The isoelectric point of this human BPA is

3.5–4.8. This BPA had a higher apparent molecular weight (45,000D) than CSF (34,000D) when analyzed using gel filtration with AcA-44. However, the BPA and CSF peaks overlapped too much to allow complete separation by this technique. The BPA in this source has a remarkable heat stability, in that 75% of the activity is retained after boiling for 30 minutes. Human BPA has been purified 300-fold from BMCM by ion-exchange chromatography using DEAE Sephadex and hydroxyapatite ultragel. Marrow BPA appears to have different characteristics than the BPA in Mo CM. For example, the marrow BPA is more heat sensitive than Mo BPA with a 50% loss in activity after treatment at 80 °C for 10 min (62) and has a higher apparent molecular weight (unpublished observations).

Since Burgess *et al* (70) were not able to separate BPA from CSF, they proposed that one molecule may be able to stimulate all four colony types: erythrocyte, eosinophil, granulocyte/macrophage and megakaryocyte. Initially they observed that when added together, purified granulocyte/macrophage CSF and purified EPO were able to support the growth of early erythrocytic precursors, whereas neither were effective when added alone (24). If we assume that their CSF was in fact pure, this would indicate an effect of CSF on erythrocytic precursors. Subsequently, the effect of preincubation with granulocyte/macrophage CSF on erythrocytic precursor cells was examined (71). Preincubation of fetal liver cells for two days in saline results in the loss of both nonerythrocytic and erythrocytic colony forming cells. This loss can be partially prevented by preincubation with very high concentrations of CSF. When cells were cultured for two days with purified CSF and the developing clones transferred to dishes containing SCM, several types of colonies were seen — granulocyte/macrophage, erythrocytic and mixed erythrocytic. If, however, clones were transferred to dishes containing only purified CSF, granulocytic colonies developed but no erythrocytic or mixed erythrocytic colonies developed. They concluded that CSF was able to directly stimulate up to five cell divisions for multipotential and early erythrocytic precursor cells. Although the CSF used in the preincubation studies (71) was highly purified, it may not be homogeneous. Determination of whether or not this CSF is completely free of BPA is critical to the interpretation of these results.

The question of the identity of BPA and CSF can also be examined by a comparison of the biochemical characteristics of BPA and CSF. Arguments for their identity include; (a) the same molecular weight was observed for BPA and CSF in PWM-SCM (70) and (b) similar elution profiles were seen for CSF and BPA on blue sepharose and phenyl sepharose (70). On the other hand, several arguments against this hypothesis can be raised. (a) BPA appears to be more labile than CSF (70). (b) Although incompletely resolved, some separation of erythrocytic and granulocyte/macrophage CSF was obtained using preparative isoelectric focusing (70). (c) Using T-lymphocyte cell line,

Mo'CM, Golde *et al* (34) found differences in the heat stability of CSF and BPA. (d) Mo CM BPA showed a broad profile on gel filtration which overlapped with CSF, but the peak of erythrocytic activity was distinct from the peak of CSF activity (34). (e) A final argument is the presence of BPA in some sources such as BMCM, in which CSF was not detectable (30). A definitive answer to this question must await purification and more complete characterization of BPA. However, using current data, it seems reasonable to conclude that BPA and CSF are similar but not identical. Interpretation is complicated by the fact that CSF is not a single factor but different factors with different specificities (72–75), and the same may be true for BPA. There may be factors specific for granulopoiesis or erythropoiesis as well as factors which act on pluripotential precursors. CSF and/or BPA at very high levels may have some activity on pluripotential CFU, but also have specificity at lower levels, with CSF acting preferentially on CFU-C and BPA acting preferentially on BFU-E.

VIII. ACTIONS OF BPA

An important question is whether or not BPA influences commitment. If BPA affected commitment, it would increase the production of BFU-E from CFU-S. A liquid culture system has been developed by Dexter and colleagues which supports the proliferation of CFU-S and the production of CFU-C and BFU-E for several weeks. In this culture system, granulopoiesis predominates over erythropoiesis. Colony stimulating activity was absent in the cultures, and the addition of exogenous CSF caused a rapid decline in the number of stem cells and reduced granulopoiesis (76). However, in later studies purified CSF had no appreciable effect (77, 78). Only a very limited erythropoiesis occurs in these cultures; however, BFU-E remain for a few weeks (79). Experiments have been carried out to determine the effect of EPO on erythropoiesis in long-term liquid cultures (80). EPO had no effect on the production of BFU-E from CFU-S, but did allow the maturation of BFU-E into CFU-E. Recently, Dexter *et al* (81) examined the effect of serum from anemic mice. Within twelve days, erythroblasts, hemoglobinized cells and CFU-E appeared. The anemic contained EPO, but EPO alone was not sufficient. These results were interpreted to mean that anemic mouse serum contains a second factor which promotes erythrocytic development. Whether or not this factor is BPA is not known. CFU-C levels were unaffected by the addition of anemic mouse serum, which indicates the absence of competition at the progenitor cell level. A DNA synthesis inhibitor from freshly isolated normal adult mouse bone marrow and a stimulatory one from regenerating bone marrow which is specific for CFU-S have been partially characterized (82). Separation of these factors is requisite to a determination of how they may affect commitment.

An alternative possibility is that the process of commitment is a stochastic process and that factors like CSF and BPA stimulate the division of early committed progenitors. According to this model, very small bursts would develop at low BPA levels and larger ones at higher BPA levels. This is analogous to a model developed for the mechanism of action of CSF (83). When early four-cell clusters were separated and replated with and without CSF, the size of the colonies that ultimately developed was dependent on the CSF concentration. Ogawa *et al* (63) compared the size of bursts that developed in the presence of BPA to the size of bursts in cultures without BPA. The size of rabbit marrow bursts varied over a wide range, and the addition of BPA resulted in a shift in the size distribution toward larger bursts. These results are consistent with the original observation that SCM increased the size of bursts even under conditions where there was no increase in burst number (26). The mechanism by which BPA increases the size of bursts could be to increase the number of cell divisions between BFU-E and hemoglobinized cells.

Under most culture conditions, various sources of BPA increase both the number and size of bursts. The increase in burst number may come from recruitment of BFU-E into proliferation in culture. Stated in another way, BPA could influence the departure of BFU-E from the G_0 phase (26). An additional effect of BPA may be the recruitment of BFU-E from an earlier pluripotential population. This possibility is supported by the effect of PHA-LCM, a source of BPA and CSF, on the observed incidence of mixed colonies (65). Recruitment by BPA could be thought of in either an active or in a passive sense. According to the first model, BPA would induce the initial events of erythropoiesis. According to the second, BPA would play a passive role by simply allowing BFU-E to develop into bursts. It is currently impossible to distinguish between these possibilities. However, the survival of BFU-E is known to depend on the composition of the culture medium. Iscove (54) observed that if BPA was absent during the first two days of culture, the number of bursts that ultimately developed was substantially reduced. The urinary factor described by Dukes *et al* (84) increased the survival of both CFU-S and BFU-E in culture. Similarly, a human fibroblast factor has been described which supports the survival of CFU-S (85, 86).

The biological significance of what has been called BPA, burst feeder activity, burst enhancing activity or ESA is not known. Thus far, BPA has been defined and assayed exclusively in cell culture systems. The development of an *in vivo* assay is necessary in order to determine its biological function. The possibility of some biological significance has been raised by the presence of BPA in the serum of patients with aplastic anemia (67, 68). In contrast, BPA was not detectable in sera from normal adults or from patients with mild anemia.

Since BPA has been under investigation for only four years, many questions remain unanswered: (a) Is BPA one factor or several? (b) What is the specificity of BPA? (c) Does it play a role in commitment? (d) Does it play a regulatory role in erythrocytic development?

IX. ACKNOWLEDGMENTS

This work was supported by NIH grants AM27040, AM22170, HL20913 and the Veterans Administration. Dr Ogawa is a VA Medical Investigator.

X. ABBREVIATIONS

EPO:	erythropoietin
ERC:	erythropoietin responsive cell
Hb:	hemoglobin
CFU-E:	colony forming unit — erythrocytic
BFU-E:	burst forming unit — erythrocytic
CFU-C:	colony forming unit — culture 'granulocytic'
CSF:	colony stimulating factor
BPA:	burst promoting activity
SCM:	spleen cell conditioned media
LCM:	leucocyte conditioned media
BMCM:	bone marrow conditioned media
PHA:	phytohemagglutinin
PWM:	pokeweed mitogen
HbF:	fetal hemoglobin

XI. REFERENCES

1. Korn, A. P., Henkelman, R. M., Ottensmeyer, F. P., and Till, J. E. (1973). 'Investigations of a stochastic model of haemopoiesis', *Exp. Hemat.*, **1**, 362–375.
2. Till, J. E., McCulloch, E. A., and Siminovitch L. (1964). 'A stochastic model of stem cell proliferation based on the growth of spleen colony-forming cells', *Proc. Nat. Acad. Sci. (USA).*, **51**, 29–36.
3. Trentin, J. J. (1971). 'Determination of bone marrow stem cell differentiation by stromal hemopoietic inductive microenvironments (HIM)', *Am. J. Path.*, **65**, 621–628.
4. Wolf, N. S., and Trentin, J. J. (1968). 'Hemopoietic colony studies. V. Effect of hemopoietic organ stroma on differentiation of pluripotent stem cells,' *J. Exp. Med.*, **127**, 205–215.
5. Graber, S. E., and Krantz, S. B. (1978). 'Erythropoietin and the control of red cell production', *Ann. Rev. Med.*, **29**, 51–66.
6. Bruce, W. R., and McCulloch, E. A. (1964). 'The effect of erythropoietic stimulation on the hemopoietic colony-forming cells of mice', *Blood,* **23**, 216–283.

7. Filmanowicz, E., and Gurney, C. W. (1961). 'Studies on erythropoiesis. XVI. Response to a single dose of erythropoietin in a polycythemic mouse', *J. Lab. Clin. Med.*, **57**, 65–72.
8. Jacobson, L. O., Goldwasser, E., Plzak, L., and Fried, W. (1957). 'Studies on erythropoiesis. VI. Reticulocyte response of hypophysectomized and polycythemic rodents to erythropoietin', *Proc. Soc. Exp. Biol. Med.*, **94**, 243–249.
9. Reissman, K. R., and Samorapoompichit, S. (1970). 'Effects of erythropoietin on proliferation of erythroid stem cells in the absence of transplantable colony-forming units', *Blood*, **36**, 287–296.
10. Reissman, K. R., and Udupa, K. B. (1972). 'Effect of erythropoietin on proliferation of erythropoietin-responsive cells', *Cell Tissue Kinet.*, **5**, 481–489.
11. Stephenson, J. R., Axelrad, A. A., McLeod, D. L., and Shreeve, M. M. (1971). 'Induction of colonies of hemoglobin-synthesizing cells by erythropoietin *in vitro*', *Proc. Nat. Acad. Sci. (USA).*, **68**, 1542–1546.
12. Gregory, C. J., and Eaves, A. C. (1977). 'Human marrow cells capable of erythropoietic differentiation *in vitro*: Definition of three erythroid colony responses', *Blood*, **49**, 855–864.
13. Gregory, C. J., McCulloch, E. A., and Till, J. E. (1973). Erythropoietic progenitors capable of colony formation in culture: State of differentiation', *J. Cell. Physiol.*, **81**, 411–420.
14. Ogawa, M., MacEachern, M. D. and Avila, L. (1977). 'Human marrow erythropoiesis in culture. II. Heterogeneity in the morphology, time course of colony formation and sedimentation velocities of the colony forming cells', *Am. J. Hemat.*, **3**, 29–36.
15. Hara, H., and Ogawa, M. (1977). 'Erythropoietic precursors in mice under erythropoietic stimulation and suppression', *Exp. Hemat.*, **5**, 141–148.
16. Iscove, N. N. (1977). 'The role of erythropoietin in regulation of population size and cell cycling of early and late erythroid precursors in mouse bone marrow', *Cell Tissue Kinet.*, **10**, 323–334.
17. Gregory, C. J. (1976). 'Erythropoietin sensitivity as a differentiation marker in the hemopoietic system: Studies of three erythropoietic colony responses in culture,' *J. Cell. Physiol.*, **89**, 289–302.
18. Wagemaker, G. (1978). 'Cellular and soluble factors influencing the differentiation of primitive erythroid progenitor cells (BFU-e) *in vitro*', in *In Vitro Aspects of Erythropoiesis*. (Ed. M. J. Murphy) Springer-Verlag, New York, pp. 43–57.
19. Hara, H., and Ogawa, M. (1976). 'Erythropoietic precursors in mice with phenylhydrazine-induced anemia', *Am. J. Hemat.*, **1**, 453–458.
20. Seidel, H. J., and Kreja, L. (1980). 'Erythroid stem cell regeneration in normal and plethoric mice treated with cytosinarabinoside,' *Exp. Hemat.*, **8**, 541–548.
21. Seidel, H. J., and Opitz, U. (1979). 'Erythroid stem cell regeneration in normal and plethoric mice treated with hydroxyurea', *Exp. Hemat.*, **7**, 500–508.
22. Wagemaker, G., and Visser, T. P. (1980). 'Erythropoietin-independent regeneration of erythroid progenitor cells following multiple injections of hydroxyurea,' *Cell Tissue Kinet.*, **13**, 503–517.
23. van Zant, G., and Goldwasser, E. (1979). 'Competition between erythropoietin and colony-stimulating factor for target cells in mouse marrow,' *Blood,* **53**, 946–965.
24. Metcalf, D., and Johnson, G. R. (1979). 'Interactions between purified GM-CSF, purified erythropoietin and spleen conditioned medium on hemopoietic colony formation *in vitro*', *J. Cell. Physiol.*, **99**, 159–174.
25. Testa, N. G., Eliason, J. F., and Frassoni, F. (1980). 'Role of purified

erythropoietin in the amplification of the erythroid compartment', *Exp. Hemat.*, **8**, (**Suppl. 8**), 144–152.

26. Axelrad, A. A., McLeod, D. L., Suzuki, S., and Shreeve, M. M. (1978). 'Regulation of the population size of erythropoietic progenitor cells', in *Differentiation of Normal and Neoplastic Cells*. (Eds. B. Clarkson, P. A. Marks, and J. E. Till), Cold Spring Harbor, New York, pp. 155–163.

27. Aye, M. T. (1977). 'Erythroid colony formation in cultures of human marrow: Effects of leukocyte conditioned medium,' *J. Cell. Physiol.*, **91**, 69–77.

28. Johnson, G. R., and Metcalf, D. (1977). 'Pure and mixed erythroid colony formation *in vitro* stimulated by spleen conditioned medium with no detectable erythropoietin', *Proc. Nat. Acad. Sci.*, *(USA).*, **74**, 3879–3882.

29. Wagemaker, G. (1978). 'Induction of erythropoietin responsiveness *in vitro*', in *Hemopoietic Cell Differentiation*. (Eds. M. J. Cline, D. W. Golde, D. Metcalf, and C. F. Fox), Academic Press, New York, pp. 109–118.

30. Porter, P. N., Ogawa, M., and Leary, A. G. (1980). 'Enhancement of the growth of human early erythroid progenitors by bone marrow conditioned medium', *Exp. Hemat.*, **8**, 83–88.

31. Barnes, D., and Sato, G. (1980). 'Serum free cell culture, a unifying approach', *Cell*, **22**, 649–655.

32. Aye, M. T., Sequin, J. A., and McBurney, J. P. (1979). 'Erythroid and granulocytic colony growth in cultures supplemented with human serum lipoproteins', *J. Cell. Physiol.*, **99**, 233–238.

33. Rinehart, J. J., Zanjani, E. S., Nomdedeu, B., Gormus, B. J., and Kaplan, M. E. (1978). 'Cell–cell interaction in erythropoiesis: Role of human monocytes', *J. Clin. Invest.*, **62**, 979–986.

34. Gordon, L. I., Miller, W. J., Branda, R. F., Zanjani, E. S., and Jacob, H. S. (1980). 'Regulation of erythroid colony formation by bone marrow macrophages', *Blood*, **55**, 1047–1050.

35. Kurland, J. I., Meyers, P. A., and Moore, M. A. S. (1980). 'Synthesis and release of erythroid colony and burst-potentiating activities by purified populations of murine peritoneal macrophages', *J. Exp. Med.*, **151**, 839–852.

36. Nathan, D. G., Chess, L., Hillman D. G., Clarke, B., Breard, J., Merler, E., and Housman, D. E. (1979). 'Human erythroid burst-forming unit: T-cell requirement for proliferation *in vitro*', *J. Exp. Med.*, **117**, 322–339.

37. Lipton, J. M., and Nathan, D. G. (1981). 'Role of T lymphocytes in human erythropoiesis', in *The Lymphocyte, Progress in Clinical and Biological Regulation*. (Eds. K. W. Sell, and W. V. Miller) Alan R. Liss, New York, pp. 57–75.

38. Niskanen, E., Ashman, R., and Cline, M. J. (1980). 'Enhancement of murine colony formation in the presence of activated T-lymphocytes', *J. Lab. Clin. Med.*, **95**, 934–942.

39. Schreier, M. H., and Iscove, N. N. (1980). 'Hematopoietic growth factors are released in cultures of H-2-restricted helper T cells, accessory cells and specific antigens', *Nature*, **287**, 228–230.

40. Kanamaru, A., Durban, E., Gallagher, M. T., Miller, S. C., and Trentin, J. J. (1980). 'Augmentation of erythroid burst formation by the addition of thymocytes and other myelo-lymphoid cells', *J. Cell. Physiol.*, **104**, 187–197.

41. Zuckerman, K. S. (1981). 'Human erythroid burst-forming units: Growth *in vitro* is dependent on monocytes but not T-lymphocytes', *J. Clin. Invest.*, **67**, 702–709.

42. Zuckerman, K. S. (1980). 'Stimulation of human BFU-e by products of human monocytes and lymphocytes', *Exp. Hemat.*, **8**, 924–932.

43. Reid, C. D. L., Baptista, L. C., and Chanarin, I. (1981). 'Erythroid colony growth *in vitro* from human peripheral blood null cells: Evidence for regulation by T-lymphocytes and monocytes', *Brit. J. Haemat.*, **48**, 155–164.

44. Golde, D. W., Bersch, N., Quan, S. D., and Lusis, A. J. (1980). 'Production of erythroid potentiating activity by a human T-lymphoblast cell line', *Proc. Nat. Acad. Sci., (USA).*, **77**, 593–596.

45. Golde, D. W., Quan, S. G., and Cline, M. J. (1978). 'Human T-lymphocyte cell line producing colony stimulating activity', *Blood*, **52**, 1068–1072.

46. Hamberger, A. W. (1980). 'Enhancement of human erythroid progenitor cell growth by media conditioned by a human T-lymphocyte line', *Blood*, **56**, 633–639.

47. Iscove, N. N., and Schreier, M. (1979). 'Involvement of T-cells and macrophages in generation of burst-promoting activity (BPA)', *Exp. Hemat.*, **7** (**Suppl. 6**), 4. (abstract).

48. Abboud, C. N., DiPersio, J. F., Brennan, J. K., and Lichtman, M. A. (1980). 'Erythropoietic enhancing activity derived from a human cell line: Similarity to colony stimulating activity', *Clin. Res.*, **28**, 303a. (abstract).

49. Ascensao, J. L., Key, N. E., Earenfight-Engler, T., Koren, H. S., and Zanjani, E. S. (1981). 'Production of erythroid potentiating factor(s) by a human monocyte cell line', *Blood*, **57**, 170–173.

50. Sundstrom, C., and Nilsson, K. (1976). 'Establishment and characterization of a human histiocytic lymphoma cell line (U-937)', *Int. J. Cancer*, **17**, 565–577.

51. Meytes, D., Ma, A., Ortega, J. A., Shore, N. A., and Dukes, P. P. (1979). 'Human erythroid burst-promoting activity produced by phytohemagglutinin-stimulated radioresistant peripheral mononuclear cells', *Blood*, **54**, 1050–1057.

52. Werts, E. D., DeGowin, R. L., Knapp, S. K., and Gibson, D. P. (1980). 'Characterization of marrow stromal (fibroblastoid) cells and their association with erythropoiesis', *Exp. Hemat.*, **8**, 423–433.

53. DeGowin, R. L., and Gibson, D. P. (1981). 'Prostaglandin-mediated enhancement of erythroid colonies by marrow stromal cells (MSC)', *Exp. Hemat.*, **9**, 274–280.

54. Iscove, N. N. (1978). 'Erythropoietin-independent stimulation of early erythro-poiesis in adult marrow cultures by conditioned media from lectin-stimulated mouse spleen cells', in *Hematopoietic Cell Differentiation*. (Eds. D. W. Golde, M. J. Cline, D. Metcalf, and F. C. Fox), Academic Press, New York, pp. 37–52.

55. Iscove, N. N., Guilbert, L. J., and Weyman, C. (1980). 'Complete replacement of serum in primary cultures of erythropoietin-dependent red cell precursors (CFU-e) by albumin, transferrin, iron, unsaturated fatty acid, lecithin, and cholesterol', *Exp. Cell. Res.*, **126**, 121–126.

56. Belger, M. B., Bersch, N., and Golde, D. W. (1979). 'Serum-free system for growth of human erythroid progenitor cells', *Blood*, **54**, (**Suppl. 1**), 133. (abstract).

57. Humphries, R. K., Eaves, A. C., and Eaves, C. J. (1979). 'Characterization of a primitive erythropoietic progenitor found in mouse marrow before and after several weeks in culture', *Blood*, **53**, 746–763.

58. Rich, I. N., Heit, W., and Kubanek, B. (1980). 'An erythropoietic stimulating factor similar to erythropoietin released by macrophages after treatment with silica', *Blut*, **40**, 297–303.

59. Rich, I. N., Anselstetter, V., Heit, W., Zanjani, E. S., and Kubanek, B. (1981). 'Release of erythropoietin from macrophages by treatment with silica,' *J. Supramol. Struc. Cell Biochem.*, **15**, 169–176.

60. Wagemaker, G., Peters, M. F., and Bol., S. J. L. (1979). 'Induction of erythropoietin responsiveness *in vitro* by a distinct population of bone marrow cells', *Cell Tissue Kinet.*, **12**, 521–537.

61. Eliason, J. F., van Zant, G., and Goldwasser, E. (1979). 'The relationship of hemoglobin synthesis to burst formation', *Blood*, **53**, 935–945.
62. Porter, P. N., and Ogawa, M. (1980). 'Characterization of human erythroid burst-promoting activity obtained from bone marrow conditioned media', *Exp. Hemat.*, **8**, **(Suppl. 8)**, 302–304.
63. Ogawa, M., Porter, P. N., Terasawa, T., and Brockbank, K. G. M. (1980). 'Effects of burst-promoting activity (BPA) on hemoglobin synthesis in culture', *Exp. Hemat.*, **8**, **(Suppl. 8)**, 90–102.
64. Kidoguchi, K., Ogawa, M., Karam, J. D., and Martin, A. G. (1978). 'Augmentation of fetal hemoglobin (HbF) synthesis in culture by human erythropoietic precursors in the marrow and peripheral blood: Studies in sickle cell anemia and non-hemoglobinopathic adults', *Blood*, **52**, 1115–1124.
65. Fauser, A. A., and Messner, H. A. (1979). 'Identification of megakaryocyte, macrophages and eosinophils in colonies of human bone marrow containing neutrophilic granulocytes and erythroblasts', *Blood*, **53**, 1023–1027.
66. Terasawa, T., Ogawa, M., Porter, P. N., Golde, D. W., and Goldwasser, E. (1980). 'Effect of burst-promoting activity (BPA) and erythropoietin on hemoglobin biosynthesis in culture', *Blood*, **56**, 1106–1110.
67. Nissen, C., Iscove, N. N., and Speck, B. (1979). 'High burst-promoting activity (BPA) in serum of patients with acquired aplastic anemia', in *Experimental Hematology Today*. (Eds. S. J. Baum, and G. D. Ledney), Springer-Verlag, New York, pp. 79–87.
68. Kigasawa, H., and Nishihira, H. (1980). 'High human erythroid burst-forming activity in sera from childhood aplastic anemia in semi-solid agar', *Brit. J. Haemat.*, **46**, 303–305.
69. Alter, B. P. (1979). 'Fetal erythropoiesis in bone marrow failure syndromes', in *Cellular and Molecular Regulation of Hemoglobin Switching* (Eds. G. Stamatoyannopoulos, and A. W. Nienhuis), Grune and Stratton, New York, pp. 87–105.
70. Burgess, A. W., Metcalf, D., Russel, S. H. M., and Nicola, N. A. (1980). 'Granulocyte/macrophage-megakaryocyte-eosinophil and erythroid-colony-stimulating factors produced by mouse spleen cells', *Biochem. J.*, **185**, 301–314.
71. Metcalf, D., Johnson, G. R., and Burgess, A. W. (1980). 'Direct stimulation by purified GM-CSF of the proliferation of multipotential and erythroid precursor cells', *Blood*, **55**, 138–147.
72. Nicola, N. A., Metcalf, D., Johnson, G. R., and Burgess, A. W. (1979). 'Separation of functionally distinct human granulocyte-macrophage colony stimulating factors', *Blood*, **54**, 614–627.
73. Staber, F. G., and Burgess, A. W. (1980). 'Serum of lipopolysaccharide-treated mice contains two types of colony-stimulating factor, separable by affinity chromatography', *J. Cell. Physiol.*, **102**, 1–10.
74. Das, S. K., Stanley, E. R., Guilbert, L. J., and Forman, L. W. (1980). 'Discrimination of a colony stimulating factor subclass by a specific receptor on a macrophage cell line', *J. Cell. Physiol.*, **104**, 359–366.
75. Wu, M. C., Miller, A. W. and Yunis, A. A. (1981). 'Immunological and functional differences between human Type I and II colony-stimulating factors', *J. Clin. Invest.*, **67**, 1588–1591.
76. Dexter, T. M., Allen, T. D., and Lajtha, L. G. (1977). 'Conditions controlling stem cells *in vitro*', *J. Cell. Physiol.*, **91**, 335–344.
77. Dexter, T. M., and Shadduck, R. K. (1980). 'The regulation of haemopoiesis in long-term bone marrow cultures: I. Role of L-cell CSF,' *J. Cell. Physiol.*, **102**, 279–286.

78. Williams, N., and Burgess, A. W. (1980). 'The effect of mouse lung granulocyte-macrophage colony-stimulating factor and other colony-stimulating activities on the proliferation and differentiation of murine bone marrow cells in long-term cultures', *J. Cell. Physiol.*, **102**, 287–295.

79. Testa, N. G., and Dexter, T. M. (1977). 'Long-term production of erythroid precursor cells (BFU) in bone marrow cultures,' *Differentiation*, **9**, 193–195.

80. Eliason, J. F., Testa, N. G., and Dexter, T. M. (1979). 'Erythropoietin-stimulated erythropoiesis in long-term bone marrow culture', *Nature*, **281**, 382–384.

81. Dexter, T. M., Testa, N. G., Allen T. D., Rutherford, T., and Scolnick, E. (1981). 'Molecular and cell biologic aspects of erythropoiesis in long-term bone marrow cultures', *Blood*, **58**, 699–707.

82. Tokosoz, D., Dexter, T. M., Lord, B. I., Wright, E. G., and Lajtha, L.G. (1980). 'The regulation of hemopoiesis in long-term bone marrow cultures. II. Stimulation and inhibition of stem cell proliferation', *Blood*, **55**, 931–936.

83. Metcalf, D. (1980). 'Clonal analysis of proliferation and differentiation of paired daughter cells: Action of granulocyte-macrophage colony-stimulating factor on granulocyte-macrophage precursors', *Proc. Nat. Acad. Sci., (USA).*, **77**, 5327–5330.

84. Dukes, P. P., Ma, A., and Meytes, D. (1980). 'Biological properties of a human urinary protein fraction with burst promoting activity', *Exp. Hemat.*, **8, (Suppl. 8)**, 128–143.

85. Blackburn, M. J., and Goldman, J. M. (1981). 'Increased haemopoietic cell survival *in vitro* induced by a human marrow fibroblast factor', *Brit. J. Haemat.*, **48**, 117–125.

86. Blackburn, M. J., and Patt, H. M. (1977). 'Increased survival of haemopoietic pluripotent stem cells *in vitro* induced by a marrow fibroblast factor', *Brit. J. Haemat.*, **37**, 337–343.

Current Concepts in Erythropoiesis
Edited by C. D. R. Dunn

CHAPTER 5

Computer modeling of erythropoiesis*

H. E. WICHMANN
Medizinische Universitätsklinik Köln,
West Germany

Contents

*Supported by the Deutsche Forschungsgemeinschaft (Wi 621/1)

I. INTRODUCTION

For many experimentalists and clinicians a mathematical model is a mysterious creation. It obviously deals with fundamental questions in their field of interest but is often described in a language and by symbols with which they are unfamiliar. Since a model uses an unknown tool — mathematics — these bioscientists have several problems in assessing the validity and importance of the results. As a consequence one finds two groups. The first group ignores mathematical models believing that they only reformulate the biological knowledge in a complicated way but are not able to improve the scientific understanding. The members of this group do not appreciate the fundamental difference between model results and a data simulation (1). The second group tends to accept model results uncritically because they have been derived by 'precise mathematical formulae'. This review attempts to reduce the membership in these two extreme groups and to strengthen the group in between which has a more realistic view. The published papers will be translated from their specific model language into biological terms (if necessary) and the essential results will be elucidated. In parallel the method of model formulation and model testing is illustrated by examples.

'Mathematical models of erythropoiesis' shall be considered. The term 'mathematical' is understood without limitations on certain techniques. However, only a small collection of technical papers is cited. The term 'models' is not limited to regulatory models (although these are the focal point) but shall have a more general meaning. Therefore, papers in which the authors formulated biological assumptions mathematically and calculated their consequences are included. 'Erythropoiesis' also is used in a general way and models dealing with pluripotential stem cells or erythrocytic progenitors are considered as well as models dealing only with the morphologically-recognizable red blood cell (RBC) precursors and erythrocytes.

The papers are discussed in a unique terminology which is not necessarily the same as in the original papers. If the presentation of a model is spread over several publications only the most important are mentioned. To be as up to date as possible, preliminary results of some very new models, which are so far only published in part, are also reviewed.

II. REGULATORY MODELS OF STEM CELL PROLIFERATION AND ERYTHROCYTIC DIFFERENTIATION

A. Review

Many mathematical models of stem cell regulation have been decribed (2–38). Most of them consider pluripotential stem cells (CFU-S) and erythrocytic differentiation in the bone marrow. Stem cell models dealing only with granulocytic differentiation are outside the scope of this chapter. Models on growth of stem cells in spleen colonies are reviewed later in Section VI.

The first mathematical approach for stem cell regulation was reported by Lajtha *et al*. in 1962 (14). It considered only the stem cell pool which was subdivided into resting cells ('available stock') and cells in active cycle ('triggered stock'). The authors assumed that the stem cells differentiated from the resting compartment. For each resting cell that differentiated a second entered the active cycle from where the two daughter cells returned to the resting pool after a constant cell cycle time. The differentiation rate was considered variable and regulated by erythropoietin (EPO). A deficiency in the stem cell population resulted in an extra number of resting cells being activated.

With a simple choice of their model parameters and with simple formulae, the authors were able to qualitatively simulate the reaction of the stem cell system to altered demand for differentiation and to reduced stem cell numbers after irradiation. The concept embodied in the model of Lajtha *et al*. (14) has influenced further models to the extent that some of the details have been incorporated into later systems. In several reports (4, 5, 7, 9, 18, 19, 24, 25, 31, 34, 38) the same subdivision into resting and proliferating stem cells was chosen; in others (12, 13, 23) the proliferative compartment was further subdivided into the four phases of the cell cycle, while in others (24, 25) a subdivision into an even larger number of age classes was used. Differentiation was considered to be possible only from the resting state (4, 7, 9, 12, 13, 18, 19, 23–25, 31) or from the G2 phase (13). A different group of models mixes all phases together considering only one stem cell compartment (2, 3, 6, 15–17, 22, 26, 27, 29, 30, 32, 35, 37) where differentiation can occur anywhere in the cell cycle.

One might get the impression that this classification of models by their compartment structure has biological relevance. Conceptually, there appear to be important differences as to whether differentiation can occur from resting or cycling cells or whether 'asymmetric divisions' can take place. However this is not necessarily true. Mathematically one can easily comprehend subcompartments and arrive at an equivalent one-compartment description. It is also possible to obtain a different 'biological structure' only by reformulating the regulatory dependences. This has already been demonstrated in one of the first mathematical models (14). Lajtha *et al* investigated the alternative hypotheses that differentiation should only be possible from resting cells or from both resting and cycling cells. They found that both assumptions resulted in almost the same model properties. Thus, the characteristics of a model are not specified by the compartment structure so much but by the quantitative feedback assumptions. These normally are described by the direct influence of the regulators on the model parameters. Activation of resting cells and control of the rate of differentiation play the most important roles.

Activation of stem cells in most models is considered to be regulated directly by the stem cell number; either through the resting (4, 9, 14, 18, 19) or the active (5) population, the S-phase cells (23) or the total stem cell population, (2, 3, 6, 7, 10–13, 15–17, 26–28, 30, 32, 34, 35, 37, 38). In some models, activation of stem cells also depended on erythrocytic progenitors or precursors (6, 15–17, 26, 27, 29, 30, 35, 37) or on RBC and EPO (14, 21, 22).

In most models an increasing demand for differentiated cells increases the rate of differentiation from the stem cell pool. However, here it is important to distinguish whether the RBC number (6, 9–11, 13, 14, 24, 25, 28, 31, 34, 35, 38) or the number of early erythrocytic cells (2, 3, 5, 7, 12, 15–17, 29, 37, 38) regulates the differentiation rate. Some workers (2, 3, 6, 12, 15–17, 35, 37) considered that the differentiation rate in addition was directly regulated by the stem cell number, while others (21, 26, 27, 30, 32) considered that a constant fraction of stem cells differentiates.

Additional influences are considered in some models. Cell death of stem cells or post-stem cells can occur physiologically in the absence of EPO (2, 3, 12). Alternatively, cell death is considered pathological (4, 8, 18, 19) and to occur only in hematological disorders. Stem cells may differentiate into both erythrocytic and granulocytic progenitors at the same level of maturity (17, 37) or differentiation into the erythrocytic cell line may take place at an earlier maturation stage (24, 25). The interaction of bone marrow and spleen in stem cell regulation has been considered (34, 38) and attempts have been made (33) to simulate the biochemical basis of cell commitment.

The description of the direct regulatory influences on cell proliferation within a model needs to be absolutely clear in order that the behaviour of the model in 'stress' situations can be understood. Unfortunately, in several models these direct influences are not sufficiently specified. Furthermore, the indirect influences also play an important role. This can be seen for the interaction of activation and differentiation of cells. Activation of resting cells need not necessarily change the stem cell number; stem cell number will only be increased if, on average, less than 50% of the post-mitotic cells differentiate. If 50% or more differentiate, even an activated stem cell population remains unchanged or decreases. Therefore, stem cell recovery also depends on the feedback influences which regulate differentiation. On the other hand, the differentiation rate is influenced by the activation of stem cells since from a highly proliferating stem cell population more cells can differentiate than from a slowly proliferating population.

One way which allows a clear characterization of the model behavior is to consider the dose/response curves of the 'production rate' and the 'differentiation rate' of stem cells as functions of the regulators. The 'production rate' characterizes the velocity of the increase (positive rate) or decrease (negative rate) of the stem cell number while the 'differentiation rate' describes the magnitude of cellular influx into the pools of differentiated progenitors. However, since nearly all published models decibe only their specific parameters in their specific model language, it is very difficult, and in many cases impossible, to elucidate the net influence of the regulators on production and differentiation of stem cells.

The 'production rate' may depend on the stem cells, on differentiated cells or on both. For a stable model it must depend on the stem cell number by negative feedback otherwise recovery to the normal steady state after perturbations is not possible. Qualitatively this has already been shown by Lajtha *et al* (14). Quantitative dose/response curves have been reported by many authors (2, 3, 4, 10, 11, 15, 18, 19, 23, 26–28, 30, 37), but in only a few of their papers are they presented explicitly.

The dependence of stem cell production on differentiated cells (if considered) has generally been thought of as an inverse relationship (2–4, 10, 11, 14, 15–19, 28, 37) although there have been exceptions (26, 27, 30). An inverse relationship means that the demand for differentiated cells and the demand for stem cells are in competition so far as stem cell recovery is concerned. Thus, despite totally different 'biological assumptions' most models are very similar in this crucial property.

The 'differentiation rate' may also depend on stem cells, on differentiated cells or on both. Since this rate in most models is proportional to the stem cell number it is better to consider the factor of proportionality which shall be called the 'differentiation fraction'. In nearly all models the differentiation fraction decreases if the number of differentiated cells is high. However, if the number of stem cells is high, this fraction has been considered to increase (2, 3), to decrease (15–17, 26, 27, 30, 37) or to be unaffected (4, 10, 11, 14, 18, 19, 26–28, 30). Thus there appears to be no general consensus as to whether a parallel demand on stem cells and differentiated cells reduces or increases the differentiation fraction.

Many models have been used to simulate experimental situations. The response to irradiation has been considered extensively (2, 3, 5, 7, 9–12, 14, 15, 23, 26–28, 30, 32, 34, 37, 38). In most models radiation injury reduces the number of stem cells and the early differentiated cells. However, in others (14, 26, 27, 30) it is presumed that irradiation kills some stem cells, sterilizes others and leaves the rest unaffected. With both concepts, experimental data can be reproduced (2, 3, 7, 10, 11, 15, 23, 26–28, 30, 34, 37, 38). Criteria for the death of the population have been identified (32) and stem cell transfusion after otherwise lethal irradiation analyzed (7, 12).

The application of drugs represents another experimental situation where stem cells are killed. Chemotherapy in general (2, 3, 5) or the specific effects of cyclophosphamide or busulfan (4, 18, 19) have been simulated. In other papers, model results are compared with data from experiments with hydroxyurea (12, 23, 37) phenylhydrazine (37), vinblastine (12), or colchicine (23).

The theoretical influence of erythrocytic stimulatory factors on the stem cells has been considered (6, 12–14, 24, 25, 31, 35), but in only a few reports (15, 17, 29, 37), dealing with stem cells and erythrocytic progenitors in anemia, hypertransfusion, hypoxia, and post-hypoxia, have the model results been compared directly to the experimental data. The influence of EPO injections on stem cell regulation has been investigated (2, 3, 13, 15, 37), and the increasing sensitivity of EPO-responsive cells (ERC) to repeated application of the hormone, analyzed (2, 3, 13). The influence of ^{55}Fe (16, 37) and combined experiments of irradiation and either anemia or hypertransfusion have also been quantitatively simulated (10, 11, 16, 28, 37).

The phenomenon of cyclic hematopoiesis, which is closely related to the question of (asymptotic) stability of a model system, has been extensively discussed (4, 8, 10–12, 18–22, 28, 36, 37, 39). However, most of these reports are only theoretical. The qualitative step from stable to oscillatory hematopoiesis can be understood by quantitative modifications (sometimes only small) of the regulatory parameters. The origin of the oscillations can be three-fold. It can be a more 'rigid' feedback (21, 36, 37) where the system reacts to stimulation and suppression in a more extreme manner than normal, a possible example being the grey collie dog. It can be an enlarged time delay (4, 8, 18, 19, 21) following from a prolonged cell cycle time or marrow transit time (e.g., cyclic chronic granulocytic leukemia), or it can be cell death either of stem cells (4, 8, 18, 19) or mature cells (39) (e.g., cyclic neutropenia after busulfan).

One can transform a stable stem cell model into a cycling system simply by making the dose-response curves a little steeper without changing the compartment structure or regulatory mechanisms. This fact shows once again that stem cell models can only be evaluated if the quantitative feedback assumptions are considered. If these are not specified a model cannot be fully appraised.

Among the most interesting conclusions which can be drawn from work with stem cell models are the following;

1. If stem cells and early differentiated cells are reduced to similar extents, recovery of differentiated cells takes priority (2, 3, 15, 17, 37).

2. In anemia, differentiation from the stem cell pool increases and the stem cell number decreases if EPO regulates the differentiation rate (14). Differentiation would decrease if the early erythrocytic cells regulate the differentiation rate since the early erythrocytic cells are increased in anemia due to their stimulation by EPO (15–17, 37).

3. A stable model that reproduces the regrowth characteristics of CFU-S could only be found if the differentiation rate was controlled by both stem cells and early differentiated cells (12).

4. General accordance with the data could only be achieved if the G_0 state was part of the cell cycle (23).

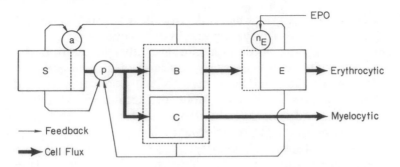

Figure 1. Block diagram of a mathematical model of (erythrocytic) stem cell regulation. S, pluripotential stem cells; B, EPO-independent erythrocytic progenitors; E, EPO-dependent erythrocytic progenitors; C, granulocytic progenitors; EPO, erythropoietin; a, proliferative fraction of S; p, probability of self-renewal in S; n_E, number of divisions in E. This model represents a generalized version of that reported earlier (15)

5. The modeling of stem cell regulation in the bone marrow and spleen seems to support the hypothesis of negative feedback between both organs (34, 38).
6. Loss of pluripotential stem cells at a low rate produces mild pancytopenia, loss at a higher rate results in periodic hematopoiesis and loss at an even higher rate causes severe pancytopenia (4, 18, 19).

B. Example

Details of this model were first described in 1980 (15) and, in a generalized version, more recently (16, 17, 37). The basic assumptions are the following (see Figure 1);

1. The biological is system influenced by stem cells, erythrocytic and granulocytic cells and regulation probably depends on all these variables. Since most of these dependences are unknown the model is constructed in steps of increasing complexity.
2. The hematopoietic cells develop from pluripotential stem cells which are identified as compartment S. These cells are self-replicative and replenish the early differentiated cells of erythropoiesis, granulopoiesis and thrombopoiesis. Of these pluripotential cells, only the fraction 'a' is in an active, proliferative cycle and the rest are in a quiescent phase. Under normal conditions 'a' is small (10–20%). It increases with increased proliferative requirements to a maximum of 100% and decreases to a minimum of 5% in the absence of stimulation.
3. After each mitosis, the fraction 'p' of the post-mitotic cells remains in the stem cell compartment while the fraction '$1 - p$' differentiates and is thereby lost to the stem cell pool. Under steady state conditions $p = 0.5$.

For $p > 0.5$, S increases, while S decreases for $p < 0.5$ since in this case more than 50% of the newly formed cells differentiate.

4. From S most of the cells differentiate into either the erythrocytic or the granulocytic cell line. Megakaryocytopoiesis is neglected here because its contribution to the total bone marrow cell population is small. The erythrocytic progenitor cells are subdivided into erythropoietin-independent cells in B and erythropoietin-dependent cells in E. The granulocytic progenitors are denoted by compartment C.

5. The fraction 'a' of active cells in S depends on S, E, and C. If the cell number in one of these compartments is reduced, the quiescent cells in S are activated.

6. The fraction 'p' of stem cells which remains in S during the next cell cycle also depends on S, E, and C. Here a reduction of S increases 'p' while a reduction of E or C decreaes 'p'. Thus we have a competition of S and the differentiated compartments for the newly formed cells.

7. EPO influences only the number of divisions in E. The pluripotential stem cells are not directly influenced by EPO but indirectly *via* the feedback of E which acts on 'a' and 'p'.

8. S corresponds to CFU-S, B to BFU-E, E to CFU-E, and C to CFU-C. However, the model results are not changed significantly if E and C are used to respresent all erythrocytic and granulocytic bone marrow cells respectively.

Two typical model results are shown in Figures 2 and 3. In Figure 2 recovery after acute irradiation of different doses is simulated. The erythrocytic progenitors recover first while the stem cell number remains small due to $p < 0.5$. After E has reached or exceeded its normal value, the system switches to $p > 0.5$ and now S recovers at the expense of the early differentiated cells. When S is nearly normal, E increases again. In total we find a typical double-peaked recovery curve for E and an early plateau for S. Both have been found experimentally.

In Figure 3 the influence of an anemic stimulus is simulated. The high EPO level leads to about two additional mitoses in E. The increased cell number in E signals to the system that enough erythrocytic progenitors are available. Thus $p > 0.5$, S increases and the efflux from S is reduced. In total we find increased cell numbers in S and E and a reduced number in B.

By means of this model it is possible to understand most of the published experimental data. In the generalized version (37) more than 120 data curves have been analyzed, for stem cells and erythrocytic progenitors after acute and chronic irradiation, anemia, hypertransfusion, hypoxia, post-hypoxia, EPO injections, [55]Fe-incorporation, hydroxyurea, phenylhydrazine, and combinations of irradiation plus anemia or hypertransfusion. Furthermore, suggestions for new experiments have been made and the optimal experimental designs identified.

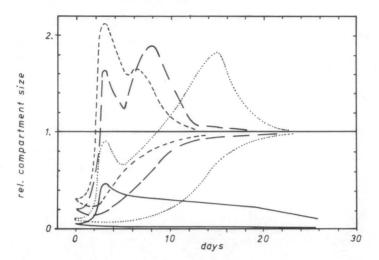

Figure 2. Model simulation of hematopoietic recovery after acute irradiation of different doses to mice. The curves show a typical biphasic and overshooting recovery of the erythrocytic progenitors in E (upper curves) and a slower normalization of the pluripotential cells in S (lower curves). From (15). Reproduced by permission of Blackwell Scientific Publications from *Cell and Tissue Kinetics*, vol. 13, 1980

III. REGULATORY MODELS OF NORMAL ERYTHROPOIESIS

A. Review

In this section, mathematical models of the later stages of erythropoiesis will be considered (9–12, 28, 29, 34, 38, 39, 40–53). In general these deal with the simulation of erythrocytic progenitors (committed cells such as BFU-E, CFU-E and ERC) or precursors (proerythroblasts, basophilic, polychromatic, orthochromatic erythroblasts and reticulocytes) by the hormone EPO. Levels of EPO depend, in turn, on the demand for RBC. Some models also include stem cells (CFU-S) (9-12, 28, 29, 34, 38). In only two (34, 38) is erythropoiesis in the bone marrow and spleen distinguished by separate compartments.

Models have been designed to simulate erythropoiesis in both man (47, 49, 50) and in rodents (10, 11, 28, 29, 34, 38, 39, 44, 45, 48, 52, 53) and their complexity ranges from one compartment (and one differential equation) (39) to ten compartments (and 42 differential equations) (29).

To clarify the discussion, the feedback loop will be separated into two parts. Part 1 represents stimulation of RBC production and part 2, the production of EPO.

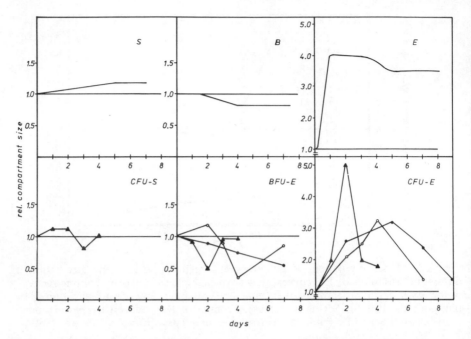

Figure 3. Acute severe anemia in model (top) and experiment (bottom). Experimental data for mice taken from references 115 (▲), 116 (○), and 117 (●) (15). Reproduced by permission of Blackwell Scientific Publications from *Cell and Tissue Kinetics*, Vol. 13, 1980

Production of RBC has been characterized by 1–4 EPO influences, depending on the complexity of the model. In models without bone marrow compartments the feedback directly controls the influx of young RBC into the blood (39, 44, 45, 47, 48). Marrow transit time is decribed by a constant (39, 44, 45, 47) or variable (48) time delay. In other models EPO controls the influx into the first precursor compartment (proerythroblasts). Stimulation of erythrocytic stem cell differentiation (9–12, 28, 34, 38), of CFU-E proliferation (12, 40–43, 52, 53) or of differentiation from BFU-E and CFU-E (12, 29) were considered responsible for this influx. Additional EPO influences included the regulation of the number of mitoses in the proliferative erythroblasts (29, 49, 50, 52, 53) and of the marrow transit time (48, 49, 50, 52, 53). The shift of reticulocytes from the bone marrow into the blood during stimulated erythropoiesis depends on EPO (49, 50, 52, 53) or directly on the RBC number (29). RBC themselves were not considered to be under direct regulatory control. However, some models considered stress erythrocytes (which are formed during high stimulation) to have a shortened lifespan (48, 53, 54, 126). In several models (39–45, 47, 49, 50, 52, 53) a random destruction was assumed either for mathematical simplification or because stress erythrocytes and hemolysis were considered. In others (9–11, 28, 34, 38, 48) RBC 'disappeared' due to an age function which, in most cases, was represented by a constant time delay.

Part 2 of the feedback loop deals with the production of EPO considered to depend on total RBC number (or total hemoglobin mass) (10–12, 28, 29, 34, 38, 39, 49, 50) or on hematocrit (or hemoglobin concentration) (44–48, 52, 53). This regulation could be direct (10–12, 28, 34, 38) or indirect based, possibly, on the arterial oxyhemoglobin concentration (48) or the venous (or tissue) oxygen tension in the kidney (44–47, 49, 50, 52, 53). Other parameters, such as cardiac output, blood viscosity, plasma volume, mean cell volume of the RBC and the hemoglobin affinity for oxygen, could also influence EPO production. These parameters are mentioned in many papers but quantitatively considered in only a few (47, 48, 52, 53).

As usual, each model has its own language and its own feedback parameters which makes direct comparisons difficult. However, in some papers the critical dose/response curves are documented.

Production of RBC has generally been made to depend on EPO (or RBC) by an exponential or sigmoidal relationship (10, 11, 34, 38, 39, 44–50, 52, 53). If no EPO was available, the production decreased to a minimum rate between zero (10, 11, 34, 38, 44–47) and 50% of normal (48). For high EPO levels, RBC production was assumed to reach a maximum between six- and ten-times normal (10, 11, 39, 44–50, 52, 53). EPO production has been considered to depend, hyperbolically, on RBC mass (10, 11, 28, 34, 38) or, exponentially, on oxygen tension (44–50, 52, 53) and to increase maximally to 100 to 1000 times normal (10, 11, 44, 45, 47–50, 52, 53). By combining these relationships with further assumptions it is possible to derive dose/response curves for RBC production as a function of RBC number, hemoglobin concentration or RBC lifespan (39, 46, 47, 49, 50, 52, 53).

Most of the mathematical models of normal erythropoiesis have been constructed in order to better understand experimental results. The effects of irradiation, chemotherapy and EPO on stem cells and erythrocytic progenitors have already been mentioned. Model simulations of the later stages of erythropoiesis have been performed in response to EPO injections (2, 3, 53), hypoxia (40–45, 47–50, 52, 53), post-hypoxia (47, 52, 53), dehydration (44, 45, 53), bleeding (29, 38, 40–43, 52), hemolysis (10, 11, 28, 39, 47, 49, 50), dilution anemia (52, 53), and hypertransfusion (29, 47, 52, 53). Direct comparison with experimental recovery curves for erythroblasts, reticulocytes or RBC numbers have been presented (10, 11, 28, 44, 45, 47–50, 52, 53) and some theoretical analyses of model stability reported (9, 10, 12, 34, 38, 39, 40–45, 47, 49, 51).

Among the interesting conclusions which have arisen from these simulations are;
1. The most realistic model behavior has been found for man and rodents (39,

46, 47, 49, 50, 52, 53) if the following assumptions were made;
  (a) The dose/response curve relating RBC production to RBC number (or hematocrit) has a sigmoidal form;
  (b) For RBC numbers of 60% to 80% of normal, RBC production increases to three to five times normal; and
  (c) For RBC numbers below 50% the production rate reaches its maximum at six to ten times normal.
2. The shift-to-the-right of the oxyhemoglobin dissociation curve (ODC) and the plasma loss, both found experimentally during hypoxia, have a minor effect on plasma EPO titers (44, 45, 49, 50, 52, 53).
3. Factors, such as, EPO responsiveness, oxygen utilization and bone marrow transit times, which could be related to energy balance, were more important to the erythrocytic suppression seen in dehydrated mice than those factors (e.g., plasma volume and blood flow) related to water balance (45).
4. For a sufficiently short RBC lifespan, model calculations could reproduce the oscillatory erythropoiesis found experimentally (10, 11, 28, 39).
5. For accurate simulations of experimental data it was not necessary to assume ineffective erythropoiesis as a normal, physiological mechanism, or other humoral regulators in addition to EPO (29).
6. The return of EPO to near baseline levels after a few days of hypoxia could not be simulated without the incorporation of some important, but poorly understood, additional influences (44, 47–50). The rapid fall in EPO titers could be reproduced by assuming some adaptational effects in oxygen supply to the kidney (52, 53), by consumption of EPO by the stimulated cells (52, 53) or by changes in the sensitivities of the ERC and of the EPO-producing mechanism (44).
7. The data on dilution anemia can be reproduced if hematocrit (or hemoglobin concentration), but not total RBC number or hemoglobin mass, regulates EPO production (52, 53).

B. Example

This example is based primarily on a mathematical model of erythropoiesis in man (49, 50) and, secondly, on a model of erythropoiesis in rodents (52,53). The results of the latter are preliminary. Similar model assumptions to those now included have been used by other authors (47, 48).

Normal erythropoiesis can be symbolized by the block diagram of Figure 4. Six compartments are considered which represent EPO-sensitive erythrocytic progenitors (CFU-E or ERC), proliferative erythroblasts, non-proliferative precursors (non-dividing blasts plus marrow reticulocytes), circulating reticulocytes, RBC and EPO.

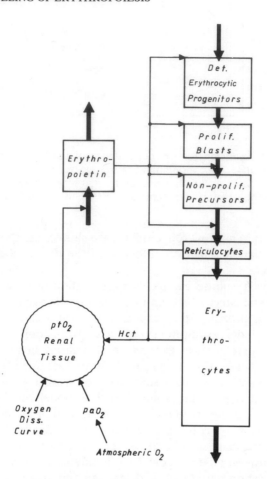

Figure 4. Block diagram of a mathematical model of normal erythropoiesis.
▶ = transition between the compartments, ➤ = regulatory influences

1. Assumptions about the influence of EPO on RBC production

The stimulatory effect of EPO may act to varying degrees at different stages of
the erythrocytic cell line. In the model the following influences are assumed;

1. EPO increases CFU-E up to three to five times normal at maximum
   stimulus. CFU-E are reduced to 25% of normal or less in the absence of
   EPO.
2. High EPO levels lead to one additional mitosis of the erythroblasts. In the
   absence of the hormone, one mitosis is omitted.
3. The marrow transit time is approximately halved under maximum
   stimulation and is increased only slightly when EPO is absent.

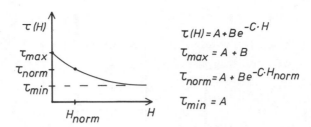

Figure 5. Model formulation for the dependence of the maturation time τ on the regulatory hormone H. An exponential, saturating form is assumed in which the model parameters A, B, and C can be determined by the three measurable values τ_{max}, τ_{norm}, and τ_{min}. From (1). Reproduced by permission of Springer-Verlag

4. The most mature marrow reticulocytes are shifted into the blood by a high EPO concentration. Thus, the lifespan of the blood reticulocytes can be nearly doubled.

5. The EPO dose/response curves for proliferation rate and transit times in the erythrocytic precursor compartments (both assumed to depend on EPO) can be approximated by exponential functions.

The first four model assumptions and the corresponding kinetic parameters can be derived directly from experimental measurements. However, data regarding the influence of EPO on proliferation rate and transit times of the recognizable erythrocytic precursors are not available. Nevertheless the amount of speculation which comes into the model can be reduced as is indicated in Figure 5. Let τ be the maturation time of the erythroblasts. We know that τ depends on EPO or in general on the feedback hormone H. In practice only three values can be measured; in suppressed erythropoiesis the prolonged maturation time τ_{max} can be estimated; after severe stimulation, a shortened maturation time (τ_{min}) is calculated and under normal conditions, τ_{norm} is found. Using these three data points and assuming a simple mathematical form for $\tau(H)$ as shown on the right in Figure 5, one can express all model parameters by measured values. In our case, A, B, and C can be calculated from τ_{max}, τ_{norm}, and τ_{min}. Thus, for the feedback function $\tau(H)$, which was at first totally unknown, only the shape of its decrease remains hypothetical.

2. Assumptions about the regulation of EPO production

Today it is generally accepted that the kidney is the major site of production of EPO. Whether EPO is produced directly or is formed as a result of the action of a renal erythropoietic factor (REF) on a plasma substrate (erythropoietinogen) is still not clear. Nevertheless, the production of EPO and/or REF seems to be regulated by the oxygen supply to the kidney, possibly in the juxtaglomerular apparatus. This implies that erythrocytic proliferation is not determined only by the number of circulating RBC but that factors such as oxygen transport, the mechanism of oxygen release and consumption in the kidney, need to be considered.

For the mathematical formulation of this part of the feedback loop the following model assumptions are made;

1. The ODC can be characterized by the parameters of the Hill equation.

Hill (55) showed that the oxyhemoglobin dissociation curve (ODC) can be described by;

$$SO_2/(100 - SO_2) = (PO_2/P_{50})^n \tag{1}$$

the so-called Hill equation. This formula connects the percent saturation of hemoglobin, SO_2, to the oxygen tension, PO_2. It has two parameters; P_{50} and n. The P_{50} is the partial pressure of oxygen corresponding to the 50% saturation of hemoglobin, i.e., at $SO_2 = 50\%$, and determines the position on the curve. Hill's coefficient (n) is an index of the slope of the curve. Such curves adequately describe the interaction of oxygen with hemoglobin (Figure 6). As average normal values one finds for man, rats, and mice $P_{50} = 26.5$, 38.0, and 40 mm Hg and $n = 2.65$, 2.50, and 3.00 respectively.

2. The venous oxygen tension is closely related to the regulation of erythropoiesis.

This also can be seen in Figure 6 where three perturbations of the normal steady state are shown. The arrows indicate the influence of these perturbations on the venous point.

A shift of P_{50} to the right (Figure 6, top right) leads to a decrease of the arterial and venous saturation but to an increase of the venous oxygen pressure. This situation is realized for abnormal hemoglobins like HbS in sickle cell anemia with an oxygen affinity lower than for normal HbA.

A reduction of the RBC mass in anemia (Figure 6, bottom left) can lead to a decrease of both venous pressure and saturation, but keeps the arterial values constant.

At altitude, (Figure 6, bottom right) the arterial and venous values are both decreased as a consequence of the reduced atmospheric oxygen pressure. Here the additional shift of the curve to the right is of minor influence.

From these curves it can be concluded that a reduction of the venous oxygen tension correlates well with stimulation of erythropoiesis. The arterial oxygen tension or saturation cannot be the stimulus because then in anemia the erythrocytic proliferation would be normal when it is usually found to be enlarged. The decreased venous saturation also cannot be the regulatory stimulus because this would cause a higher RBC proliferation rate in sickle cell anemia than in comparable anemias with normal

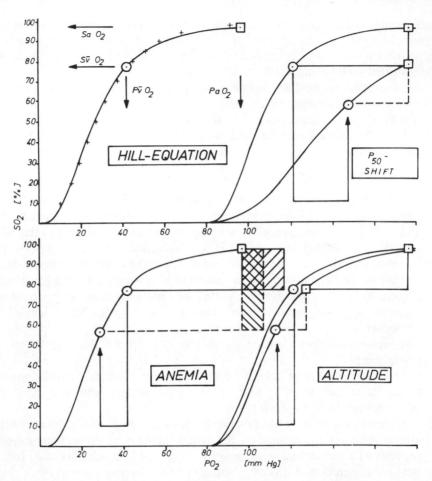

Figure 6. Oxygen dissociation curve in the model. □ = the arterial point, ⊙ = the venous point. Top left; the data for normal individuals from (118) are reproduced by the Hill equation (55). The average venous oxygen tension $P_{\bar{v}}O_2$ is closely correlated with the production of erythropoietin. Top right; a shift of the curve to the right leads to an increased venous tension (arrow) and thus to a reduced stimulus for erythropoietin production. Bottom left; reduction of the oxygen transport capacity in anemia leads to higher desaturation. The venous tension is reduced (arrow) and erythropoietin production is stimulated. Bottom right; lower atmospheric pressure also reduces the venous oxygen tension (arrow) and stimulates erythropoietin production. The additional shift of the dissociation curve to the right is of minor importance

hemoglobin. In point of fact the opposite generally occurs. However, the venous oxygen tension is reduced in anemia and hypoxia and is higher in HbS-type anemias than in HbA-associated anemias. Thus the increase in

erythropoiesis correlates most closely with a decrease in venous oxygen tension.
3. The tissue oxygen tension of the kidney is responsible for the production of EPO and this dependence is exponential.

As shown, the venous oxygen tension closely correlates with the regulation of erythropoiesis. Since the kidney is the organ which determines the production (or activation) of EPO we assume that the tissue oxygen tension of the kidney denoted by P_tO_2, (which is very similar to the venous oxygen tension of this organ) is the regulator of EPO production) EPO_{prod}. This correlation shall be assumed to be exponential and is, therefore, expressed by;

$$EPO_{prod} = A \exp(-B P_tO_2) \tag{2}$$

A and B are constants which symbolize the maximum production (A) and the sensitivity (B) of EPO_{prod} to changes in P_tO_2. EPO_{prod} increases by 100 to 1000 times normal for high stimulation (in severe anemia) and is reduced to nearly zero in hyperoxic situations.

The tissue oxygen tension, P_tO_2, depends only indirectly on the RBC and must be calculated from the arterial oxygen parameters and the desaturation of hemoglobin in the kidney.
4. The arterial oxygen saturation is determined by the arterial oxygen tension and the Hill parameters.

Re-arranging equation (1) gives:

$$S_aO_2 = 100/((P_{50}/P_aO_2)^n + 1) \tag{3}$$

where P_aO_2 and S_aO_2 are the arterial values. For the dependence of P_aO_2 on the atmospheric oxygen pressure, $P_{atm}O_2$, the proportionality:

$$P_aO_2 = \text{constant} \times P_{atm}O_2 \tag{4}$$

is assumed. Since the normal values for P_aO_2 for man, rats, and mice at sea level are 97, 95, and 80 mm Hg respectively, the corresponding S_aO_2 values (from equation 4) are 97, 91, and 89% assuming the P_{50} and n values given above. These average arterial values are also assumed for the kidney.
5. The tissue saturation is determined by the arterial saturation and the desaturation of hemoglobin.

The oxygen values in a tissue are very similar to the corresponding venous values. Therefore the desaturation of hemoglobin (ΔSO_2, or the arteriovenous difference) can be approximated by:

$$S_tO_2 \approx S_vO_2 = S_aO_2 - \Delta SO_2 \tag{5}$$

Thus, the desaturation in the kidney needs to be known.
6. The average desaturation per hemoglobin molecule is determined by the

available hemoglobin, the blood velocity and the oxygen utilization.

Before discussing the situation in the kidney, the total body needs to be considered. The oxygen utilization of the body per unit time, O_{2util}, depends on the available number of hemoglobin molecules per unit time and the average desaturation per molecule. As can easily be seen, this leads to the formula;

$$\Delta SO_2 \times Hb_{mass} \times v_{blood} = \text{constant} \times O_{2util}(\text{body}) \tag{6}$$

where Hb_{mass} denotes the total hemoglobin mass and v_{blood} the average blood velocity. From the normal values for man, rats, and mice of $\Delta SO_2 = 20\%$, 40% and 30% corresponding average venous saturation values can be calculated at 77%, 51% and 59% respectively.

For a constant oxygen utilization, equation 6 suggests that in an anemia with a hemoglobin mass of 50% of normal, the reduced capacity for oxygen transport will be compensated either by a doubled desaturation (as shown in Figure 6, bottom left) or a doubled blood velocity or by a combined reaction of both where the product ($\Delta SO_2 \times v_{blood}$) is doubled.

Expressing Hb_{mass} by the hemoglobin concentration, Hb_{conc}, and the blood volume, Bl_{vol};

$$Hb_{mass} = Hb_{conc} \times Bl_{vol} \tag{7}$$

and substituting in equation (6) and re-arranging;

$$\Delta SO_2 = \frac{(\text{constant} \times O_{2util})}{(Hb_{conc} \times Bl_{vol} \times v_{blood})} \tag{8}$$

This formula holds true for the total body but can also be applied to a single organ using the oxygen consumption, the blood volume and the blood velocity appropriate for that organ. In the kidney, blood volume times velocity corresponds to the renal blood flow (RBF) such that:

$$RBF = \text{constant} \times Bl_{vol} \times v_{blood} \tag{9}$$

and we find

$$\Delta SO_2 = \frac{(\text{constant} \times O_{2util})}{(Hb_{conc} \times RBF)} \tag{10}$$

Hemoglobin concentration, Hb_{conc}, and hematocrit, Hct, are connected by the mean corpuscular hemoglobin concentration (MCHC):

$$Hb_{conc} = MCHC \times Hct \tag{11}$$

If MCHC is constant, we can also write;

$$\Delta SO_2 = \frac{(\text{constant} \times O_{2\text{util}})}{(\text{Hct} \times \text{RBF})} \tag{12}$$

7. The quotient of oxygen utilization and blood flow in the kidney is approximately constant during mild anemia and hypoxia.

Mathematically, this leads to;

$$\Delta SO_2 = \text{constant}/Hb_{\text{conc}} = \text{constant}/\text{Hct} \tag{13}$$

as follows from equations 10 and 12.

If this assumption is correct, renal Hb desaturation is inversely proportional to the concentration of RBC. The constant in equation 13 is specific for the kidney but is unknown.

The above hypothesis (equation 13) seems to be realistic for moderate stresses. In these cases, autoregulation by the kidney ensures that RBF and oxygen consumption are stable. However, in severe anemia and hypoxia as well as after stimulation by catecholamines, renal (preglomerular) vasoconstriction is found. As a consequence, during these stresses the arterio-venous oxygen difference shows a much larger increase in the renal cortex (near the presumptive sites of EPO or REF production) than in the total kidney or the total body, as the few available measurements of ΔSO_2 demonstrate.

8. The tissue oxygen tension is determined by the tissue saturation and the Hill parameters.

We find directly from the Hill equation (1);

$$P_t O_2 = P_{50} \times \left(\frac{S_t O_2}{(100 - S_t O_2)} \right)^{1/n} \tag{14}$$

For the average tissue oxygen tension of the body, this formula leads to normal values of $P_{\bar{t}}O_2 = P_{\bar{v}}O_2 = 42$, 39 and 45 mm Hg for man, rats and mice respectively. The corresponding tissue tension at the sites of EPO (or REF) production in the kidney is speculative.

By a combination of equations 2–5, 10, and 12–14, the dose/response relationship of EPO production to Hct or Hb_{conc} can be derived. Moreover it can also be determined how atmospheric pressure or hemoglobin–oxygen affinity influence the production of the hormone.

In total, one needs to know the Hill parameters (P_{50} and n), the atmospheric pressure ($P_{\text{atm}}O_2$), Hct or Hb_{conc} and the renal constant in equation 13 which characterizes the ratio of oxygen consumption, $O_{2\text{util}}$, and RBF.

For the model simulations which are presented in the following section, P_{50}, n, and $P_{\text{atm}}O_2$ are taken from the direct measurements. Hct or Hb_{conc} are computed from the cell numbers in the reticulocyte and RBC

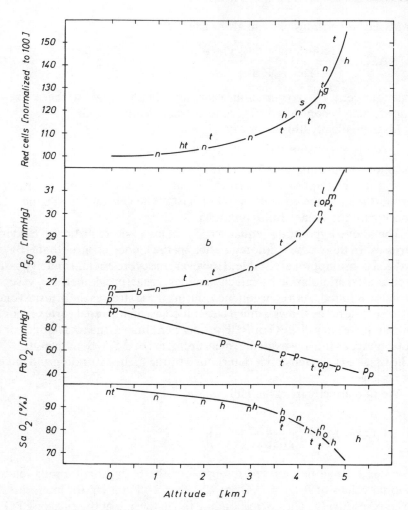

Figure 7. Red blood cells, P_{50} and arterial PO_2 (P_aO_2) and arterial SO_2 (S_aO_2) in residents at different altitudes. Comparison of model results (−) with data from several authors. From (5). Reproduced by permission of Springer-Verlag

compartments and the plasma volume. The renal constant has been chosen arbitrarily but has been kept unchanged in all calculations.

3. Model results

In Figure 7 hypoxia is simulated and the model curves are compared with steady state values of residents at different altitudes. Atmospheric pressure and P_{50} values were used as input parameters and the other oxygen parameters

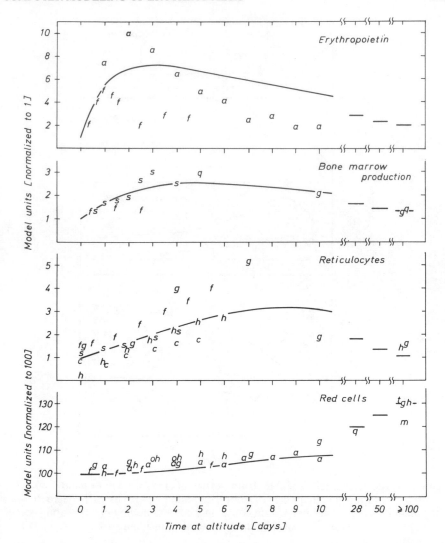

Figure 8. Changes in erythropoiesis after ascent from sea level to 4.5 km altitude. Comparison of model results (−) with data from several authors. From (50). Reproduced by permission of Springer-Verlag

(of which only P_aO_2 and S_aO_2 are shown), as well as RBC numbers were received as output.

In Figure 8 changes in erythropoiesis after ascent of volunteers from sea level to 4.5 km are considered. This situation is simulated in the model using the atmospheric pressure and the P_{50} of that altitude. The EPO curve of the model reaches its peak within three days and decreases slowly to twice the normal

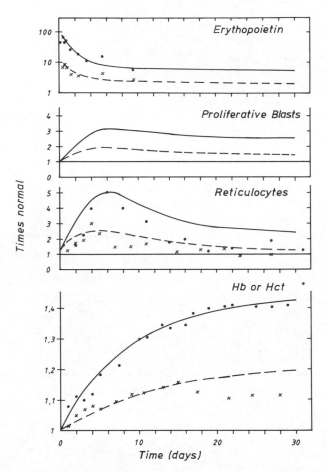

Figure 9. Hypoxia in mice. The data from (48) and (117) for 6 km (●) and 3.2 km (x) are compared with preliminary curves from the model (−,--). The early decrease seen in the model curves for erythropoietin could only be obtained by incorporating one of the additional hypotheses discussed in Figure 10

value after 100 days. In contrast, measured EPO concentrations increase in a similar way but they decrease much more rapidly. Better agreement is found for the changes in cell numbers. The maximum of bone marrow production is reached within three to five days, followed by a peak reticulocytosis after seven to ten days. These parameters return to nearly normal values after 100 days, when the steady state of RBC production is reached.

Because of the unsatisfactory reproduction of the EPO curve, different degress of hypoxia were analyzed in more detail. These simulations are summarized in Figure 9. Here the model curves are compared with experimental data derived from mice.

Part 1 of the feedback loop, which represents the influence of EPO on RBC production, can be tested if we use the EPO curve as input for the model and compare the output, i.e., the changes in the cellular compartments, with the data. Doing this, we find that the high EPO peak leads to a broad maximum for the proliferative blasts and a steeper one for the reticulocytes, followed by an increase of the hematocrit. As can be seen from Figure 9, the curves correspond quite well to the measured cell numbers. Therefore, as a first result we find that the model assumptions for the action of EPO on the erythrocytic cells are sufficient to understand the data.

Let us now consider Part 2 of the feedback loop, i.e., the influence of RBC on EPO. Because of the lowered atmospheric pressure in hypoxia, the arterial tension and, thus, the tissue tension, decreases. This increases EPO production dramatically. But now the problems begin; if nothing additional happens during the first few days, the concentration of the hormone would decrease only slowly and stay at a high level for weeks as shown in Figure 7. This result has also been found in other simulations (44, 48). Furthermore, additional model calculations show that the shift-to-the-right of the ODC (often considered important in the adaptation to altitude) as well as the plasma volume loss (both of which are found experimentally), have only a minor influence on the production of EPO. They cannot be responsible for the rapid fall in EPO titers even if they change dramatically. Thus, we find the second result: The above model assumptions for Part 2 of the feedback loop are not sufficient to explain the results—there must be additional influences.

In Figure 10 once more the data points for 6 km altitude from Figure 9 are redrawn. The curves represent two modifications in which additional assumptions about EPO production or destruction are made.

Alternative hypothesis 1. During the first days of acute anemia or hypoxia an additional stimulus for the production of EPO is effective.

This assumption might be interpreted by adaptational phenomena. As already discussed renal vasoconstriction, which is experimentally found after a severe anemic or hypoxic stimulus, might enlarge hemoglobin desaturation in the kidney and thus stimulate EPO production. If this effect is only transient (which is not known) reversal of the vasoconstriction during adaptation may partially alleviate renal hypoxia and lead to falling EPO titers. However no quantitative knowledge is available and other adaptational processes might also be effective. Therefore this simulation includes a poorly defined additional stimulus on EPO production which vanishes exponentially within three to four days.

Alternative hypothesis 2. The half-life of EPO depends on the number of erythrocytic precursors.

This hypothesis corresponds to the old and controversial contention that

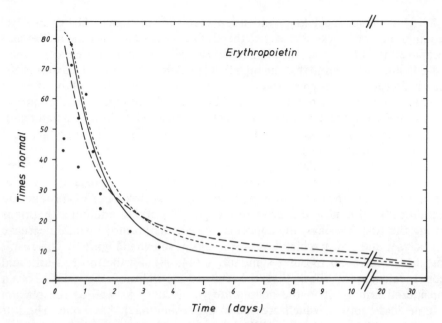

Figure 10. Additional simulations regarding the production or destruction of erythropoietin during hypoxia. The data from Figure 9 (●, 6 km altitude) are reproduced including additional hypotheses of an adaptational process influencing the production of erythropoietin (—) or of a variable lifespan of the hormone due to utilization by CFU-E (— —) or by all proliferating erythroid cells (– –)

EPO might be utilized by a hyperactive erythrocytic bone marrow. Mathematically it can be formulated by;

$$EPO_{loss} = const_1 \times EPO \times E_{prec} + const_2 \times EPO \tag{15}$$

The first term, $const_1 \times EPO \times E_{prec}$, corresponds to the utilization of EPO by the erythrocytic precursors E_{prec}. The second term, $const_2 \times EPO$, represents the loss of EPO from the plasma due to excretion and catabolism.

For the half life of EPO one finds in this situation;

$$\tau_{1/2}^{EPO} = \ln 2/(const_1 \times E_{prec} + const_2) \tag{16}$$

It is shortened for an increased value of E_{prec} and the amount of shortening depends also on the two constants.

In the following we have alternatively used either the committed erythrocytic stem cells (CFU-E) or all proliferative cells (CFU-E plus proliferative erythroblasts) for E_{prec}. The normal half-life of EPO is 2 h (for mice) and for simplicity $const_1 = const_2$ has been assumed.

In Figure 10, the full line corresponds to alternative hypothesis 1. The curve shows a high initial EPO production which is reduced exponentially. With this hypothesis, the initial adaptational influences disappear with a half-life of approximately one day.

The dashed curves in Figure 10 represent simulations using alternative hypothesis 2, one for EPO consumption by CFU-E, the second for EPO consumption by all proliferative erythrocytic cells. Under this hypothesis, utilization of EPO increases to about 3 times normal. This value is reached within one week and is nearly unchanged thereafter due to the increased number of erythrocytic precursors.

As Figure 10 shows, all three curves decrease in about the same way. Thus, as a third result, the hypothesis of adaptation or EPO consumption both allow us to reproduce the peak and rapid decline of EPO titers during hypoxia.

In Figure 11 is shown a simulation of bleeding anemia. The data are collected from three experiments where rats were bled approximately one-third of their blood volume. Here the origin of the erythrocytic stimulus is different from hypoxia. The arterial oxygen tension is unchanged but the tissue oxygen tension decreases due to a higher desaturation. Together with either of the two mechanisms for the early EPO decrease during hypoxia, the model results correspond quite well to the data in all five compartments of the figure.

Proliferative and non-proliferative blasts need a special comment. The theoretical curves represent the average increase of all erythroblasts corresponding to the increase of reticulocytes and hematocrit found in the blood. As the full circles show (Figure 11), proliferation of bone marrow blasts is smaller than in the model. Better agreement is found if the sum of erythroblasts in the bone marrow and spleen are considered assuming that the spleen produces 50% of all blasts on the day of its maximum proliferation. This corresponds to a normal splenic production of 6% of total erythropoiesis.

Figure 12 shows the simulation of an experiment in rabbits where neither the RBC mass nor the oxygen supply were changed. Only the plasma volume was doubled by infusion of 'Macrodex' for eight days.

This simulation again raises the question of whether the concentration of RBC, represented by the hematocrit or hemoglobin concentration, or the RBC mass or a third factor is responsible for the feedback. If the RBC mass was responsible, 'dilution anemia' would have no influence on erythropoiesis, i.e., the percentage of reticulocytes would not change although the hematocrit would be reduced, due to the increased plasma volume, and return to normal without an overshoot at the end of the experiment. The data show that this appears not to be correct. 'Dilution anemia' obviously has a strong stimulatory effect which leads to a nearly five-fold increase in reticulocytes experimentally and a similar pattern follows from the modal calculations. Although the data are for rabbits and the model curves for rats, the characteristics of the experimental outcome are reproduced by the model.

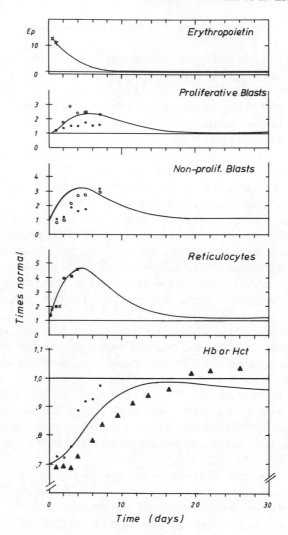

Figure 11. Bleeding anemia in rats with the hemoglobin being reduced to 0.7 times normal. x = data from Millar (personal communication); ⊙, ● = data from (120) (●, blasts in the bone marrow, ⊙, blasts in the bone marrow plus spleen where the spleen is assumed to contain 50% of all blasts on day 3); ▲ = data from (121), — = preliminary model results

The preliminary model results presented here are only part of the investigations which are in progress and will be published in the near future (53). In total, more than 60 experimental curves for bleeding anemia, dilution anemia, hypoxia, post-hypoxia, hypertransfusion, hyperoxia, dehydration, and injections of EPO in mice and rats have been analyzed.

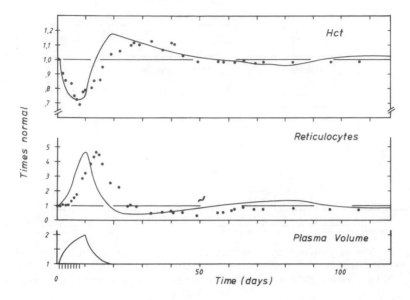

Figure 12. 'Dilution anemia' in rabbits induced by daily infusions of 'Macrodex' for eight days. ● = data from (122): — = preliminary model results using the parameters for rats

IV. REGULATORY MODELS OF ABNORMAL ERYTHROPOIESIS

A. Review

Only a few models have been employed to simulate feedback influences in erythrocytic disorders or during therapy (40–43, 47, 49, 50). Aplastic anemia, cyclic erythroleukemia and polycythemia have been simulated but the results not compared with clinical data (40–43). Steady state control in hemolytic anemia has been discussed (47) and dose/response curves for RBC production depending on a shortened RBC lifespan given. Several disorders and therapies are analyzed in two reports (49, 50) and these will be described in the following examples.

B. Examples

1. Disorders

In Figure 13 the block diagram of a mathematical model of abnormal erythropoiesis in man is presented (49,50) which considers a limited number of defects. These are;

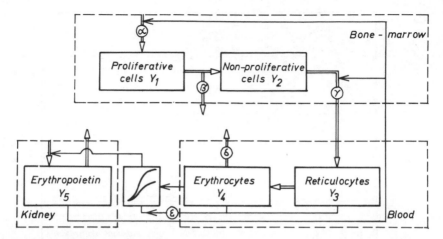

Figure 13. Model of human erythropoiesis considering some hematological disorders.
(◊ =   transitions   of   cells   and   hormones; → = regulatory   mechanisms;
α β, γ, δ, ε = disease parameters. From reference 50. Reproduced by permission of
Springer-Verlag

α: reduced (or increased) proliferation of erythrocytic progenitor and
   precursor cells;
β: death of erythroblasts ('ineffective erythropoiesis');
γ: prolonged erythrocytic marrow transit time;
δ: shortened lifespan of RBC;
ε: shift of the ODC.

α to ε are called 'disease parameters'. Combinations of these can be used to
quantitatively characterize some disorders of erythropoiesis, e.g., aplastic
anemia (α, γ), pernicious anemia (β, γ, δ), hemolytic anemia (δ), and sickle
cell anemia (δ, ε).

   With this mathematical model two questions will be addressed. First, is it
possible to quantitatively reproduce the known clinical data? Second, can we
estimate unknown clinical parameters which are difficult to measure?

   A positive answer to the first question implies that the following points are
fulfilled;

1. The model hypothesis regarding regulation of normal erythropoiesis (as
   described above) corresponds to the biological feedback mechanisms.
2. The diseases in question can be characterized sufficiently by their 'disease
   parameters'.
3. The normal model parameters have a small inter-individual variance and
   can be used for all patients.
4. The disease parameters which are specific for each individual patient
   change slowly with the progression or regression of a disease and therefore
   can be considered as constant during the time of observation.

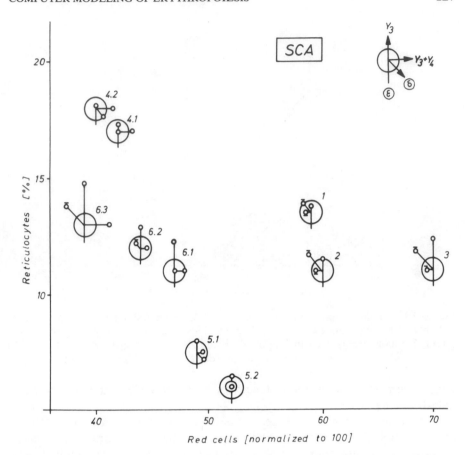

Figure 14. Simulations of the clinical status of six patients with sickle cell anemia (SCA). The form of a wind rose has been chosen to compare the model results with the measured data (top right, symbols as in Figure 13). The patients' values are localized in the center of the wind rose and the model values are drawn in the different directions. The length of the arms is normalized to the accuracy of the experimental method. The large circle represents the 95% confidence limits, the small circle represents the calculated values. For patients 4 and 6 the disease is progressing (4.1 to 4.2 and 6.1 to 6.3) while for patient 5 the situation is improving (5.1 to 5.2)

The methodology for a comparison of the clinical data, from patients, with model results will be illustrated by the following examples.

In Figure 14 the states of disease for six patients with sickle cell anemia (SCA) are shown. The way of presentation is explained in the figure legend. As can be read off the wind roses (Figure 14, top right), the variables Y_3 (reticulocytes), $Y_3 + Y_4$ (number of RBC) and the disease parameters (RBC lifespan) have been measured. The second disease parameter (P_{50} of the ODC) has been estimated. We find a good agreement of model results and measured

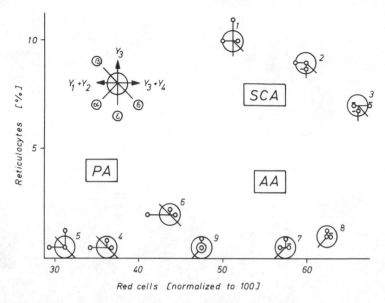

Figure 15. A comparison of model results with the clinical data, from (123), of nine patients with sickle cell anemia (SCA), pernicious anemia (PA), or aplastic anemia (AA). Symbols are as used in Figure 13. From (50). Reproduced by permission of Springer-Verlag

data. Figure 15 shows a similar result for SCA, pernicious anemia (PA) and aplastic anemia (AA).

In total more than 60 disease states have been investigated (49, 50). In approximately 75%, the measured data could be satisfactorily reproduced. However, only data from men could be used. Results from women had to be excluded because their erythrocytic parameters showed too large inter-individual variances.

Thus, the first question can be answered: a number of clinical situations exist in which erythropoiesis of the patients can be understood quantitatively by a regulatory model.

The described mathematical procedure can be inverted. Thus in principle, cell numbers in the bone marrow (generally unknown in clinical situations) can be calculated from cell numbers in the blood if the type of disease is known. The method is limited only by the accuracy of measurement and the variance of the parameters.

2. Therapies

As has been shown (49, 50), it is also possible to simulate therapeutic manipulations in a model. The necessary condition is that the point of action of the therapy on the feedback system can be clearly identified.

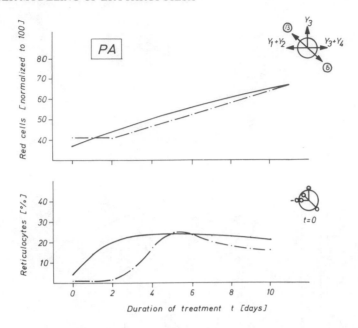

Figure 16. A simulation of the hematological response of a patient with pernicious anemia (PA) to therapy with vitamin B_{12}. Model predictions (—) are compared with clinical data from (124) (–·–). The state of the disease before therapy (t = 0) is shown on the right. Symbols are as used in Figure 13. From(50). Reproduced by permission of Springer-Verlag

A first example is shown in Figure 16. A patient with PA is treated with vitamin B_{12}. This therapy stops the death of erythrocytic precursor cells due to the lack of the vitamin. The therapy shows an effect within a few hours but it influences only the formation of new cells. This causes a time delay for the increase in the reticulocytes. In the model, this special property of vitamin B_{12} is not considered and therefore the calculated reticulocyte curve increases immediately. Apart from this difference, the curves agree both before and during therapy.

In Figure 17 the data from a patient with SCA treated with 50% oxygen are shown. As oxygen supply to the tissues is increased by this therapy, the production of EPO is suppressed and bone marrow production of RBC is reduced. The observable effect in the blood is a steep decrease of the reticulocyte number within a few days and a slower decrease of the RBC mass. After cessation of the therapy the cell numbers increase again and the clinical status of the patient improves. As Figure 17 shows, the consequences of this treatment could have been predicted using the model and the therapy could have been avoided. This is a simple example of how the consequences of therapeutic actions can be tested on a computer. Thus, these could be

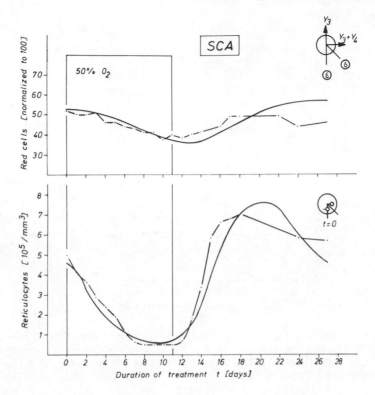

Figure 17. A simulation of the hematological response of a patient with sickle cell anemia (SCA) to oxygen therapy. Model predictions (—) are compared with clinical data from reference 125 (–·–). The state of the disease before therapy (t = 0) is shown on the right. Symbols are as used in Figure 13. From (50). Reproduced by permission of Springer-Verlag

optimized by means of a mathematical model before the therapy is applied to the patient. However, this use of a model is restricted to those therapies for which the mode of action is known and can be quantified.

V. MODELS FOR STEADY STATE KINETICS

A. Review

In this section papers are reviewed in which feedback is not considered but only the flux of erythrocytic cells in steady state.

The first group of models (56–66) deals with the analysis of isotope labeling curves of erythrocytic precursors (proerythroblasts, basophilic, polychromatic, and orthochromatic erythroblasts). Some of the models also take into account stem cells and erythrocytic progenitors (62, 63), reticulocytes and RBC (62) or granulocytic precursors (58–61). Since in principle there are only two alternatives for cell transitions between compartments, namely by age or at random, nearly all papers consider both possibilities and investigate the consequences. More precisely, 'transition by age' means that the cells within each morphological category go sequentially through the cell cycle phases and enter the next compartment after mitosis. However, morphological boundaries at an arbitrary position in the cell cycle are also considered (58, 59). 'Transition at random' means that cell flux between the phases of adjacent 'downstream' compartments is possible. Mixed assumptions have also been investigated (60, 61).

These models have been applied to the analysis of mitotic indices (58–61), ^{55}Fe labeling indices (56, 57, 62, 64–66) and ^{3}H-TdR or ^{14}C-TdR labeling curves (56, 57, 60, 61, 63–66). Cell kinetic parameters such as influx and efflux rates, transit times, cell cycle times and division numbers for the morphologically recognizable cell stages have been derived for normal and for moderately and maximally stimulated erythropoiesis (56, 57, 64–66). However, some model results are contradictory;

1. Some authors find that the experimental data favor cell transitions occurring at random (56, 57, 64–66) while for others the mathematical analysis of the data supports the hypothesis that the flux is sequential (63).
2. Cell kinetic parameters for the recognizable proliferating erythrocytic and neutrophilic granulocyte precursors are not consistent with any existing proliferation–maturation model (60, 61).

The second group of steady state models is used for the analysis of ferrokinetic data. These models are of increasing practical importance and many of them are applied clinically to localize disorders of iron metabolism. Important papers are referenced (67–87). One example is discussed below.

The third group deals with models of RBC in steady state or after different stresses. They are used primarily for the analysis of RBC survival curves and the estimation of RBC lifespan. Most of them consider random labeling curves (using ^{51}Cr or DF-^{32}P) or cohort labeling curves (using ^{15}N- or ^{14}C-glycine). Several important papers (53, 84, 88–94, 126) have been reviewed (95).

B. Example

Numerous applications of a distributed model of iron kinetics in man have been described (67–76, 86). The authors considered compartments of radio-iron in plasma, in the erythrocytic bone marrow, the RBC, in the hemoglobin catabolic system and in the non-erythrocytic tissues. As a combination of these compartments, radio-iron in liver, spleen and marrow can also be analyzed. The hemoglobin catabolic system receives radio-iron from the RBC (by cell death) or from the erythrocytic marrow (by ineffective erythropoiesis). It replenishes the plasma pool from which the radio-iron enters the erythrocytic marrow and the non-erythrocytic storage compartments. With this type of model it is possible to determine transfer constants, plasma iron turnover, daily hemoglobin synthesis, RBC lifespan and ineffective iron turnover of individual patients. These parameters are derived from the curves of ^{59}Fe in plasma and RBC and from activity measurements in liver, spleen and bone marrow. Aplastic anemia, primary acquired sideroblastic anemia, Fanconi's anemia, heterozygous β-thalassemia, hereditary spherocytosis, and autoimmune hemolytic anemia, have been analyzed in detail.

VI. SPECIAL TOPICS

A. Review

In 1961 the CFU-S technique for stem cell measurement was reported. Three years later, the first mathematical model on the growth of stem cells and erythrocytic cells in spleen colonies was published (96). This was followed by several other reports (97–101). A Monte Carlo simulation of colony growth (96) with constant cell birth and death probabilities, predicted that the number of CFU-S per colony would be γ-distributed. In a stochastic model (99–101) this approach was generalized. Self-renewal probability, doubling time, generation time and the number of erythrocytic divisions (and the coefficients of variation of these parameters) could be derived from experimental cell numbers in bone marrow, spleen and spleen colonies. Using these results, the biphasic growth of spleen colonies has been analyzed (98). Finally, differentiation to the erythrocytic and granulocytic cell lines has been considered (97).

A quite different model has been developed for the kinetics of embryonic cells (102). Maturation times for the erythrocytic precursors in fetal mice during the hepatic phase of erythropoiesis have been calculated. These times seem to be significantly shorter for comparable cells in the bone marrow of adult animals.

In vitro differentiation has also been simulated mathematically (103). The addition of inducer to Friend erythroleukemia cells increases the probability for differentiation. This probability can be calculated from the numbers of colonies derived from uncommitted and committed cells.

A first order reaction of hemoglobin and glucose and a fixed lifespan of RBC has been assumed to simulate glycosylated hemoglobin levels for normal, increased and periodic glucose concentrations in patients with diabetes mellitus (104).

VII. MATHEMATICAL TECHNIQUES

The vast majority of models on erythropoiesis use difference equations or differential equations with or without a time delay. For some ferrokinetic models, the equations are linear but for most regulatory models the equations are non-linear. Partial differential equations (4, 8, 15–19, 36, 37, 67–76), stochastic models (62, 96, 99–101), and algebraic formulae (48, 56–61, 64–66, 97, 98) have also been used. Some of the models are applied on analog computers (5, 7, 9, 13, 26, 27, 30, 40–43, 46). A simple introduction to these mathematical techniques has been given (105). Further theoretical papers with applications in hematopoiesis are listed (106–114).

How to handle mathematical models: A short guideline for biologists and physicians

The following short summary of the essentials of 'model building' should help non-mathematicians to more realistically assess mathematical models. It is restricted to regulatory models of cell kinetics and even then only to the most frequent applications.

What information is needed to construct a model?

For a mathematical model of a cellular feedback system one needs;

1. The normal steady state values for the cell numbers, the transit times and the number of divisions in the different cellular compartments. The half-lives of the feedback hormones are also required.
2. The mode of transition between compartments or of cell death (by age or at random).
3. The number of mitoses, transit times and production rates under maximum and minimum stimulation of cell production.
4. Realistic hypotheses about the regulatory influences. (Where do they act? What are the dose–response curves of the regulators? etc.)
5. Alternative hypotheses if parts of the feedback system are controversial.

How does a model work?

With the above information regarding the parameters and with some clear hypotheses about the role of the regulators, it is possible to derive the mathematical formulae (in most cases in the form of deterministic or stochastic differential equations). Then, several applications of the model are possible. Some examples are;

1. Experiments with manipulated cell numbers. These are simulated by a corresponding modification of the initial values in the affected model compartments. Then the reaction in all compartments is calculated and compared with the data (e.g., bleeding anemia, hypertransfusion, single or

repeated injections of EPO). Characteristically the cell numbers and hormones return to normal steady state after some dampened oscillations.

2. Experiments in which external 'environmental' conditions are changed. These are simulated by modification of the corresponding model parameters. Then the responses in all compartments are calculated and compared with the data (e.g., hypoxia, hyperoxia, by a modified oxygen pressure). Characteristically the cell numbers and hormones approach a new steady state.

3. States of disease are simulated by modification of the 'disease parameters'. Then the new steady states in model compartments are compared with the data.

4. Therapies are simulated by modification of the corresponding initial values or model parameters which correspond to the therapy (e.g., reduced cell numbers in chemotherapy, enlarged oxygen parameters in oxygen therapy). Here the starting point is not the normal steady state but the pathological steady state of the disease.

5. Dose/response curves for indirectly correlated variables are derived from the steady state values in the corresponding compartments (e.g., steady state correlations between RBC number and altitude, between marrow transit time and hematocrit, between bone marrow production and RBC lifespan).

What is the practical use of a model?

1. It condenses the physiological knowledge about a feedback system.

2. It can be used to test different hypotheses about unknown regulatory influences. Thus incorrect hypotheses could be excluded and the most probable theories extracted.

3. Quantitative information about the regulatory mechanisms, which might not be amenable to direct measurement, can be obtained.

4. If a model is able to reproduce experimental data from different stress situations, it might be applied to predict the results of experiments not yet performed.

5. Model predictions allow one to suggest the optimal design for new experiments (time of measurement, variables to be measured, etc.)

6. The defects in special animal strains can be investigated quantitatively.

What are the criteria for a 'good' regulatory model?

1. The model parameters and the regulatory dependences should be interpretable in biological terms.

2. High complexity does not necessarily mean high quality. The complexity must be orientated to the biological knowledge of the regulatory system. It is important that as many model parameters as possible be known.

3. The number of parameters which must be assumed should be as small as possible. This is probably the most important point since each unknown parameter reduces the value of a model and makes it more speculative. Thus a

model which incorporates too many unknown values only transforms the problem of data interpretation to the problem of the interpretation of the speculative model parameters.

4. The model should be able to simulate different types of experiments.
5. The model results should be comparable with experimental data quantitatively and the model should reproduce the characteristics of the data.
6. The quality of a model is the higher if the data are reproduced simultaneously in a large number of compartments.
7. The quality of a model is the higher if it can simulate the data from many different stresses without changing the model parameters.
8. The model should be predictive, i.e., it should help in the design of new experiments.

VIII. ACKNOWLEDGMENTS

I wish to acknowledge the technical assistance of Mr S. Gontard and would like to thank Markus Loeffler and Heinz Wulff for reading the manuscript and for helpful comments.

IX. REFERENCES

1. Wichmann, H. E., and Gross, R. (1981). 'How mathematical models can interpret and predict experimental results in hematology', *Klin. Wochenschr.*, **59**, 1–4.
2. Aarnaes, E. (1977). *'Some aspects of the control of red blood cell production; a mathematical approach'*, University of Oslo thesis, pp. 1–101.
3. Aarnaes, E. (1978). 'A mathematical model of the control of red blood cell production', in *Biomathematics and Cell Kinetics*, (Eds. A. J. Valleron, and P. D. M. MacDonald), Elsevier/North-Holland Biomedical Press, Amsterdam, pp. 309–321.
4. Glass, L., and Mackey, M. C. (1979). 'Pathological conditions resulting from instabilities in physiological control systems', *Ann. N.Y. Acad Sci.*, **316**, 214–235.
5. Grudinin, N. M., Klochko, A. V., Lukshin, Y. V., and Klochko, E. V. (1978). 'Study of the kinetics of the functioning of a population of haemopoietic stem cells using analogue modelling devices', *Biophysics*, **23**, 343–349.
6. Hirschfeld, W. J. (1970). 'Models of erythropoiesis', in *Regulation of Hematopoiesis, vol. 1 Red Cell Production*, (Ed. A. S. Gordon), Appleton-Century-Crofts, New York, pp. 297–316.
7. Hradil, J., and Smid, A. (1971). 'A model of relationships between the stem cell and proerythroblast compartments', in *The Regulation of Erythropoiesis and Hemoglobin Synthesis*, (Eds. T. Travnicek and J. Neuwirth), The University Press, Prague, pp. 147–155.
8. Kazarinoff, N. D., and van den Driessche, P. (1979). 'Control of oscillations in hematopoiesis', *Science*, **203**, 1348–1349.
9. Kiefer, J. (1968). 'A model of feedback-controlled cell populations', *J. Theoret. Biol.*, **18**, 263–279.
10. Kirk, J., Orr, J. S., and Hope, C. S. (1968). 'A mathematical analysis of red blood cell and bone marrow stem cell control mechanisms', *Brit. J. Haemat.*, **15**, 35–47.

11. Kirk, J., Orr, J. S. Wheldon, T. E., and Gray, W. M. (1970). 'Stress cycle analysis in the biocybernetic study of blood cell populations', *J. Theoret. Biol.*, **26**, 265–276.
12. Koschel, K. (1975). *'Studies of Controlled Cell Populations'*. University of Melbourne thesis, pp. 1–250.
13. Kretchmar, A. (1966). 'Erythropoietin: Hypothesis of action tested by analog computer', *Science*, **152**, 367–370.
14. Lajtha, L. G., Oliver, R., and Gurney, C. W. (1962). 'Model of a bone-marrow stem-cell population', *Brit. J. Haemat.*, **8**, 442–460.
15. Loeffler, M., and Wichmann, H. E. (1980). 'A comprehensive mathematical model of stem cell proliferation which reproduces most of the published experimental results', *Cell Tissue Kinet.*, **13**, 543–561.
16. Loeffler, M., and Wichmann, H. E. (1980). 'How to plan experiments by use of a mathematical model of stem cell proliferation', *Exp. Hemat.*, **8**, **(Suppl. 7)**, 102.
17. Loeffler, M., Herkenrath, P., and Wichmann, H. E. (1981). 'Do erythropoiesis and granulopoiesis interact at the stem cell level? — A first mathematical model calculation', *Exp. Hemat.*, **9**, **(Suppl. 9)**, 53.
18. Mackey, M. C. (1978). 'Unified hypothesis for the origin of aplastic anemia and periodic hematopoiesis', *Blood*, **51**, 941–956.
19. Mackey, M. C. (1979). 'Dynamic haematological disorders of stem cell origin'. In *Biophysical and Biochemical Information Transfer in Recognition*, (Eds. J. G. Vassileva-Popova and E. V. Jensen), Plenum Publishing Co., New York, pp. 373–409.
20. Mackey, M. C., and Lasota, A. (1980). 'The extinction of slowly evolving dynamical systems'. (in press).
21. Monichev, A. Y. (1978). 'Conditions for the appearance of auto-fluctuations in the haemopoietic system', *Biophysics*, **23**, 697–701.
22. Nazarenko, V. G. (1978). 'Modification of the model of a cell population depressing its mitotic activity', *Biophysics*, **23**, 337–342.
23. Necas, E., Hauser, F., and Neuwirt, J. (1980). 'Computer model of haemopoietic stem cell population testing a possible role of DNA-synthesizing cells in proliferation control', *Blut*, **41**, 335–346.
24. Newton, C. (1965). 'Computer simulation of stem cell kinetics', *Bull. Math. Biophys.*, **27**, 275–290.
25. Newton, C. M. (1966). 'Modelling the stem cell system—current status', *Ann. N.Y. Acad. Sci.*, **128**, 781–789.
26. Okunewick, J. P., and Kretchmar, A. L. (1967). *'A mathematical model for post-irradiation recovery'*, Rand Corporation Memorandum, RM-5272-PR, pp. 1–32.
27. Okunewick, J. P., and Kretchmar, A. L. (1968). 'Mathematical model for post-irradiation haemopoiesis', in *Effects of Radiation on Cellular Proliferation and Differentiation*, I.A.E.A., Vienna, pp. 259–273.
28. Orr, J. S., Kirk, J., Gray, K. G., and Anderson, R. J. (1968). 'A study of the interdependence of red cell and bone marrow stem cell populations', *Brit. J. Haemat.*, **15**, 23–35.
29. Pabst, G., Kreja, L., and Seidel, H. J. (1981). 'Regulation of erythropoiesis—a mathematical model', *Exp. Hemat.*, **9**, **(Suppl. 9)** 52.
30. Ranft, U. (1978). 'Ein Simulationsmodell der Hämatopoese nach Strahlenschädigung, In *Simulationsmethoden in der Medizin und Biologie. Medizinische Information und Statistik*. Volume 8, (Eds. B. Schneider, and U. Ranft) Springer-Verlag, Berlin, pp. 335–350.

31. Reincke, U., and Slatkin, D. N. (1979). *Elementary model of a cell renewal population controlled by differentiated cell demand*. Fifth meeting of the International Society of Haematology, Hamburg, Abstracts p. 11.
32. Sacher, G. A., and Trucco, E. (1966). 'Theory of radiation injury and recovery in self-renewing cell populations', *Rad. Res.*, **29**, 236–256.
33. Svetina, S. (1981). 'Protein induction process and stochastic nature of cell commitment to proliferation and differentiation', *J. Theoret. Biol.*, **90**, 151–158.
34. Vacha, J., and Znojil, V. (1975). 'The application of the mathematical model of erythropoiesis to the dynamics of recovery after acute x-irradiation in mice', *Biofizika*, **20**, 872–879.
35. Weiss, P., and Kavanau, J. L. (1957). 'A model of growth and growth control in mathematical terms', *J. Gen. Physiol.*, **41**, 1–47.
36. Wichmann, H. E. (1980). 'Das allgemeine Stammzellproblem und seine mathematische Behandlung', *Math. Forschungsinst. Oberwolfach. Medizinische Statistik*, pp. 17–18. (in German).
37. Wichmann, H. E., and Loeffler, M. (1983). *Mathematical Modeling of Cell Proliferation, Volume 1, Stem Cell Regulation in Hemopoiesis'.* CRC Press, Boca Raton, FL, (in press).
38. Znojil, V., and Vacha, J. (1975). 'Mathematical model of the cytokinetics of erythropoiesis in the bone marrow and spleen of mice', *Biophysics*, **20**, 671–679.
39. Mackey, M. C. (1979). 'Periodic auto-immune hemolytic anemia: An induced dynamical disease', *Bull. Math. Biol.*, **41**, 829–834.
40. Duechting, W. (1973). 'Entwicklung eines Erythropoese-regelkreismodells zur Computer-Simulation', *Blut*, **27**, 342–350.
41. Duechting, W. (1975). 'Computersimulation von Zellerneuerungssytemen', *Blut*, **31**, 371–388.
42. Duechting, W. (1976). 'Computer simulation of abnormal erythropoiesis—an example of cell renewal regulating systems', *Biomed. Techn.*, **21**, 34–43.
43. Duechting, W. (1978). 'Control models in hemopoiesis', in *Biomathematics and Cell Kinetics*, (Eds. A. J. Valleron, and P. D. M. MacDonald), Elsevier/North-Holland Biomedical Press, Amsterdam, pp. 297–308.
44. Dunn, C. D. R., Smith, L. N., Leonard, J. I., Andrews, R. B., and Lange, R. D. (1980). 'Animal and computer investigations into the murine erythroid response to chronic hypoxia', *Exp. Hemat.*, **8, (Suppl. 8)**, 259–282.
45. Dunn, C. D. R., Leonard, J. I., and Kimzey, S. L. (1981). 'Interactions of animal and computer models in investigations of the "anemia" of space flight', *Aviat. Space Environ. Med.*, **52**, 683–690.
46. Hodgson, G. (1970). 'Application of control theory to the study of erythropoiesis', in *Regulation of Hematopoiesis, Volume I, Red Cell Production*, (Ed. A. S. Gordon), Appleton-Century-Crofts, New York, pp. 327–337.
47. Leonard, J. I., Kimzey, S. L., and Dunn, C. D. R. (1981). 'Dynamic regulation of erythropoiesis: A computer model of general applicability', *Exp. Hemat.*, **9**, 355–378.
48. Mylrea, K. C., and Abbrecht, P. H. (1971). 'Mathematical analysis and digital simulation of the control of erythropoiesis', *J. Theoret. Biol.*, **33**, 279–297.
49. Wichmann, H. E. (1976). *Untersuchung eines nichtlinearen Differentialgleichungssystems und seine Anwendung auf den Regelkreis der Bildung roter Blutzellen (Erythropoese) beim Menschen.* University of Köln thesis, pp. 1–106. (in German).
50. Wichmann, H. E., Spechtmeyer, H., Gerecke, D., and Gross, R. (1976). 'A mathematical model of erythropoiesis in man', in *Mathematical Models in*

Medicine, Lecture Notes in Biomathematics Volume 11, (Eds. J. Berger, W. Buehler, R. Repges, P. Tautu), Springer-Verlag, Berlin, pp. 159–179.

51. Wichmann, H. E., and Koeppen, L. (1978). 'Stability of non-linear systems', *EDV in Med. U. Biol.*, **9**, 118–123.

52. Wichmann, H. E., Wulff, H., and Gross, R. (1981). 'Regulation of erythopoiesis in rats and mice—a mathematical analysis', *Exp. Hemat.*, **9**, (**Suppl., 9**), 51.

53. Wulff, H. (1982). *Ein mathematisches Modell des erythropoetischen Systems von Ratte und Maus*, (in press). (In German).

54. Zajicek, G. (1968). 'A computer model simulating the behavior of adult red blood cells. Red cell model', *J. Theoret. Biol.*, **19**, 51–66.

55. Hill, A. V. (1910). 'The possible effects of the aggregation of the molecules of hemoglobin on its dissociation curve', *J. Physiol.*, **40**, IV–V.

56. Hanna, I. R. A., Tarbutt, R. G., and Lamerton, L. F. (1969). 'Shortening of the cell-cycle time of erythroid precursors in response to anaemia', *Brit. J. Haemat.*, **16**, 381–387.

57. Hanna, I. R. A., and Tarbutt, R. G. (1971). 'The relationship between cell maturation and proliferation in the erythroid system of the rat', *Cell Tissue Kinet.*, **4**, 47–59.

58. Killmann, S. A., Cronkite, E. P., Fliedner, T. M., and Bond, V. P. (1963). 'Mitotic indices of human bone marrow cells. II. The use of mitotic indices for estimation of time parameters of proliferation in serially connected multiplicative cellular compartments', *Blood*, **21**, 141–163.

59. Killmann, S. A., Cronkite, E. P., Fliedner, T. M., and Bond, V. P. (1964). 'Mitotic indices of human bone marrow cells. III. Duration of some phases of erythrocytic and granulocytic proliferation computed from mitotic indices', *Blood*, **24**, 267–280.

60. Mackey, M. C. (1980). *The connection between recognizable erythroid cell proliferation and maturation in humans*. Abstracts of the eighteenth Congress of the International Society of Hematology, p. 141.

61. Mackey, M. C. (1981). 'Random maturation in the recognizable proliferating hemopoietic precursors?' *Exp. Hemat.*, **9**, (**Suppl. 9**), 81.

62. Mary, J. Y., Valleron, A. J., Croizat, H., and Frindel, E. (1980). 'Mathematical analysis of bone marrow erythropoiesis: Application to C3H mouse data', *Blood Cells*, **6**, 241–254.

63. Prothero, J., Starling, M., and Rosse, C. (1978). 'Cell kinetics in the erythroid compartment of guinea pig bone marrow: A model based on ^{3}H-TdR studies', *Cell Tissue Kinet.*, **11**, 301–316.

64. Tarbutt, R. G. (1967). 'A study of erythropoiesis in the rat', *Exp. Cell. Res.*, **48**, 473–483.

65. Tarbutt, R. G., and Blackett, N. M. (1968). 'Cell population kinetics of the recognizable erythroid cells in the rat', *Cell Tissue Kinet.*, **1**, 65–80.

66. Tarbutt, R. G. (1969). 'Erythroid cell proliferation in hypertransfused rats', *Brit. J. Haemat.*, **17**, 191–198.

67. Barosi, G., Berzuini, C., Cazzola, M., Colli-Franzone, P., Morandi, S., Stefanelli, M., Viganotti, C., and Perugini, S. D. (1976). 'An approach by means of mathematical models to the analysis of ferrokinetic data obtained by liquid scintillation counting of Fe59', *J. Nucl. Biol. Med.*, **20**, 8–22.

68. Barosi, G., Cazzola, M., Marchi, A., Morandi, S., Perani, V., Stefanelli, M., and Perugini, S. (1978). 'Iron kinetics and erythropoiesis in Fanconi's anaemia', *Scand. J. Haemat.*, **21**, 29–39.

69. Barosi, G., Cazzola, M., Stefanelli, M., and Perugini, S. (1978). 'Erythropoiesis and iron kinetics', *Brit. J. Haemat.*, **40**, 503–504.

70. Barosi, G., Cazzola, M., Stefanelli, M., and Ascari, E. (1979). 'Studies of ineffective erythropoiesis and peripheral haemolysis in congenital dyserythropoietic anaemia type II', *Brit. J. Haemat.*, **43**, 243–250.
71. Berzuini, C., Colli-Franzone, F., Stefanelli, M., and Viganotti, V. (1978). 'Iron kinetics; Modelling and parameter estimation in normal and anemic states', *Comp. Biomed. Res.*, **11**, 209–227.
72. Cazzola, M., Alessandrino, P., Barosi, G., Morandi, S., Stefanelli, M. (1979). 'Quantitative evaluation of the mechanisms of the anaemia in heterozygous beta-thalassemia', *Scand. J. Haemat.*, **23**, 107–114.
73. Cazzola, M., Barosi, G., Orlandi, E., and Stefanelli, M. (1980). 'The plasma ^{59}Fe clearance curve in man', *Blut*, **40**, 325–335.
74. Colli-Franzone, P., Stefanelli, M., and Viganotti, C. (1978). 'Identification of distributed model for ferrokinetics', in *Distributed Parameter Systems: Modelling and Identification*, (Ed. A. Ruberti), Lecture Notes in Control and Information Sciences, Vol. 1, pp. 221–235. Marcel Dekker, New York.
75. Colli-Franzone, P., Stefanelli, M., and Viganotti, C. (1979). 'Parameter estimation of a distributed model of ferrokinetics: Effects of data errors on parameter estimate accuracy', in Identification and System Parameter Estimation, (Ed. R. Iserman), Proceedings of the Fifth I.F.A.C. Symposium. Pergamon Press, Oxford, pp. 827–834.
76. Colli-Franzone, P., Stefanelli, M., and Viganotti, C. (1979). 'A distributed model of iron kinetics for clinical assessment of normal-abnormal erythropoietic activity', *I.E.E.E. Trans. Biomed. Eng.*, **26**, 586–596.
77. Cook, J. D., Marsaglia, G., Escbach, J. W., Funk, D. D., and Finch, C. A. (1970). 'Ferrokinetics; A biologic model for plasma iron exchange in man', *J. Clin. Invest.*, **49**, 197–205.
78. Garby, L., Schneider, W., Sundquist, O., and Vuille, J. C. (1963). 'A ferro-erythro-kinetic model and its properties', *Acta Physiol. Scand.*, **59**, **Suppl. 216**, 4–29.
79. Groth, T., Schneider, W., Sandewall, E., and Vuille, J. C. (1970). 'Computer simulation of ferrokinetic models', *Compt. Prog. Biomed.*, **1**, 90–104.
80. Kutzim, H., and Wellner, U. (1972). 'Quantitative determination of iron turnover and iron pools in diseases of the erythropoietic system and their significance in differential diagnosis', *Excerpta Medica, International Congress Series*, **285**, 79–84.
81. Monot, C., Najean, Y., Dresch, C., and Martin, J. (1975). 'Models of erythropoiesis and clinical diagnosis', *Math. Biosci.*, **27**, 145–154.
82. Nooney, G. C. (1966). 'An erythron-dependent model of iron kinetics', *Biophys. J.*, **6**, 601–609.
83. Pollycove, M., and Mortimer, R. (1961). 'The quantitative determination of iron kinetics and hemoglobin synthesis in human subjects', *J. Clin. Invest.*, **40**, 755–782.
84. Ricketts, C., Jacobs, A., and Cavill, I. (1975). 'Ferrokinetics and erythropoiesis in man: The measurement of effective erythropoiesis, ineffective erythropoiesis and red cell lifespan using ^{59}Fe', *Brit. J. Haemat.*, **31**, 65–75.
85. Sharney, L., Wasserman, R. L., Schwartz, L., and Tendler, D. (1963). 'Multiple pool analysis as applied to erythro-kinetics', *Ann. N.Y. Acad. Sci.*, **108**, 230–249.
86. Stefanelli, M., Barosi, G., Cazzola, M., and Orlandi, E. (1980). 'Quantitative assessment of erythropoiesis in haemolytic disease', *Brit. J. Haemat.*, **45**, 297–308.
87. Wellner, U. (1981). *Tracer in Lebewesen, Mathematische Modelle und Quantitative Bestimmungen*. Hippokrates, Stuttgart, (in German).

88. Bentley, S. A., Lewis, S. M., and White, J. M. (1974). 'Red cell survival in patients with unstable haemoglobin disorders', *Brit. J. Haemat.*, **26**, 85–92.
89. Bergner, P. E. (1965). 'On stationary and non-stationary red cell survival curves', *J. Theoret. Biol.*, **9**, 366.
90. Callender, S. T., Powell, E. O., and Witts, L. J. (1945). 'The life-span of the red cell in man', *J. Path.*, **57**, 129–139.
91. Dornhorst, A. C. (1951). 'The interpretation of red cell survival curves', *Blood*, **6**, 1284–1292.
92. Eadie, G. S., and Brown, I. W. (1953). 'Analytical review. Red Blood cell survival studies', *Blood*, **8**, 1110–1136.
93. Garby, L., Groth, T., and Schneider, W. (1969). 'Determination of kinetic parameters of red blood cell survival by computer simulation', *Compt. Biochem. Res.*, **2**, 229–241.
94. I.C.S.H. Panel, (1971). 'Recommended methods for radioisotope red-cell survival studies', *Brit. J. Haemat.*, **21**, 241–256.
95. Bentley, S. A. (1977). 'Red cell survival studies reinterpreted', in *Radioisotopes in Haematology*. (Ed. S. M. Lewis), *Clin. Haemat.*, **6**, 601–624.
96. Till, J. E., McCulloch, E. A., and Siminovitch, L. (1964). 'Stochastic model of stem cell proliferation based on the growth of spleen colony-forming cells', *Proc. Nat. Acad. Sci.*, **51**, 29–36.
97. Korn, A. P., Henkelman, R. M., Ottensmeyer, F. P., and Till, J. E. (1973). 'Investigations of a stochastic model of haemopoiesis', *Exp. Hemat.*, **1**, 362–375.
98. Lajtha, L. G., Gilbert, C. W., and Guzman, E. (1971). 'Kinetics of haemopoietic colony growth', *Brit. J. Haemat.*, **20**, 343–354.
99. Matioli, G., Vogel, H., and Niewisch, H. (1968). 'The dilution factor of intravenously injected hemopoietic stem cells', *J. Cell. Physiol.*, **72**, 229–234.
100. Vogel, H., Niewisch, H., and Matioli, G. (1968). 'The self renewal probability of hemopoietic stem cells', *J. Cell. Physiol.*, **72**, 221–228.
101. Vogel, H., Niewisch, H., and Matioli, G. (1969). 'Stochastic development of stem cells', *J. Theoret. Biol.*, **22**, 249–270.
102. Wheldon, T. E., Kirk, J., Orr, J. S., Paul, J., and Conkie, D. (1974). 'Kinetics of development of embryonic erythroid cells', *Cell Tissue Kinet.*, **7**, 181–188.
103. Gusella, J. (1976). 'Commitment to erythroid differentiation by Friend erythroleukemia cells: A stochastic analysis', *Cell*, **9**, 221–229.
104. Beach, K. W. (1979). 'A theoretical model to predict the behavior of glycosylated hemoglobin levels', *J. Theoret. Biol.*, **81**, 547–561.
105. Simon, W. (1972). *'Mathematical Techniques for Physiology and Medicine*, Academic Press, New York.
106. Coe, F. L. (1968). 'Mean life in steady-state populations', *J. Theoret. Biol.*, **18**, 171–180.
107. Creekmore, S. P., Aroesty, J., Willis, K. L., Morrison, P. F., and Lincoln, T. L. (1978). 'A cell kinetic model which includes heredity, differentiation and regulatory control', in *Biomathematics and Cell Kinetics*, (Ed. A. J. Valleron and P. D. M. MacDonald), Elsevier/North-Holland Biomedical Press, Amsterdam, pp. 255–267.
108. Rubinow, S. I. (1969). 'A simple model of a steady state differentiating cell system', *J. Cell. Biol.*, **43**, 32–39.
109. Rubinow, S. I., and Lebowitz, J. L. (1975). 'A mathematical model of neutrophil production and control in normal man', *J. Math. Biol.*, **1**, 187–225.
110. Trucco, E. (1965). 'Mathematical models for cellular systems. The von Foerster Equation. Part I', *Bull. Math. Biophys.*, **27**, 285–304.

111. Valleron, A. J., and MacDonald, P. D. M. (1978). *Biomathematics and Cell Kinetics*, Elsevier/North-Holland Press, Amsterdam.
112. von Foerster, H. (1959). 'Some remarks on changing populations', in *The Kinetics of Cellular Proliferation*, (Ed. F. Stohlman), Grune and Stratton, New York, pp. 382–407.
113. Wheldon, T. E., Kirk, J., and Orr, J. S. (1974). 'Non-steady-state analysis of cellular development', *Cell Tissue Kinet., 7*, 173–179.
114. Wichmann, H. E., Gerhardts, M. D., Spechtmeyer, H., and Gross, R. (1979). 'A mathematical model of thrombopoiesis in rats', *Cell Tissue Kinet., 12*, 551–567.
115. Adamson, J. W., Torok-Storb, B., and Lin, N. (1978). 'Analysis of erythropoiesis by erythroid colony formation in culture', *Blood Cells, 4*, 89–103.
116. Iscove, N. N. (1977). 'The role of erythropoietin in regulation of population size and cell cycling of early and late erythroid precursors in mouse bone marrow', *Cell Tissue Kinet., 10*, 323–334.
117. Hara, H., and Ogawa, M. (1977). 'Erythropoietic precursors in mice under erythropoietic stimulation and suppression', *Exp. Hemat., 5*, 141–148.
118. Arturson, G., Garby, M., Robert, M., and Zaar, B. (1974). 'Determination of the oxygen affinity of human blood *in vivo* and under standard conditions', *Scand. J. Clin. Lab. Med., 34*, 15–18.
119. Abbrecht, P. H., and Littell, J. K. (1972). 'Plasma erythropoietin in men and mice during acclimatization to different altitudes', *J. Appl. Physiol., 32*, 54–58.
120. Lord, B. I. (1967). 'Erythropoietic cell proliferation during recovery from acute haemorrhage', *Brit. J. Haemat., 13*, 160–167.
121. Tribukait, B. (1960). 'Verhalten von Gesamthaemoglobin und Blutvolumen der Ratte bei akuter Blutungsanaemie', *Acta Physiol. Scand., 49*, 148–154. (in German).
122. Becker, J. H., and Spengler, D. (1966). 'Die Verduennungsanaemie', *Acta Haemat. (Basle)., 35*, 1–29. (in German).
123. Bothwell, T. H., Hurtado, A. V., Donohue, D. M., and Finch, C. (1957). 'Erythrokinetics, IV. The plasma iron turnover as a measure of erythropoiesis', *Blood, 12*, 409–427.
124. Hillman, R. S., Adamson, J. W., and Burka, E. (1969). 'Characteristics of vitamin B_{12} correction of the abnormal erythropoiesis of pernicious anemia', *Blood, 31*, 419–433.
125. Tinsley, J. C., Moore, C. V., Dubach, R., Minnich, V., and Grinstein, M. (1949). 'The role of oxygen in the regulation of erythropoiesis. Depression of the rate of delivery of new red cells to the blood by high concentrations of inspired oxygen', *J. Clin. Invest., 28*, 1544–1564.
126. Weiss, G. H., and Zajicek, G. (1969). 'Kinetics of red blood cells following hemolysis,' *J. Theoret. Biol., 23*, 475–491.

Current Concepts in Erythropoiesis
Edited by C. D. R. Dunn

CHAPTER 6

Erythropoiesis in dogs and humans with cyclic hematopoiesis

ROBERT D. LANGE and JIMMY B. JONES
Department of Medical Biology
University of Tennessee Center for the Health Sciences/Knoxville Unit

CONTENTS

I. INTRODUCTION

In 1910 Leale (1) described the case of an infant who had recurrent furunculosis and a leukopenia with an extreme relative lymphocytosis. It remained for Rutledge *et al* (2) to ascertain in this same patient, that recurrent agranulocytosis was present and the condition was subsequently termed cyclic neutropenia (CN). A somewhat similar condition in grey collie dogs was described by Lund and his co-workers in 1967 (3). In dogs the condition is inherited and when it was shown that reticulocytes and platelets also cycled it was more aptly called cyclic hematopoiesis (CH). Early on it was shown that changes in the bone marrow preceded the changes in the peripheral blood and

143

subsequently bone marrow transplantation studies demonstrated that the condition could either be caused or abrogated by appropriate bone marrow grafting (4–7).

The rigorously recurring cycles lend themselves to investigations of the progenitor cell populations and studies of blood cell controlling factors. Indeed, if the pathogenic mechanisms of CN and CH are ascertained it will most certainly give us clues regarding the controlling factors of normal differentiation of blood cells.

The great majority of the studies of these fascinating conditions have been concerned with the dramatic changes in neutrophils. However, changes in erythrocytic parameters have also been described and it is the purpose of this review to focus on those perturbations. First in the dog, since more information is available, and then the observed changes in human patients. Finally, the pathogenesis of these disorders will be discussed with emphasis on the likely heterogeneity of their origin.

II. ERYTHROPOIESIS IN CANINE CYCLIC HEMATOPOIESIS

Cyclic neutropenia in grey collie dogs was first recognized and described by Lund *et al* (3). From later studies which elucidated many aspects of the grey collie syndrome, it was correctly surmised that the disease was inherited as an autosomal recessive gene (8, 9). The grey collie syndrome can be genetically transferred to other breeds of dogs; in every case, the diluted coat color and hematopoietic abnormalities occur at the same time (5). A similar association has been noted in two mouse models of anemic disorders (10, 11).

The early studies of the grey collie revealed the presence of inter-current cycles of all the formed elements of the blood and each element's cycle was precise in its relationship to the cycles of each of the other elements (3, 12). Cycles of reticulocytosis and thrombocytosis occurred at regular 11–13 day intervals, and the disease was appropriately called CH (12). Figure 1 illustrates a typical cycle. The onset of neutropenia, usually designated as day 1 of a twelve-day cycle, was accompanied by thrombocytosis and reticulocytosis. Invariably, as the neutropenia abated, a monocytosis preceded the rise in neutrophil counts.

Repetitive cycles of reticulocytosis suggested surges of erythropoiesis. Since the lifespan of the CH dog's erythrocytes did not differ from that of controls, hemolysis could be eliminated as a cause of the reticulocytosis (13). As other possible causes of reticulocytosis were explored, the CH puppy's total erythron development was found generally to lag behind that of normal litter mates (Figure 2) (14); erythrocytic values varied from distinctly lower than normal to just within the lower end of the normal range. These variations were related to the CH dog's over-all health and if the puppy's health remained quite good for many weeks, erythrocytic values reached the lower end of the normal range.

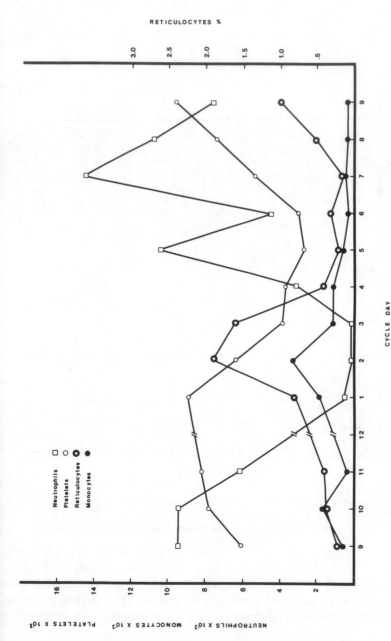

Figure 1. Cycles of neutrophils, platelets, reticulocytes and monocytes in a CH dog. Day 1 of the cycle is the day the absolute neutrophil count is less than $1600/mm^3$.

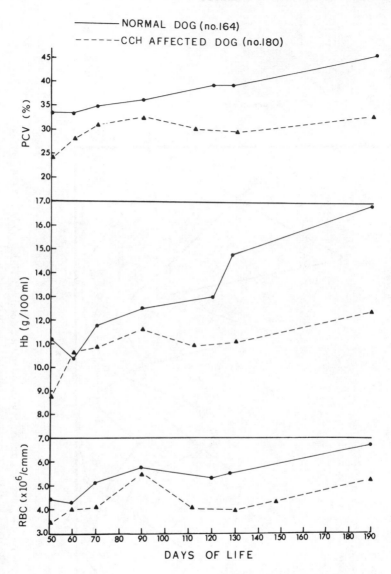

Figure 2. Changes with age of erythrocyte (RBC), hemoglobin (Hb), and packed cell volume (PCV) values in a CCH-affected and a normal dog. Reproduced with permission of the *Journal of the American Veterinary Medical Association* from Jones *et al* (14)

The iron supply and kinetics of the CH dog showed that the iron disappearance was not different from that of controls (13). Although serum iron values cycled, they were related to cycles of erythrocytic activity and thus

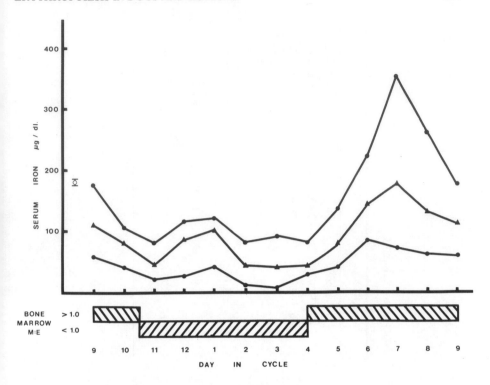

Figure 3. Serum iron values in four dogs with CH over an entire cycle period. Samples were collected for 14 days but since the cycles varied from twelve to 14 days, only the values for the twelve days (in which four values were obtained) are included. Solid line and '▲' represents average results of four dogs and (●–●) represents the minimal–maximal results on any given day. The serum iron value of $177 \pm 9.6 \ \mu g/dl$ for the 14 determinations in a normal dog is represented by the symbol 'Φ' at the left hand portion of the graph. The lower cross-hatched horizontal bars indicate when the bone marrow is in either a myelocytic or erythrocytic phase. M:E represents the myelocytic:erythrocytic ratio. Reproduced with permission of the *American Journal of Veterinary Research from Lange et al* (13)

appeared to be compatible with the prevailing marrow activity (Figure 3).

The normal erythrocyte lifespan, together with normal iron metabolism, indicated that erythropoiesis was not being perturbed by either of these two common avenues of anemia. Further studies were then conducted to evaluate the erythrocyte diphosphoglyceric acid (2,3-DPG) levels and the blood gases in two CH dogs and a normal dog over a period of several weeks as well as single determinations on six normal dogs. The CH dogs' 2,3-DPG and P_{50} values were different from those of the normal dogs (Table 1) (15). This finding indicated an abnormality that might be linked to the slowed erythron development of the CH dog. However, the 2,3-DPG values were not cyclic

Table 1. Blood gas and 2,3-DPG results in normal and CH dogs

	Normal dogs†	Normal 524‡	CH 863	CH 911
Hct %, mean ± s.D.	N.D.	51.5 ± 1.9	38.0 ± 0.92	31.0 ± 1.8
pH, mean ± s.D.	N.D.	7.42 ± 0.02	7.45 ± 0.02	7.44 ± 0.01
PCO_2 mm Hg mean ± s.D.	N.D.	28.6 ± 2.02	28.6 ± 2.9	31.4 ± 3.16
PO_2 mm Hg mean ± s.D.	N.D.	91.1 ± 9.3	90.0 ± 7.2	86.9 ± 6.2
% O_2 Sat. mean ± s.D.	N.D.	97.1 ± 1.0	97.4 ± 0.7	97.0 ± 0.6
2,3-DPG µg/g Hgb mean ± s.D.	16.3 ± 0.3	16.6 ± 1.8	24.125* ± 2.5	25.85* ± 2.6
P_{50} mm Hg mean ± s.D.	29.5 ± 1.2	29.6 ± 0.7	32.15* ± 1.2	31.2* ± 0.08

* $p < 0.0005$, CH 863, and CH 911 vs. normal controls
†Single determination on six normal dogs
‡Ten determinations, dog 524

and, therefore, were not directly related to the cyclic reticulocytosis and erythropoietin (EPO) fluctuations (6).

The cyclic reticulocytosis, when considered together with the normal erythrocyte lifespan, iron metabolism, and blood gases, seemed to be caused by waves of erythropoiesis occurring in the bone marrow rather than to peripheral cell destruction or malfunction. Since the nature of the CH dog's anemia appeared to be related primarily to the dog's general health, the question becomes; what initiates or controls the waves of marrow erythropoiesis?

As a convenient marker to time and plot the events of the cyclic phenomena in CH, the day that the absolute peripheral neutrophil count decreased to 1600 mm^3 was designated as day 1. Using this designation, repetitive events in several cycles are easily compared. In terms of actual events, day 9 of the twelve-day cycle seems critical. On day 9 the bone marrow was still predominantly myelocytic in character and had a plethora of mature neutrophils. However, when studies were carried out with an underlayer of bone marrow adherent cells obtained from CH dogs, on day 9 the underlayer did not cause stimulation of colony forming units—culture (CFU-C) of normal dog non-adherent cells. Furthermore, the conditioned medium (CM) prepared from this marrow inhibited the proliferation of murine colony forming units—spleen (CFU-S) (16). At this time the cyclic 3',5' guanosine monophosphate (cGMP) activity of CM from CH adherent cells was nearing its apogee and stayed at high activity through day 3.

From day 10 to day 2 (days 10, 11, 12, 1, 2) the bone marrow was predominantly erythrocytic in character; early erythroblasts were seen first, then progressed to more mature forms. Electron microscopic studies did not disclose any abnormal morphologic features in the erythrocytic cells (17). A myelocytic phase then began, and a day-by-day progression from myeloblasts and promyelocytes to the late myelocytic cells peaking on day 7 and 8. The cycle then repeated itself.

Studies have been carried out to measure the ability of CH bone marrow cells to form erythrocytic colonies and to proliferate in diffusion chambers implanted in the peritoneal cavities of irradiated mice.

The colony forming units—erythrocytic (CFU-E) of CH marrow were measured on each day of the cycle for their response to dog EPO. The CFU-E fluctuated from four to five times above normal to less than 0.1 times normal. The highest numbers found were measured during the erythrocytic phase of the bone marrow (i.e. days 10, 11, 12, 1, 2), and the lowest numbers occurred on days 6 to 8 during the peak of the peripheral neutrophil count (18). The EPO responsive cells (ERC) fluctuated in the same phase as CFU-C (19). The ERC cycle in one study was preceded three or four days by an increase of EPO, as measured in the fetal mouse liver cell assay (FMLC). An elevation of reticulocytes usually followed, although it sometimes coincided with the CFU-E peak. The proliferation rate of CFU-E was measured by using tritiated thymidine and no change was evident throughout the cycle (Figure 4) (18).

Bone marrow cells have been found to proliferate in diffusion chambers implanted into lethally irradiated mice. Some investigators have suggested that this system supports the growth of pluripotential stem cells (20). Dunn *et al* (21) measured the cytopoietic potential (CP) of CH dog bone marrow. (The CP was defined as the slope of the regression line relating the number of cells harvested from the diffusion chambers to the number of cells in the inoculum.) The CP fluctuated from near normal levels during neutropenia to below normal when neturophils were increased. Thus again, when marrow was obtained on cycle days 12, 1, 2, and 3, cellularity in diffusion chambers was greatest during the marrow erythrocytic phase.

The long-range stimulators of hematopoiesis (EPO, thrombopoietin (TSF) and the putative leukopoietin, colony stimulating factor (CSF)), conceivably could be important in the regulation of CH. Dale *et al* (22) reported that the levels of CSF in the urine of CH dogs peaked during the neutropenic phase and were not detectable when the blood neutrophil counts reached normal levels. TSF was found to cycle (23). Serum EPO in CH dogs was found to cycle when profound anemia was produced by phlebotomy (24).

Two types of EPO bioassays were carried out in our laboratory. The first utilized exhypoxic polycythemic mice and the second employed the FMLC assay as modified by Dunn *et al* (19). In our original EPO investigations we were unable to detect any cycling in the levels of the hormone in non-phlebotomized dogs. However, when CH and normal dogs were exposed to constant hypoxia over a prolonged period of time, a spike of EPO activity was found at one to three days, just as occurs in all normal mammals (25). In the normal dogs, the EPO level then returned to near normal for the duration of the hypoxia period. However, in spite of rising hematocrits and a constantly low O_2 level, the CH dogs had bursts of serum EPO activity at eleven- to twelve-day intervals. Characteristically the highest activity was found five days after the onset of neutropenia with minor peaks of serum EPO activity occurring mid-cycle in some dogs. In one dog, 1600 ml of blood were removed in a 32-day period of constant hypoxia. The reticulocytes were present at a higher level but still appeared to respond to bursts of EPO activity. Interestingly, the granulocyte cycles continued uninterrupted. The sustained erythropoiesis and the continued granulocyte cycles indicated no limitation in the number of "stem" cells and no evidence of competition at the stem cell level.

After the dogs had received a bone marrow transplantation and then were exposed to hypoxia, EPO levels were measured (6). The EPO response to hypoxia in CH dogs engrafted with normal bone marrow was the same as for a normal dog in that an initial elevated level of EPO returned to near normal and remained there for the duration of the hypoxia. However, in normal dogs engrafted with CH marrow, cycles of EPO occurred just as in the CH dogs

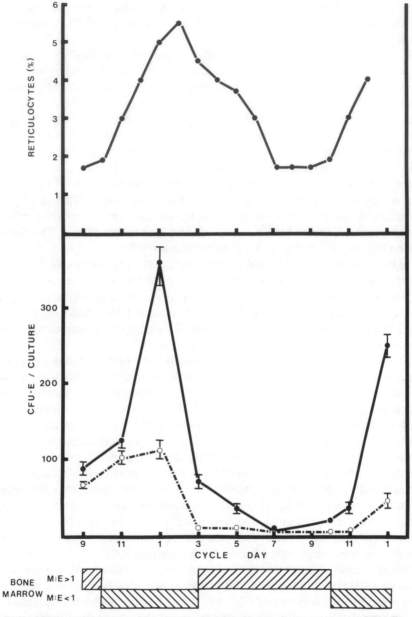

Figure 4. Relationship between peripheral blood reticulocyte values, CFU-E and bone marrow in CH dogs. CFU-E are reported per 2.4×10^5 nucleated bone marrow cells in CH dog 596. Solid symbols and lines, CFU-E in untreated marrows; open symbols and broken line, CFU-E surviving a 20-min incubation with high specific activity ^{3}H-TdR. Vertical bars indicate $\pm$ s.e.m. Reproduced with permission of *Experimental Hematology* from Dunn *et al* (18)

described previously. Thus, the distinct possibility arises that a marrow produced substance was acting as a stimulator of EPO production—a 'poietin-poietin'.

EPO levels, as measured in the FMLC assay, were cyclically elevated three to four days before the ERC cycle which, in turn, was followed by an elevation of reticulocytes (19). The same assay was used to measure EPO activity in CM produced from the bone marrow cells of CH dogs. The CM prepared with marrow obtained on day 10 contained erythropoiesis stimulating activity (16). This day was the one following the critical events occurring on day 9.

Cyclic nucleotides have possible involvement in erythropoiesis. Thus, the conditions known to lead to an increase in EPO levels can be associated with prior increases in cyclic $3',5'$ adenosine monophosphate (cAMP) and cGMP. The serum of CH dogs exposed to hypoxia was assayed by White et al (26) for its ability to affect hemoglobin synthesis by normal dog bone marrow cells. The varying levels indicated the presence of an agent which cycled. The timing of action indicated that the agent probably was not EPO.

In later studies of cAMP and cGMP levels in the plasma of CH dogs, cAMP levels showed no consistent change during the twelve-day cycle. However, when the percentage change of cGMP was measured, a net elevation appeared on day 3 and day 4 of the cycle. The cGMP levels in CM of adherent cells of CH dogs reached a low point on day 6 followed by rising titers and elevated levels during day 10 to day 3 (days 10, 11, 12, 1, 2, 3).

The possibility that CH could be caused by an organ dysfunction, e.g., the pituitary, or an abnormal bone marrow response to the total body environment presented researchers with a large number of possible experiments aimed at elucidating the interactions between the marrow and various organs. Appropriate allograft experiments pinpointed the marrow as the site of the disease. The disease was both induced and eliminated through appropriate bone marrow grafts. A report describing the cure effected by a bone marrow transplant (4) was closely followed by another reporting the induction of the disease with a marrow transplant (7). In our laboratory, we transplanted normal marrow into a CH dog and eliminated the disease, then transplanted CH marrow into a normal dog and induced the disease (27). Platelet and reticulocyte counts, made before and after the transplantations, showed that the disease was completely effected by the marrow itself.

We also studied EPO levels. Cycles of EPO were detected in a normal dog bearing a CH transplant but not the converse, thereby showing that the marrow was primary to the cycles of EPO (27). Furthermore, the transplanted dogs showed packed cell volumes characteristic of the allografted marrow in that CH dogs receiving normal marrow showed increased hematocrits while the reverse was true of normal dogs bearing CH marrow allografts (Figure 5) (28).

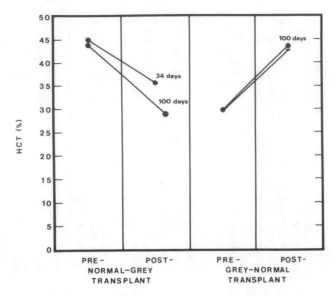

Figure 5. Hematocrit values of bone marrow chimeras before and after transplant. Normal-grey transplant refers to a normal dog transplanted with bone marrow from a CH grey litter mate. Grey-normal refers to a CH grey dog transplanted with bone marrow from a normal-colored littermate. Reproduced with permission of M. Shifrine and F. Wilson, editors of *The Canine as a Biomedical Research Model* from Lange and Jones (28)

III. ERYTHROPOIESIS IN HUMAN CYCLIC HEMATOPOIESIS

The first case of cyclic neutropenia (CN) in a human patient was reported by Leale (1) in an article entitled 'Recurrent furunculosis in an infant showing an unusual blood picture'. Rutledge and co-workers (2) later documented the cyclic nature of the disorder in Leale's patient. In all, about 130 patients have been described in the medical literature although some of the information is very fragmentary (29).

Two-thirds of the cases have been reported as starting in infancy or childhood. In some instances a definite familial history can be documented (e.g., cases 7 and 17, Table 2). Typically, the human cycle is 21 days with a neutropenic period of approximately five days. During the neutropenic period the patient is frequently febrile and may note lassitude, oral ulcerations, sore tongue and gums as well as sore throats and minor skin infections. Children with CN are particularly prone to ear infections. The course of the disease has been described as benign (46), and in many patients it is relatively benign (Leale's patient lived to age 37 before he succumbed to pneumonia). However, serious infections can occur and can be life threatening. Records document at

Table 2. Data on patients with cyclic neutropenia who demonstrated erythrocytic abnormalities

Case	Senior author (reference)	Sex	Age at study (years)	Age at onset (years)	Cycle time (days)	Splenectomy (weight)	Remarks
1	Doan 1932 (30) Kitchen 1934 (31)	F	18	—	20–21	+	Represented second case reported. Had compensatory monocytosis. Therapy included liver extract, nucleotide injections, and splenectomy without effect. Had marked gingivitis and oral ulcers. Hemolytic icterus reported by Coventry.
2	Embleton 1936 (33) Embleton 1937 (34)	F	43	26	17–36		Had attacks of buccal ulceration that occurred during a period of 10–17 years prior to observation. Had a rise and fall of red blood cells (RBC) associated with rise and fall of leucocyte count.
3	Coventry 1953 (32) Becker 1959 (35)	F	16	1	17–22	+ 250 g	Admitted to dermatology service because of severe furunculosis. Hb 9.5 g % with RBC of 3,400,000. Monocytosis present.
4	Duane 1958 (36)	F	28	21	16–29		Patient was black and was the first recorded case of that race. Had monocytosis and an eosinophilia which was not cyclic. Hb was 10.5 g %.
5	Henley 1959 (37) Telsey 1962 (38)	F	12 14	0.3	17–21	+ (?)	Onset at age of 4 months with repeated ear infections, pharyngitis, and gingivitis. Hb of 8.2 g % with RBC of 3.72 million. Had eosinophilia and monocytosis. Neither splenectomy nor three-year course of steroids resulted in significant improvement.
6	Alestig 1961 (39)	F	58	56	14		Monocytosis. Patient had a fairly moderate hypochromic anemia, was treated with cortisone and prednisone without striking change in blood picture but fever and symptoms were improved.
7	Morley 1967 (40) Moore 1974 (41)	F	8 15	1	16–28 18–21		Mother had neutropenia and two sisters have cyclic neutropenia. Hb of 8.6 g % found at age 6. Monocytosis with persisting eosinophilia and mild basophilia noted. Also had decreased platelet counts.

8	Montford 1968 (42)	M	3	0.2	21		Patient had a hypochromic anemia with Hb of 5 g %. Treated with prophylactic antibiotics and short course of prednisone without affecting cycle.
9	Guerry 1973 (43) Guerry 1974 (44) Wright 1978 (45) Wright 1981 (46)	F	67 70	63	21	+ (?)	See text
10	Hansen 1973 (47)	M	68	66	20	+ 212 g	Spleen had normal histology. Splenectomy was without effect. Chromosomes were normal. Subsequently developed aplastic anemia with neutropenia, thrombocytopenia and anemia. Died as a result of septicemia.
11	Degnan 1973 (48)	M	67	65			Possible case. Patient had moderate neutropenia but definite cycles not demonstrated. Also had 'slight anemia' for which iron therapy was initiated.
12	Brandt 1975 (49)	M	18	16	21		See text
13	Pachman 1975 (50)	M	2.5	0.75	21		See text
14	Greenberg 1976 (51)	M	8	Early childhood	20		Patient had monocytosis. Serial platelet and reticulocyte levels fluctuated without evidence of periodicity. CSF levels high when neutrophil count was low.
15	Greenberg 1976 (51)	F	32	Childhood	21.4		Patient had oral ulcers, skin abscesses and 'flu-like' symptoms (fever, headaches, myalgias, and URI). Monocytosis present. Reticulocytes and platelets fluctuated without periodicity. CSF varied inversely with neutrophil count.
16	Uyama 1976 (52)	F	7	0.1	α 21		See text
17	Andrews 1979 (53) Lange 1981 (54)	F	18	Infancy	21–25		Father has leukopenia. One sister and two nephews have cyclic neutropenia. Monocytosis present and there was possible cycling of erythropoietin.
18	Roozendaal 1981 (55)	F	62	52?	38.5		See text

least 15 deaths, the most frequent complication being with pulmonary involvement. At least two patients had amyloidosis (29, 54, 56), a disorder which has also been described in CH dogs (57).

When peripheral blood counts are monitored, the *sine qua non* is the demonstration of a regularly recurring fall in absolute neutrophil count. Frequently a drop in the total white blood cell count also occurs. Of the definite cases of CN, 50% have a recorded monocytosis which typically is present during the neutropenic period just before the onset of an increase in absolute neutrophil count. The other formed elements of the blood are not as frequently involved.

Anemia has been described in 18 patients (Table 2). In 13 patients anemia was probably an incidental finding, i.e., an accompanying iron deficiency or development of aplastic anemia. However, in five patients, the cycling of erythrocytic (reticulocytic) elements was recorded. Brief case histories of those patients follow:

1. Case number 9, (43, 45). The patient, when first studied, was 67 years old. Neutropenia was discovered when she was 63 and undergoing treatment for pneumonia. Her history showed recurrent fever, oral ulcers, and minor skin infections. Splenectomy had produced no apparent benefit. The patient demonstrated cyclic fluctuation of her neutrophil, monocyte, lymphocyte, platelet, and reticulocyte counts. Subsequent studies showed that CSF levels increased during the neutropenic periods concomitantly with monocytosis. EPO levels in the urine were also increased during the period of neutropenia preceding the periodic reticulocytosis. Later treatment with etiocholanolone and prednisolone every other day led to a gradual decrease in cyclic fluctuations of neutrophils but the patient relapsed when treatment was stopped. Prednisolone alone every other day reproduced these results but neutrophil counts were in the range of $1500 \times 10^9/l$. Symptomatically the patient improved and the cycling of monocytes, platelets, and reticulocytes were eliminated. In this study lymphocyte cycles were apparently not recorded.

2. Case number 12, (49). An 18-year-old male who during early childhood had frequent episodes of otitis, tonsillitis, and bronchitis was studied. He had been well between the ages of ten and 16 years but then, at three-week intervals and lasting four to five days, he had fever, oral ulcers, cervical adenitis, dysphagia, and sometimes conjunctivitis. He had a sore throat on some febrile occasions. On one occasion, a pleural effusion was noted.

   A true monocytosis was present during profound neutropenia. His lymphocyte counts fluctuated without relation to neutrophil counts but eticulocytes exhibited cyclic changes with a cycle period identical to but out-of-phase with neutrophils.

   Bone marrow cells had a normal level of colony-forming cells. Neutrophil function studies gave normal results and bone marrow karotype analyses displayed normal patterns.

3. Case number 13, (50). This two and a half-year-old boy had been noted to have recurrent apthous stomatitis, otitis media, and cervical adenitis at the age of nine months. Neutropenia with periodic elevations of the absolute mature polymorphonuclear count at 21-day intervals were documented. Cyclic fluctuations were also found in monocytes, platelets, and reticulocytes. When neutrophil function was evaluated at the peak of the neutrophil cycle, myeloperoxidase was present, the ability to normally reduce nitroblue tetrazolium dye was present following incubation with latex particles, and hexose monophosphate activity was adequately stimulated by phagocytosis.

The patient's neutrophil cycles were not altered by infusions of normal plasma or by injections of epinephrine or typhoid vaccine. However, an out-of-phase rise in polymorphonuclear cells resulted after he received an injection of plasma from donors reactive to typhoid vaccine.

4. Case number 16, (52). Since the age of two weeks, this seven-year-old girl had temperature elevations to 30 °C, stomatitis, lymphadenitis, and furunculosis at three-week intervals. A cycle of 19 days was found. Monocytes, lymphocytes, eosinophils, basophils, and red blood cells (RBC) also showed cyclic fluctuations. Serum protein electrophoresis revealed a hypergammaglobulinemia.

5. Case number 18, (55). This 62-year-old patient demonstrated recurrent fluctuations of neutrophil, monocyte, reticulocyte, and platelet counts with a cycle time of 38.5 days. Cycling of bone marrow granulocytic, erythrocytic, and megakaryocytic elements was also apparent.

The disease had an onset of tiredness, dyspnea, and anorexia due to the patient's progressive anemia. Her hemoglobin was 3.4 g%, platelets $5 \times 10^9/l$, and white blood cells (WBC) $1.4 \times 10^9/l$. Aplastic anemia was diagnosed and treatment with prednisone was started. The patient relapsed and, over a six-month interval, her blood cells had a periodicity of 38.3 days for platelets, 39.5 days for reticulocytes, 36.6 days for neutrophils, and 39 days for monocytes.

Later treatment with oxymetholone for six years resulted in a reduced magnitude of cyclic fluctuations. Her hemoglobin became normal, and her WBC and platelet counts were at low normal and subnormal levels respectively.

Two studies of the long-range stimulator of RBC production, EPO, in patients with CN have been carried out. In the first study, Guerry et al. (44) (patient number 8, Table 2) measured EPO in the urine of a patient through three cycles. EPO, unmeasurable on 17 of the 20 days when neutrophil counts were highest, usually was detectable in urine early during the period of neutropenia. In the study of Andrews et al. (53), EPO was measured in the FMLC bioassay; some evidence of cycling was obtained with levels being elevated during periods of neutropenia. As detailed above, definite cycling of EPO is demonstrable in CH dogs.

Table 3. Suggested causes of cyclic hematopoiesis

1. Increased destruction of mature neutrophils.
2. Elaboration of a toxic factor (60).
3. Competition at the stem cell level (61).
4. Cycling of short-range or long-range stimulators (62).
5. Deficiency or damage of pluripotential stem cells (63).
6. Monocyte–macrophage control (41).
7. Cycling of hematopoietic stem cells probably due to a defect in regulation at the stem cell level (64).

Treatment of CN is still unsatisfactory. Many hematinics (including iron, liver extract, and B_{12}) have been without obvious benefit. Splenectomy frequently has not affected the over-all cycling of blood elements (Table 2, cases 1, 3, 5, 9, 10). Recent reports indicate that two patients benefitted from prednisolone (45) (Table 2, case 9) and oxymetholone (55) (Table 2, case 18). However, many other patients who have received corticosteroid therapy and oxymetholone showed no amelioration of clinical symptoms or blood counts. Reports of the stimulation of neutrophil production by lithium (58) and a favorable response in CH dogs (59) led us to treat one of our patients with a course of lithium (54). Although our patient symptomatically may have improved, a constant neutropenia and muted monocyte cycles developed and the medication was discontinued. This patient has since had an unsuccessful trial of prophylactic antibiotic therapy and is currently being treated with oxymetholone without apparent benefit.

IV. PATHOGENESIS

The cause of CH is unknown although, in the dog, it is genetically transmitted as an autosomal recessive gene. A number of theories, proposed to explain this intriguing disorder, are listed in Table 3. In general, they fall into two classes:
1. A disorder of pluripotential stem cells (PSC).
2. A disorder of regulatory substance. It is, of course, possible that both mechanisms may be involved.

Any theory of the pathogenesis of CH must take into consideration the following factors:
1. CH syndromes can be produced or abrogated by bone marrow transplantation. EPO not only cycles in CH dogs but also in normal dogs bearing CH marrow allografts.
2. Platelets and reticulocytes reach their apogee near the nadir of the neutrophil counts, and a monocytosis occurs as neutrophil counts rise.
3. The highest levels of CSF occur at the nadir of the granulocyte count.

4. In erythrocytic stress experiments, the highest levels of EPO are seen starting five to six days after the onset of neutropenia; a secondary midcycle peak may also occur.

5. Each of the cycles of neutrophils, platelets, and erythrocytic elements is independent of the cycles of the other two elements in relation to peripheral stimulation by phlebotomy, hypoxia, and endotoxin.

6. The progenitor cells (CFU-C, CFU-E, and diffusion chamber progenitor cells (DCPC)) appear to cycle synchronously.

7. The cells of CH bone marrow vary in the elaboration cGMP and factors which:
   (a) inhibit or stimulate murine bone marrow CFU-S proliferation rate, and
   (b) support or inhibit cyclically the CFU-C formation of normal dog non-adherent marrow cells.

Since transplantation experiments have shown that the CH syndrome can be either abrogated in CH dogs by transplantation with normal dog bone marrow or initiated in normal dogs by transplantation with CH bone marrow, the syndrome's pathogenesis must reside in the bone marrow. Although the particular type of cell involved is still not known, the invariable cycling of granulocytes, monocytes, reticulocytes, and platelets (Figure 1) would seem to point at an early progenitor cell. The CH marrow cells have been shown to elaborate factors into culture media (CM). These factors can influence the proliferation or inhibition of murine CFU-S, and adherent cell preparations alternately stimulate or inhibit the colony forming activity of normal dog bone marrow cells (Figure 6). The adherent cells cyclically elaborate cGMP on different days of the cycle when incubated with CM. These findings agree with the theory that bone marrow macrophages, through alternate production or non-production of prostaglandin E, may profoundly effect the proliferation of marrow elements. Toksoz et al (65), who isolated DNA stimulatory and inhibitory substances in long-term cultures containing proliferating and non-cycling CFU-S, suggest that a balance between these factors determines CFU-S proliferation in long-term cultures.

The CFU-C, CFU-E, and DCPC in CH all reach their highest levels during the cycle period days 10 through 2 (days 10, 11, 12, 1, 2) with the highest levels occurring near days 12 and 1. These peak levels follow the apparently critical events occurring on cycle days 9 and 10 (Figure 6). Day 9 bone marrow CM inhibits mouse CFU-S proliferation rate, and immediately following on day 10 CFU-S stimulating activity and also an erythrocytic stimulating factor in the CM of CH dog bone marrow are seen (16). Further, adherent day 9 CH bone marrow cells completely inhibit CFU-C formation by normal dog bone marrow non-adherent cells. In spite of a critical day 9 followed by synchronous proliferation of CFU-C, CFU-E, and DCPC (in human CN, Jacobson and Broxmeyer (66) have shown that DCPC and CFU-C denote different cell types), the apogees of peripheral cells differ in that reticulocytes and

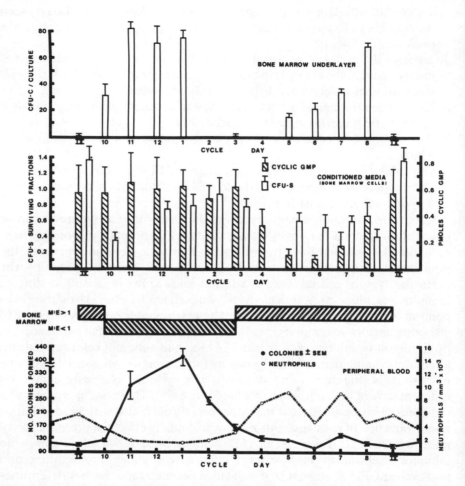

Figure 6. Inter-relationships of events in peripheral blood and bone marrow through a cycle of twelve days in the CH dog. The lower graph represents the absolute neutrophil counts and colony stimulating factor in peripheral blood, indirectly measured as the number of colonies formed by normal dog bone marrow cells overlaid with serum from a CH dog on each day of the cycle. Bone marrow myelo-cytic: erythrocytic ratio is schematically portrayed above the peripheral blood values. The third graph represents the cyclic GMP in supernatant fluid conditioned media prepared by incubating bone marrow on each day of the cycle in culture media. Also portrayed are results of exposure of mouse marrow cells to this conditioned media and subsequent ability to form spleen colonies after exposure to ^{3}H-TdR. The conditioned media was thus affecting the CFU-S proliferation rate. The upper panel represents the number of CFU-C formed by normal dog bone marrow with an underlayer of CH marrow on each day of the cycle. Note inhibition present on days IX and 3 of the cycle

platelets peak on days 1 and 2 of the cycle, monocytes on days 4 and 5, and neutrophils on days 7 to 9. It is difficult to understand why the peripheral reticulocytosis occurs simultaneously with the peak of CFU-E since the latter represent an early progenitor which is active before the identifiable early erythroblast is seen. Perman *et al* (67) thought that a period of approximately 96 hr transpires from the onset of a stimulation to the appearance of reticulocytes in the peripheral blood. Thus, a surge of erythropoiesis on day 10 could result in the reticulocytosis occurring on day 2. It is, however, difficult to understand why the highest values for granulocytic progenitor cells are found when the bone marrow is in its erythrocytic phase. Morphologically, the bone marrow then goes through a wave of myelopoiesis, culminating in an increase of neutrophil components in the peripheral blood.

CH bone marrow has the ability to respond to appropriate stimulation by the long-range stimulators (18, 19). Results from early studies of both the urine (12) and serum (68) of CH dogs showed that CSF levels varied inversely with neutrophil counts, thus suggesting a feedback control mechanism. Similarly, a spike of erythropoiesis stimulating activity, found in media produced by incubation of day 10 CH bone marrow cells, appeared to be EPO (16).

Our early studies were concerned with measuring EPO in CH dogs. Our *in vivo* exhypoxic mouse assay did not show any significant EPO activity in unstimulated CH dogs although cycles were found when an FMLC assay was used. On the other hand, cyclic spikes of EPO were found by the exhypoxic mouse assay when the CH dogs were exposed to constant hypoxia (26) and in normal dogs which had been transplanted with CH dog bone marrow (6). Since oxygen stimulus was constantly low and the hematocrit was rising, a stimulus for a second peak in EPO activity did not appear to be present. On this basis, we postulated that the bone marrow was in some way controlling the production of EPO (25).

We have recently reviewed the concepts regarding the pathogenesis of CN in humans and CH in dogs (28) and proposed a new hypothesis. This hypothesis envisions that CN is a heterogeneous group of disorders but that both CN and CH are disorders at the stem cell level. Depending on the progenitor cell involved, one may see cycling of only;
1. Granulocytes
2. Granulocytes and monocytes
3. Granulocytes, monocytes, reticulocytes, and platelets; and
4. Granulocytes, monocytes, reticulocytes, platelets, and lymphocytes.
The long-range stimulators also cycle and may undoubtedly influence the over-all picture. In CH a major event must occur on day 9 or 10 of the cycle which would correspond to day 17 of a 21-day cycle in human CN. On these critical days stem cell production may cease and an erythrocytic phase of bone marrow activity is instituted to be followed by myelocytic activity. The

cycle(s) then start again and the oscillations in peripheral blood counts are once more demonstrable.

The relationship of the progenitor cell levels to the bone marrow morphological picture is not clear, and so the complete picture of this jigsaw puzzle awaits solution. Hopefully, a few pieces have been put into place although much more needs to be done. When the picture is completed we should have a better understanding of the factors which control the normal differentiation of hematopoietic cells.

V. ACKNOWLEDGMENTS

These studies were supported in part by the National Heart, Lung, and Blood Institute grants number HL 10567–15 and HL 15647–07. The assistance of present and former colleagues who include C. D. R. Dunn, E. A. Machado, J. E. Fuhr, T. P. McDonald, and T. J. Yang is gratefully acknowledged. Mrs Janet Jolly and Mrs Dianne Trent rendered technical and artistic assistance. The editorial and stenographic help of Mrs Marty Evers and Mrs Doris Long is very much appreciated.

VI. REFERENCES

1. Leale, M. (1910). 'Recurrent furunculosis in an infant showing an unusual blood picture', *J. Am. Med. Assoc.,* **54**, 1854–1855.
2. Rutledge, B. H., Hansen-Pruss, O. C., and Thayer, W. S. (1930). 'Recurrent agranulocytosis', *Bull. Johns Hopkins Hosp.,* **46**, 369–389.
3. Lund, J. E., Padgett, G. A., and Ott, R. L. (1967). 'Cyclic neutropenia in grey collie dogs', *Blood,* **29**, 452–461.
4. Dale, D. C., and Graw, R. G., Jr. (1974). 'Transplantation of allogeneic bone marrow in canine cyclic neutropenia', *Science,* **183**, 83–84.
5. Jones, J. B., Lange, R. D., and Jones, E. S. (1975). 'Cyclic hematopoiesis in a colony of dogs', *J. Am. Vet. Med. Assoc.,* **166**, 365–367.
6. Jones, J. B., Lange, R. D., Yang, T. J., Vodopick, H., and Jones, E. S. (1975). 'Canine cyclic neutropenia: Erythropoietin and platelet cycles after bone marrow transplantation', *Blood,* **45**, 213–219.
7. Weiden, P. L., Robinett, B., Graham, T. C., Adamson, J., and Storb, R. (1974). 'Canine cyclic neutropenia: A stem cell defect', *J. Clin. Invest.,* **53**, 950–953.
8. Lund, J. E. (1969). *Canine cyclic neutropenia.* Washington State University Ph.D. dissertation.
9. Lund, J. E., Padgett, G. A., and Gorham, J. R. (1970). 'Additional evidence on the inheritance of cyclic neutropenia in the dog', *J. Hered.,* **61**, 47–49.
10. Russell, E. S., Smith, L. J., and Lawson, F. A. (1956). 'Implantation of normal blood-forming tissue in radiated genetically anemic hosts', *Science,* **124**, 1076–1077.
11. Russell, E., and Bernstein, S. E. (1966). 'Blood and blood formation', in *Biology of the Laboratory Mouse,* (Ed. E. L. Green) Second edition. McGraw-Hill, New York, p. 362.

12. Dale, D. C., Alling, D. W., and Wolff, S. M. (1972). 'Cyclic hematopoiesis: The mechanism of cyclic neutropenia in grey collie dogs', *J. Clin. Invest.*, **51**, 2197–2204.
13. Lange, R. D., Jones, J. B., Chambers, C., Quirin, Y., and Sparks, J. C. (1976). 'Erythropoiesis and erythrocyte survival in dogs with cyclic hematopoiesis', *Am. J. Vet. Res.*, **37**, 331–334.
14. Jones, J. B., Jones, E. S., and Lange, R. D. (1974). 'Early life hematologic values of dogs affected with cyclic neutropenia', *Am. J. Vet. Res.*, **35**, 849–852.
15. Khraisha, S., Andrews, R. B., Evans, J. H., Jones, J. B., and Lange, R. D. (1982). 'Canine cyclic hematopoiesis: Blood gas and 2,3-DPG studies', *Am. J. Vet. Res.*, **43**, 528–530.
16. Dunn, C. D. R., Jones, J. B., Lange, R. D., Wright, E. G., and Moore, M. A. S. (1982). 'Production of presumptive humoral hematopoietic regulators in canine cyclic hematopoiesis', *Cell Tissue Kinet.*, **15**, 1–10.
17. Machado, E. A., Jones, J. B., Aggio, M. C., Chernoff, A. I., Maxwell, P. A., and Lange, R. D. (1981). 'Ultrastructural changes of bone marrow in canine cyclic hematopoiesis (CH dog). A sequential study', *Virchows Arch (Pathol. Anat.).*, **390**, 93–108.
18. Dunn, C. D. R., Jolly, J. D., Jones, J. B., and Lange, R. D. (1978). 'Erythroid colony formation *in vitro* from the marrow of dogs with cyclic hematopoiesis: Interrelationship of progenitor cells', *Exp. Hemat.*, **6**, 701–708.
19. Dunn, C. D. R., Jones, J. B., Jolly, J. D., and Lange, R. D. (1977). 'Progenitor cells in canine cyclic hematopoiesis', *Blood*, **50**, 1111–1120.
20. Squires, D. J. P., and Lamerton, L. F. (1975). 'The effect of various cytotoxic agents on bone marrow progenitor cells as measured by diffusion chamber assays,' *Brit. J. Haemat.*, **29**, 31–42.
21. Dunn, C. D. R., Jones, J. B., Jolly, J. D., and Lange, R. D. (1978). 'Cell proliferation of canine cyclic hematopoietic marrow in diffusion chambers', *Proc. Soc. Exp. Biol. Med.*, **158**, 50–53.
22. Dale, D. C., Brown, C. H., Carbone, P., and Wolff, S. M. (1971). 'Cyclic urinary leukopoietic activity in gray collie dogs', *Science*, **173**, 152–153.
23. McDonald, T. P., Clift, R., and Jones, J. B. (1976). 'Canine cyclic hematopoiesis: Platelet size and thrombopoietin level in relation to platelet count,' *Proc. Soc. Exp. Biol. Med.*, **153**, 424–428.
24. Adamson, J. W., Dale, D. C., and Elin, R. J. (1974). 'Hematopoiesis in the grey collie dog. Studies of the regulation of erythropoiesis', *J. Clin. Invest.*, **54**, 965–973.
25. Lange, R. D., and Jones, J. B. (1976). 'Hormonal control of erythropoiesis in canine cyclic haematopoiesis', *Scand. J. Haemat.*, **16**, 56–65.
26. White, J. F., Jones, J. B., Lange, R. D., and Fuhr, J. E. (1978). 'Evidence for the existence of an agent in the serum of the cyclic hematopoietic dog which influences hemoglobin synthesis', *Experientia*, **34**, 1367–1368.
27. Jones, J. B., Yang, T. J., Dale, J. B., and Lange, R. D. (1975). 'Canine cyclic haematopoiesis: Marrow transplantation between littermates', *Brit. J. Haemat.*, **30**, 215–223.
28. Lange, R. D., and Jones, J. B. (1980). 'Canine cyclic hematopoiesis', in *The Canine as a Biomedical Research Model. Immunological, Hematological and Oncological Aspects.* (Eds. M. Shiffrine and F. Wilson) Department of Energy/Technical Information Center, Davis, CA, pp. 278–295.
29. Lange, R. D., and Jones, J. B. (1981). 'Cyclic neutropenia: Review of clinical manifestations and management', *Am. J. Pediatr. Hematol. Oncol.*, **3**, 363–367.

30. Doan, C. A. (1932). 'The neutropenic state. Its significance and therapeutic rationale', *J. Am. Med. Assoc.,* **99**, 194–202.
31. Kitchen, P. C. (1934). 'Oral observations in a case of periodic agranulocytosis', *J. Dent. Res.,* **14**, 315–322.
32. Coventry, W. D. (1953). 'Cyclic neutropenia. Report of a case treated by splenectomy', *J. Am. Med. Assoc.,* **153**, 28–31.
33. Embleton, D. (1936). 'Rhythmical agranulocytosis', *Brit. J. Med.,* **2**, 1258–1259.
34. Embleton, D. (1937). 'Rhythmical neutropenia with recurrent buccal ulceration', *Proc. Royal Soc. Med.,* **30**, 980–982.
35. Becker, F. T., Coventry, W. D., and Tuura, J. L. (1959). 'Recurrent oral and cutaneous infections associated with cyclic neutropenia', *Am. Med. Assoc. Arch. Dermat.,* **80**, 731–741.
36. Duane, G. W. (1958). 'Periodic neutropenia', *Am. Med. Assoc. Arch. Intern. Med.,* **102**, 462–467.
37. Henley, W. L. (1959). 'Hypogammaglobulinemia and hypergammaglobulinemia', *J. Mount Sinai Hosp.,* **26**, 138–159.
38. Telsey, B., Beube, F. E., Zegarelli, E. V., and Kutscher, A. H. (1962). 'Oral manifestations of cyclical neutropenia associated with hypergammaglobulinemia', *Oral Surg.,* **15**, 540–543.
39. Alestig, K. (1961). 'Cyclic agranulocytosis treated with steroids', *Acta Med. Scand.,* **169**, 253–257.
40. Morley, A. A., Carew, J. P., and Baikie, A. G. (1967). 'Familial cyclical neutropenia', *Brit. J. Haemat.,* **13**, 719–738.
41. Moore, M. A. S., Spitzer, G., Metcalf, D., and Pennington, D. G. (1974). 'Monocyte production of colony stimulating factor in cyclic neutropenia', *Brit. J. Haemat.,* **27**, 47–55.
42. Montford, A. (1968). 'Cyclic neutropenia', *Nurs. Times,* **64**, 1506–1508.
43. Guerry, D., IV, Dale, D. C., Omine, M., Perry, S., and Wolff, S. M. (1973). 'Periodic hematopoiesis in human cyclic neutropenia', *J. Clin. Invest.,* **52**, 3220–3230.
44. Guerry, D., IV, Adamson, J. W., Dale, D. C., and Wolff, S. M. (1974). 'Human cyclic neutropenia: Urinary colony-stimulating factor and erythropoietin levels', *Blood,* **44**, 257–262.
45. Wright, D. G., Fauci, A. S., Dale, D. C., and Wolff, S. M. (1978). 'Correction of human cyclic neutropenia with prednisolone', *N. Eng. J. Med.,* **298**, 295–300.
46. Wright, D. G., Dale, D. C., Fauci, A. S., and Wolff, S. M. (1981). 'Human cyclic neutropenia: Clinical review and long-term follow-up of patients', *Medicine,* **60**, 1–13.
47. Hansen, N. E., Andersen, V., and Karle, H. (1973). 'Plasma lysozyme in drug-induced and spontaneous cyclic neutropenia', *Brit. J. Haemat.,* **25**, 485–495.
48. Degnan, E. J., and Perlov, A. N. (1973). 'Infected oral lesions of cyclic neutropenia', *J. Oral Med.,* **28**, 29–31.
49. Brandt, L., Forssman, O., Mitelman, F., Odeberg, H., Olofsson, T., Olsson, I., and Svensson, B. (1975). 'Cell production and cell function in human cyclic neutropenia', *Scand. J. Haemat.,* **15**, 228–240.
50. Pachman, L. M., Schwartz, A. D., Barron, R., and Golde, D. W. (1975). 'Chronic neutropenia: Response to plasma with high colony-stimulating activity', *J. Pediatr.,* **87**, 713–719.
51. Greenberg, P. L., Bax, I., Levin, J., and Andrews, T. M. (1976). 'Alteration of colony-stimulating factor output, endotoxemia and granulopoiesis in cyclic neutropenia', *Am. J. Hemat.,* **1**, 375–385.

52. Uyama, Y., Mizui, M., Tanaka, H., Ninomiya, T., Yamada, T., and Miyao, M. (1976). 'A case of cyclic neutropenia with special reference to the function of neutrophil mobilization', *Jpn. J. Clin. Hemat.*, **17**, 1309–1319.
53. Andrews, R. B., Dunn, C. D. R., Jolly, J. D., Jones, J. B., and Lange, R. D. (1979). 'Some immunological and haematological aspects of human cyclic neutropenia', *Scand. J. Haemat.*, **22**, 97–104.
54. Lange, R. D., Crowder, C. G., Cruz, P., Hawkinson, S. W., Lozzio, C. B., Machado, E., Painter, P., Terry, W., and Jones, J. B. (1981). 'Cyclic neutropenia: A tale of two brothers and their family', *Am. J. Pediatr. Oncol.*, **3**, 127–133.
55. Roozendaal, K. J., Dicke, K. A., and Boonzajer-Flaes, M. L. (1981). 'Effect of oxymetholone on human cyclic hematopoiesis', *Brit. J. Haemat.*, **47**, 185–193.
56. Shiomura, T., Ishida, Y., Matsumoto, N., Sasaki, K., Ishihara, T., and Miwa, S. (1979). 'A case of generalized amyloidosis associated with cyclic neutropenia', *Blood*, **54**, 628–635.
57. Machado, E. A., Jones, J. B., and Lange, R. D. (1979). 'Ultrastructural studies on the evolution of amyloidosis in the cyclic hematopoietic (CH) dog', *Virchows Arch. (Pathol. Anat.).*, **383**, 167–179.
58. Stein, R. S., Flexner, J. M., and Graber, S. E. (1979). 'Lithium and granulocytopenia during induction therapy of acute myelogenous leukemia', *Blood*, **54**, 636–641.
59. Hammond, W. P., and Dale, D. C. (1980). 'Lithium therapy of canine cyclic hematopoiesis', *Blood*, **55**, 26–28.
60. Scott, R. E., Dale, D. C., Rosenthal, A. S., and Wolff, S. M. (1973). 'Cyclic neutropenia in grey collie dogs: Ultrastructural evidence for abnormal neutrophil granulopoiesis', *Lab. Invest.*, **28**, 514–525.
61. Patt, H. M., Lund, J. E., and Maloney, M. A. (1973). 'Cyclic hematopoiesis in grey collie dogs: A stem cell problem', *Blood*, **42**, 873–884.
62. King-Smith, E. A., and Morley, A. A. (1967). 'A computer model for the mammalian (human) leukocyte system', *Proc. 20th. Ann. Conf. Eng. Med. Biol.*, **9(19)**, 9.
63. Mackey, M. C. (1978). 'Unified hypothesis for the origin of aplastic anemia and periodic hematopoiesis', *Blood*, **51**, 941–956.
64. Dale, D. C., and Wolff, S. M. (1972). 'Cyclic neutropenia in man and grey collie dogs', *Birth Defects*, **8**, 59–62.
65. Toksoz, D., Dexter, T. M., Lord, B. I., Wright, E. G., and Lajtha, L. G. (1980). 'The regulation of hemopoiesis in long-term bone marrow cultures. II. Stimulation and inhibition of stem cell proliferation', *Blood*, **55**, 931–936.
66. Jacobson, N., and Broxmeyer, H. E. (1979). 'Oscillations of granulocytic and megakaryocytic progenitor cell populations in cyclic neutropenia in man', *Scand. J. Haemat.*, **23**, 33–36.
67. Perman, V., Sorensen, D. K., Usenik, E. A., Bond, V. P., and Cronkite, E. P. (1962). 'Hemopoietic regeneration in control and recovered heavily irradiated dogs following severe hemorrhage', *Blood*, **19**, 738–742.
68. Yang, T. J., Jones, J. B., Jones, E. S., and Lange, R. D. (1974). 'Serum colony-stimulating activity of dogs with cyclic neutropenia', *Blood*, **44**, 41–48.

Current Concepts in Erythropoiesis
Edited by C. D. R. Dunn
© 1983 John Wiley & Sons Ltd.

CHAPTER 7

In vitro *studies of erythropoiesis in polycythemia vera*

ALLEN C. EAVES and CONNIE J. EAVES
Terry Fox Laboratory
British Columbia Cancer Research Centre,
Cancer Control Agency of British Columbia,
and
Departments of Medicine and Medical Genetics
University of British Columbia,
Vancouver, B.C.

Contents

I. INTRODUCTION

Polycythemia vera (PV) was first described at the turn of the century by Vaquez (1) and Osler (2) as a condition characterized by erythrocytic hyperplasia, but it was quickly appreciated that granulopoiesis (3) and megakaryocytopoiesis (4) are also commonly increased. This elevation in the proliferative activity of several myelocytic lineages is a feature of a number of other conditions including chronic myelocytic leukemia (CML), essential thrombocytosis (ET), and myelofibrosis with myelocytic metaplasia (MF). These, together with PV, are now referred to as myeloproliferative disorders, following the suggestion by Dameshek in 1951 (5) that certain as yet undefined common underlying mechanisms are involved in their genesis. In the 1960s, the existence of a pluripotential hematopoietic stem cell (6) was conclusively established, and the Philadelphia chromosome (7) was identified as a unique marker in multiple marrow cell types in CML. More recently, analysis of the X-linked G6PD isoenzyme distribution in blood cells from heterozygous females has provided further evidence of the clonal nature and pluropotential stem cell origin of all of these conditions (8). Thus it now seems that all myeloproliferative disorders originate from a type of lesion that confers upon a single hematopoietic stem cell and its progeny an abnormal growth advantage. Although it is not known how this is achieved at the stem cell level, it seems likely that abnormalities in growth regulation are involved and that these are the result of changes in the genome of members of the malignant clone. The current challenge is to determine the precise nature of events that lead to clonal dominance and to define where and how in the differentiation hierarchy this phenomenon becomes manifest.

Over the last ten years, significant advances have occurred in the development of reproducible clonal assays for primitive hematopoietic cells, and these have permitted some insight into altered regulatory mechanisms believed to operate in the myeloproliferative disorders in general and in PV in particular. The most widely documented example is the altered erythropoietin (EPO) requirement exhibited by PV cells *in vitro*. This was first shown by Krantz (9) using short-term marrow suspension cultures and later confirmed when erythrocytic progenitor colony assays became available (10). Although the terms 'independence' and 'endogenous' or 'autonomous erythrocytic growth' have been widely used in connection with this phenomenon, it is still not clear if such growth is truly autonomous of EPO. It is also not known whether the mechanisms underlying this trait contribute to clonal dominance either in the stem cell compartment or during the production of other types of mature blood cells, both of which occur in this fascinating disease. Against this broader background, the present review will focus on recent *in vitro* studies that have contributed to our understanding of erythropoiesis in polycythemia vera.

II. TERMINOLOGY OF *IN VITRO* ERYTHROPOIESIS

Before attempting to describe perturbations of progenitor compartments in PV, we shall briefly review how various progenitor types have been operationally defined by *in vitro* colony assay procedures. The essential feature of all such assays is their indirect, retrospective nature. This is because the unit of origin or colony forming unit (CFU), usually a single cell, is defined by the final number and type of recognizable progeny generated. Since the earliest colonies obtainable *in vitro* were found to contain cells of a single lineage (in marked contrast to spleen colonies which had been shown to be mixed), the concept arose of populations of primitive, but unipotential, derivatives of the pluripotential stem cell compartment. Thus granulocyte–macrophage colony numbers provide a measure of CFU-GM (initially called CFU-C because they were the first colony type obtained in culture), erythrocytic colony numbers provide a measure of CFU-E, megakaryocyte colony numbers provide a measure of CFU-M, and lymphocyte colony numbers provide a measure of CFU-BL and CFU-TL (11). These *in vitro* assays have been discussed extensively in detail elsewhere (11).

Additional studies over the last decade have revealed a more complex hierarchical structure of progenitor types (Figure 1), and with improved culture conditions, *in vitro* assays for pluripotential CFU have been established. These progenitors have been called CFU-mix (12,13), macroscopic BFU-E (14), and CFU-GEMM (15,16). In the latter case, the suffixed letters indicate the joint presence of granulocytes, erythroblasts, megakaryocytes, and monocytes or macrophages in single colonies. Murine macroscopic BFU-E are not only pluripotential, they also generate progenitors capable of macroscopic spleen colony formation (17), and clearly undergo self-renewal as shown by replating into secondary cultures (18). Some renewal of the pluripotential feature of human CFU-GEMM has also been documented (19,20). The demonstration of pluripotentiality, extensive proliferative capacity, and self-renewal suggest that some of these progenitors are very close to or synonymous with the most primitive hematopoietic stem cells.

There are some interesting features of *in vitro* erythrocytic colony growth that facilitate the study of erythropoiesis. First, mature erythrocytic colonies can be readily distinguished from all other types of colonies in the living state because they become visibly red as they produce and accumulate hemoglobin. This makes it possible to perform sequential counts on the same cultures of different sized erythrocytic colonies, an important economy both in terms of scoring time and the number of cells required to assess different progenitor compartments. A second feature of erythrocytic colonies is the fact that the erythroblasts within them are arranged in subcolonies or clusters. This is the result of an abrupt and permanent loss of migratory ability, a phenotypic change that is used to define the transition between a BFU-E and a CFU-E. Enumeration of the clusters in each colony permits a rapid assessment of over-all colony size and hence the minimum number of divisions expressed by the original progenitor. This in turn provides a simple way to measure the location of an erythrocytic progenitor in the over-all hierarchy (Figure 1)

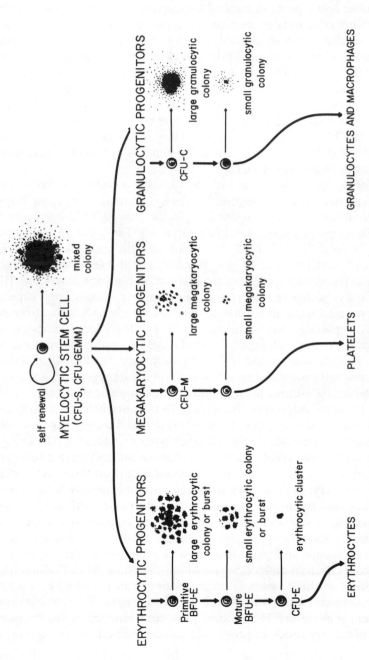

Figure 1. Diagrammatic representation of the hierarchy of hematopoietic progenitor compartments currently identified by colony assay procedures

(21), and has allowed differentiation-related changes in hormone sensitivity (21), cycle status (21), surface antigen expression (22), and other properties to be followed. Finally, early and late stages of erythrocytic cell development appear to differ markedly in their requirements for regulators (23). The early growth phase of colonies derived from primitive BFU-E *in vitro* is strongly dependent on the presence of certain non-EPO factors released by leukocytes or marrow adherent cells (BEF, BPA, BFA) (24–27). Only the later phases of erythrocytic colony development (post-mature BFU-E) appear to be crucially dependent on the presence of significant quantities of EPO (14). Unlike BPA-type factors, EPO has a clearly established regulatory role *in vivo*. Also, EPO does not appear to be released or removed by hematopoietic cells in culture (28,29). This latter feature has made it possible to vary precisely the concentration of EPO in a given culture down to very low levels, independent of the cell source assayed. It is therefore not surprising that to date most *in vitro* studies attempting to define regulatory anomalies in PV have focused on EPO responsiveness.

III. ABSOLUTE NUMBERS OF PROGENITORS

Colony assays for primitive hematopoietic progenitors have been applied to the study of PV patients in two ways: first, to evaluate quantitative changes in compartment size; and second, to look for qualitative changes in properties of progenitor cells. This section will review the results of studies designed to look at quantitative changes.

In fact, few such studies have been reported. This is partly due to the well-recognized variation in plating efficiency with different assay procedures (e.g., plasma clot, methylcellulose, agar), and even with different batches of essential components of the culture medium used in a given procedure (e.g., FCS, BSA, EPO, etc.). These sources of variation can be minimized if efforts are made to standardize reagents and procedures. However, even under such conditions, considerable variation has been encountered in the number of progenitors measured per 10^5 nucleated marrow aspirate cells for individuals used to provide control values (30). Moreover, there are significant problems inherent in extrapolating marrow compartment size estimates from measurements based on counts per 10^5 cells plated. This is due to the fact that marrow cellularity varies from site to site, dilution with peripheral blood may vary from one aspirate to another, and progenitor cell recoveries may vary from one specimen to another. In addition, the absolute number of nucleated cells may be increased (or decreased) in proportion to the number of progenitors such that, on a per cell basis, no change is noted. For peripheral blood, progenitors can be quantitated on a per ml basis, assuming variations in their recovery in the light density fraction (31) are minimal. Peripheral blood also has the advantage that measurements of truly normal individuals have been readily obtainable. However, such studies have shown that the progenitor content of normal blood also yields a relatively wide range of values (31–33), even for single individuals followed over the course of a few weeks (34). The significance of these findings is not clear, nor has any relationship between the concentration of progenitors in the blood and marrow been established. Moreover, it seems likely that myelofibrosis, not uncommon in patients with long-standing PV, might significantly alter the distribution of progenitors between marrow and blood. A few studies have suggested that myelofibrosis can lead to an increase in the number of circulating progenitors (35,36), and recent studies of our own on eight such patients provide additional support for this hypothesis (see Figure 2).

All of these considerations suggest that measurements of progenitor numbers in man are unlikely to yield useful information unless very large deviations from the norm are anticipated and/or large numbers of unselected patients and controls are available for study. Unfortunately, most published data are either for small numbers of PV and control patients or for larger series of PV patients but without adequate clinical documentation or controls. Over the course of the last five years, we have accumulated progenitor data on a large number of individuals with myeloproliferative disease, including 21 patients with PV who had elevated hemoglobins at the time of assessment but who had not yet been treated with either ^{32}P or chemotherapy. The results, shown in Figure 2, represent an extension of previously published data from this laboratory using the same or equivalently standardized culture reagents and the same colony scoring procedures. Our initial failure to obtain evidence for an increase in any progenitor compartment has been upheld. This is not unexpected for marrow where, as mentioned above, current methodology can only pick up relative changes in progenitor concentration. However, if there were significant, absolute increases in marrow progenitor compartments, it might be anticipated that corresponding changes would be detected in the blood. Since no evidence of changes in circulating progenitor numbers has emerged, it seems likely that marked changes in early compartments do not commonly occur in PV. Alternatively, there may be characteristic disease-related changes that are too small to be detected with procedures presently available. The latter point is not a trivial consideration when it is remembered that the actual number of circulating red blood cells (RBC) in PV is rarely increased more than two-fold above normal.

The findings for progenitor numbers in PV are similar to those for ET. We have recently assessed 19 untreated cases of ET and these also have shown no evidence of a change in either erythrocytic or granulocytic progenitor compartments (see again Figure 2). In contrast, several groups have shown that untreated CML patients have markedly increased numbers of all types of progenitors in the circulation (Figure 2 and references 37–42). This suggests that the lesion in CML leads to a profound absolute increase in stem cell

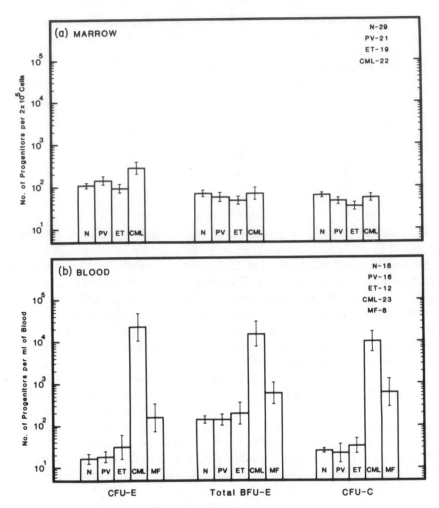

Figure 2. Progenitor concentrations in marrow and peripheral blood for groups of control individuals and patients with various types of untreated myeloproliferative disease

turnover and differentiation in the marrow, a change that assessment of marrow progenitor cell concentrations would not necessarily be expected to and in fact (Figure 2) does not reveal.

The data in Figure 2 also suggest that pluripotential stem cell commitment to particular pathways remains normal, not only in PV, but in all of the myeloproliferative diseases we have looked at to date. This conclusion is based on the use of the ratio of BFU-E to CFU-C numbers in the marrow as a measure of stem cell commitment behavior. The ratios shown in Table 1 are

Table 1. Ratio of BFU-E:CFU-C numbers in the marrow of control individuals and
in patients with untreated myeloproliferative disease

Marrow (per 200,000 cells)	Mean*	Range (± 2 s.d.)†	N‡
Normal	1.13	0.18– 7.14	29
PV	1.21	0.23– 6.49	21
ET	1.43	0.26– 7.79	19
CML	1.30	0.16–10.35	22

*Geometric mean values were calculated from the same data used to generate Figure 2. None of these values are significantly different from one another ($p = 0.05$).
†Range expected to include 95% of all ratios.
‡Number of individuals in each group.

those calculated from the same data used to generate Figure 2. As previously reported (33), this parameter shows a wide variation in control individuals without myeloproliferative disease, and a similar spread of values is apparent in each of the disease categories. In PV, in particular, this cannot be considered altogether surprising, since a shift in the level of stem cell commitment in favor of erythropoiesis would not explain the significant increase in granulocyte and platelet production that also occurs in many PV patients. In addition, there is evidence that a significant proportion of the CFU-C and BFU-E present in some PV patients may derive from normal (i.e., non-clonal) stem cells (43) whose commitment behavior might be anticipated to continue to function normally. In two patients, where it has been possible to estimate separately the abnormal (i.e., clonal) progenitors, an attempt has been made to compare the ratios of clonal BFU-E to CFU-C in the peripheral blood with those obtained for normal individuals. In one patient, it was also possible to compare this value with the ratio obtained for non-clonal (i.e., residual normal) BFU-E to CFU-C coexisting in the circulation. Again no evidence of marked variation from the norm was revealed (44).

In summary, we conclude that considerable caution must be exercised in attempting to interpret progenitor assay data in relation to groups of patients. Absolute changes in marrow compartments can only be inferred from corresponding changes in peripheral blood, and variation in normal values dictates the need for relatively large samples. In terms of explaining lineage-specific increases in terminal cell output, for example RBC in PV, our ability to discriminate absolute changes in progenitor cell numbers is probably inadequate in most instances. The notable exception to this would be the correlated and dramatic increase in circulating white blood cells in CML. Attempts to use marrow BFU-E:CFU-C ratios to provide an explanation for the imbalanced terminal cell output observed in PV or CML have also proved essentially negative. Nevertheless, these findings do strengthen the concept that simple deregulation of stem cell turnover may be a common feature of all myeloproliferative disorders, with variations in the extent to which this occurs determining at least in part the different patterns of terminal maturation observed in the various disease categories.

IV. PROGENITOR CELL CYCLING STATE

An assessment of proliferative activity can be obtained by determining the proportion of progenitors surviving a brief *in vitro* exposure to high specific-activity tritiated thymidine (45) or hydroxyurea (46). In general, this technique has shown that in human marrow CFU-E and mature BFU-E are normally proliferatively active, but that a significant proportion of primitive BFU-E (21) and most CFU-GEMM (47) are quiescent. CFU-C in the marrow resemble mature BFU-E in their active cycling characteristics (39). Curiously, all progenitors found in normal peripheral blood appear to be non-cycling (31,48,49). This includes CFU-C and BFU-E as well as CFU-GEMM. CFU-E, although detectable in the circulation, are commonly present at very low levels (33).

A recent study suggests that in PV a significant proportion of circulating BFU-E and CFU-GEMM are in S-phase, although the cycling characteristics of CFU-C remain unchanged from normal (49). At first glance, these data suggest an erythrocytic lineage-specific alteration in progenitor cell cycling properties. However, in the absence of results for marrow which houses the majority of all early progenitor cell populations, interpretation must remain guarded. Moreover, a corresponding lineage-specific alteration in progenitor cell cycling properties has not been found in CML where only quiescent CFU-C circulate (39), even though their numbers are significantly increased. Since our own studies suggest that, in PV, erythrocytic progenitor cell numbers remain within normal limits down to the CFU-E stage (Figure 2), it would seem unlikely that altered cycling characteristics at an earlier point contribute to the increased RBC output seen in this disease. On the other hand, an abnormally increased proliferative activity in early progenitor cell compartments might be envisaged to reflect either the preferential growth advantage of transformed elements, or an unusual genetically-determined phenotype which predisposes individuals to develop PV. A precedent for the latter possibility has recently been described by Axelrad and co-workers. These investigators have shown that, in mice, the Fv-2 locus determines susceptibility to Friend virus-induced polycythemia by regulating production of a factor that specifically inhibits BFU-E cycling. Resistance segregates with the presence of the inhibitor and a very low proportion of BFU-E in S-phase; susceptibility with the absence of detectable inhibitor activity and most BFU-E in cycle (50,51).

V. 'ERYTHROPOIETIN INDEPENDENCE'

The concept that erythropoiesis in PV is not regulated by EPO developed initially from a number of *in vivo* approaches. The most convincing of these was the demonstration that erythropoiesis in PV patients is not suppressed by an oxygen-rich environment (52,53) or hypertransfusion (54), procedures expected to reduce EPO levels *in vivo*. Low EPO serum levels (55,56) and urinary excretion rates (57) in PV patients are also consistent with this interpretation, although determination of true EPO levels remains a problem due to the low sensitivity of *in vivo* mouse or rat assays (58), the distortion of *in vitro* assays by non-specific inhibitors and non-EPO stimulators (58,59), and the uncertainty of the relationship between levels of EPO bioactivity and levels determined by radioimmunoassays. Thus, to date, measurements of EPO levels have not been adequate to exclude the possibility that PV cells may be hypersensitive to low levels of EPO, or that residual normal erythrocytic progenitor cells can become productive in PV patients whose EPO levels may have increased following phlebotomy.

The first *in vitro* evidence that erythrocytic cells from patients with PV have either an intrinsically altered responsiveness to, or requirement for, EPO was provided by Krantz (9,60). Suspensions of marrow cells were incubated in the presence or absence of EPO for one to three days and the amount of ^{59}Fe incorporated into heme during the last 24 hr of culture was determined. From the short duration of the assay, it can be inferred that the response measured was erythroblast maturation—a relatively late event. The results suggested that, in active PV, this compartment is composed almost exclusively of cells that can mature in the absence of added EPO. However, this situation appeared to be reversible since patients who had been extensively treated with busulfan yielded results indicating the reappearance of a significant proportion of cells with a normal EPO responsiveness. In order to test these interpretations more rigorously, it was necessary to develop assay procedures that would allow individual EPO responsive cells to be enumerated and hence characterized. This was made possible with the introduction of erythrocytic colony assays in the early 1970s, and in 1974, the first results with PV marrow cells were reported by Prchal and Axelrad (10). They found that PV cultures to which no EPO was added yielded readily identifiable colonies of erythroblasts; whereas, under the same conditions, they found that many more colonies were generated in PV cultures when EPO concentrations were increased to that required by normal progenitors. These results thus confirmed the concept of 'EPO independent' precursors in PV, but suggested that they were not the predominant type of erythrocytic colony-forming cell.

Erythrocytic colonies are not, however, derived from the same EPO responsive cells measured in the type of three-day cultures used by Krantz. Even the smallest colonies scored with the generally accepted eight-cell criterion are thought to arise from cells (CFU-E) more primitive than the first morphologically recognizable erythrocytic elements. Consistent with this concept are the longer times required for colony growth prior to the appearance of maturing erythroblasts. Nevertheless, there is some evidence that CFU-E are themselves EPO responsive (21,23). Thus, to reconcile the observations of Krantz with those of Prchal and Axelrad, it is necessary to propose a model which takes into account the belief that, during normal erythrocytic cell differentiation, contact with EPO is a continuing require- ment starting at the level of CFU-E or even earlier (21,23,24). Since cultures of PV-cells without added EPO yield whole colonies of erythroblasts, it can be assumed that such colonies derived from cells whose EPO independence was maintained through several successive daughter genera- tions. For example, in cultures without added EPO, loss of EPO independence by the progeny of CFU-E would lead to failure of detectable colony formation and all EPO independent CFU-E would fail to be detected, even though in theory some might have had the potential to yield EPO independent progeny. We therefore propose that abnormal EPO responsiveness may be viewed as a phenotype that is determined relatively early, i.e., at or before the CFU-E stage, and that once acquired, it may be maintained throughout subsequent cell divisions and maturational changes.

If this assumption is correct, then it would be expected that *in vivo* under conditions of low levels of EPO, phenotypically abnormal cells would enjoy a selective advantage over their phenotypically normal counterparts at stages of development normally subject to EPO control. Accordingly, they would be expected to become predominant at this point. Such a phenomenon is illustrated in Figure 3. This concept provides an explanation for the superficial discrepancy between the results of Krantz and the results of Prchal and Axelrad, and similarly, the difference in the absence and presence of an effect of EPO on ^{59}Fe uptake on three-day as opposed to seven- to ten-day-old suspension cultures of PV cells observed by Golde *et al* (61).

The assumption regarding fixation of phenotype also makes possible the use of EPO dose/response curve analysis to look at a number of questions pertaining to phenotype heterogeneity both within and between different clones. A number of groups (63–65) have now confirmed that colony assays of PV progenitors yield the type of hockey stick EPO dose response curve illustrated by curve B in Figure 4. This is the shape of curve predicted for a single progenitor compartment composed of a mixture of two phenotypes, one normally EPO responsive (curve A), and the other either very sensitive to EPO (B') or completely autonomous of it (B"). The major point that emerges from this general finding is that colony counts in cultures containing less than 0.01 units of EPO appear to offer a reasonable method for quantitating the representation of phenotypically abnormal progenitors in a given compart- ment in a given PV patient. Evaluation of a large number of such patients (49,63–66) has indicated that this proportion is usually detectable, but less than 50% when BFU-E type colonies are counted. This proportion is usually higher, but still less than 100% when care is taken to score CFU-E type colonies as a

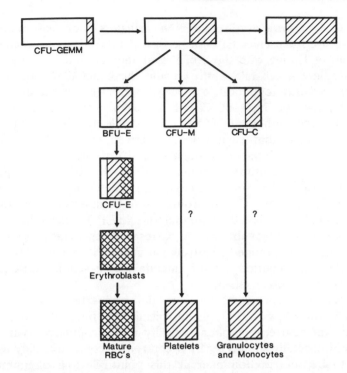

Figure 3. Evolution of clonal dominance with time (horizontal arrows) and during the course of differentiation (vertical arrows) in PV. Early compartments are envisaged to change in composition but not in over-all size (see text). Increases in the transformed component are shown by the hatched areas. G6PD isoenzyme studies suggest that when all red blood cells, granulocytes, and platelets are of the malignant clone (62), non-clonal (normal) progenitors may still be present in early progenitor compartments (43,44). EPO dose/response studies suggest that the expression of EPO independence *in vivo* (cross-hatched areas) may lead to a progressive selection in favor of transformed derivatives bearing this phenotype (9,60,61). The mechanism that confers a selective advantage on transformed progenitors of megakaryocytes and granulocytes/monocytes is unknown

separate entity. Such observations raise the question as to whether abnormal EPO responsiveness might prove a consistent property of all erythrocytic derivatives of transformed (PV type) stem cells. However, this does not appear to be the case. Analysis of colonies from two female patients with naturally occurring G6PD cellular mosaicism (43,44) showed all their phenotypically abnormal progenitors to be members of the transformed clone, but not *vice versa;* i.e., some erythrocytic derivatives of the abnormal clone did appear to respond to and require EPO to complete their maturation.

This phenomenon of phenotype heterogeneity within the transformed clone has been recently re-examined in our laboratory (67). The question asked was

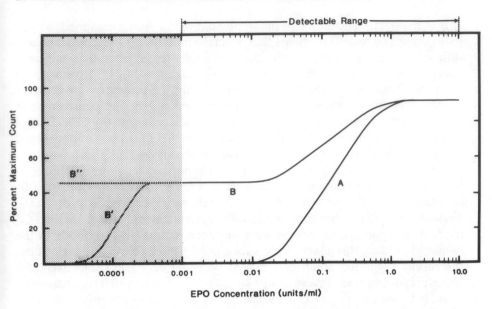

Figure 4. Typical EPO dose/response curves for erythrocytic colony formation by cells from normal individuals (curve A) and patients with PV (curve B). The clear plateau on curve B between 0.01 and 0.001 units per ml of EPO suggests the presence of two populations of progenitors: one requiring > 0.01 units of EPO per ml, the other requiring < 0.001 units of EPO per ml. Possible extrapolations of curve B below the lower limit set by the use of fetal calf serum in the culture medium are shown as B' (hypersensitivity model) and B″ (autonomous model)

whether abnormal phenotypes are randomly distributed amongst the differentiating progeny of transformed stem cells or whether they belonged to particular stem cell subclones. A large number of nine-day-old primary erythrocytic colonies were individually replated into paired secondary assays with and without added EPO. Primary colonies from all five PV patients studied appeared to fall into two categories. The most common type consisted of variable proportions of phenotypically normal and abnormal progeny (some colonies in the secondary assay without added EPO, but more in the paired assay with EPO). A much smaller number of primary colonies yielded only phenotypically normal progeny (no colonies in the secondary assay without added EPO, but some in the paired assay with EPO). No colonies contained only phenotypically abnormal progeny (equal or higher numbers of colonies in the secondary assay without added EPO). Thus, the findings are not consistent with the concept of segregation of phenotypes at the stem cell level. Rather, they support a model in which the frequency of phenotypically abnormal erythrocytic progenitors is determined at a later stage of differentiation according to a probability function that may vary from patient to patient (i.e., from clone to clone).

It is inviting to speculate that the timing of this decision corresponds to and may perhaps be related to events that normally initiate EPO responsiveness in differentiating erythrocytic cells. Present evidence suggests that this may occur at or just prior to the mature BFU-E stage (21,23,24). However, we have no idea how rigidly this part of the erythrocytic program is co-ordinated. It is conceivable that acquisition of EPO responsiveness is normally somewhat variable, being delayed in some cells until the CFU-E stage is reached. The implication for PV would then be that the timing of phenotype fixation would also be expected to show an analogous degree of variation.

A major unresolved question is whether phenotypically abnormal progenitors are truly autonomous of EPO as is known to be the case in cells transformed by Friend virus (68), or merely hypersensitive to very small amounts of EPO in other components of the culture medium (e.g., in the FCS used). One approach to this problem has been to add EPO antibody to the cultures to reduce this unavoidable background EPO level. In one such study, the results suggested abnormal cells to be exquisitely EPO sensitive (65). Clearly, confirmation of these results would be of interest, and it should now be possible to test more rigorously the specificity of any antibody effects obtained using highly purified EPO (69). A second approach has been to try to develop serum-free culture conditions (70), although again reconstitution with impure preparations of EPO that may contain other limiting growth factors could give misleading results. Finally, the possibility should be considered that phenotypically abnormal cells could be both autonomous and EPO responsive. Autonomy implies the existence of a mechanism that allows cells to by-pass their normal requirement for contact with EPO. Such a mechanism could well be envisaged to operate with varying degrees of success. This would explain why PV colonies obtained under conditions of very low EPO are commonly found to be slightly smaller and not quite as well hemoglobinized as those obtained at concentrations required to stimulate normal colonies. The prediction would then be that the EPO response mechanism itself is not affected by transformation, and in fact remains intact even in phenotypically abnormal cells. The attraction of such a model lies in the concept of a by-pass mechanism that need not be lineage-specific and might therefore be envisaged to affect other types of hematopoietic progenitors.

VI. CLONAL DOMINANCE

Studies on two female patients with PV, who were also heterozygous for the A and B isoenzymes of G6PD, have provided strong evidence in favor of the concept that this disease results from the unbalanced proliferation of a single cell. These same studies also provided the first opportunity to evaluate in PV the proportion of cells in various progenitor compartments that might belong to the malignant clone (43,44,71). When the two heterozygotes were first studied, roughly half of the BFU-E were found to belong to a residual normal population. On re-examination two and three years later, this component appeared to have progressively diminished in both patients (44). Although direct assessment of the stem cell compartment was not possible at the time these studies were undertaken, it seems likely that disease progression also involved a relative increase in the malignant clone at the stem cell level. This is depicted by the horizontal changes illustrated in Figure 3.

Clonal dominance also appears to take place during the course of differentiation. Even at the time when these two patients were first assessed, all circulating RBC, granulocytes, and platelets were clonal. Simultaneous comparison of BFU-E and CFU-E isoenzyme types suggested that a major shift in favor of clonal progenitors occurred during this transition. Similarly, significant numbers of normal granulocytic progenitors were able to penetrate as far as the CFU-C compartment, but failed to contribute a corresponding proportion of mature progeny to the circulating pool of granulocytes (43,44,71). These changes are shown vertically in Figure 3. It seems that in PV, transformed cells retain features that either enhance their ability to outgrow normal cells, or allow them to actively suppress their normal counterparts at all levels of differentiation and that this phenomenon occurs most efficiently at the more terminal stages of maturation. Clearly, this is an interesting area for future investigation.

VII. CLINICAL RELEVANCE OF *IN VITRO* STUDIES

The diagnosis of PV currently relies on a combination of stringent clinical criteria put forth by the Polycythemia Vera Study Group (PVSG) (72). The initial purpose of these criteria was to clearly exclude patients without PV so that a trial of several treatment modalities could be evaluated on a population of patients who unquestionably had PV. However, the stringency of the criteria adopted meant that some patients with PV might also be excluded. Moreover, in practice, access to all of the tests required may not be convenient for a number of patients. In a recent survey, we have found that approximately half of the PV patients in British Columbia probably fall into one of these two categories. A number of groups have found that patients with a clinical diagnosis of PV exhibited EPO independent growth *in vitro* (10,43,49,63–66). However, the very high precision and sensitivity of this approach in separating primary from both secondary erythrocytosis and Gaisböck's syndrome has only recently been established (66). In this study, 179 patients presenting with an elevated hemoglobin were evaluated. Peripheral blood and bone marrow were shown to be equally useful as a source of progenitors for this test and specimens remained assessable for many hours, thus allowing shipment from one site to another. In addition, progenitors with an altered EPO responsiveness remained in the detectable range regardless of treatment, or the degree of plethora at time of culture, or the duration of known disease. Although the presence of such progenitors clearly distinguishes PV from secondary polycythemia or Gaisböck's syndrome, this phenotype is not unique to PV. It has also been observed in other myeloproliferative disorders such as ET (74), MF (73,74), and CML (37,42), although there appear to be marked differences in the prevalence of this phenotype in each disease category.

VIII. FUTURE DIRECTIONS

Recent studies of two G6PD heterozygotes with PV indicated this disease to fit the description of a clonal neoplasm in both instances. Cytogenetic studies suggest that only a small proportion of clones carry a stable chromosomal change (75,76). Analysis of the behavior of erythrocytic progenitors in culture has provided evidence for an abnormal phenotype that allows some CFU-E and BFU-E to complete their proliferation and maturation program at non-permissive EPO concentrations. G6PD isoenzyme studies of colonies generated by cells from heterozygotes with PV have shown that not all members of the malignant clone exhibit the abnormal EPO responsive phenotype. Such studies have also shown that residual normal progenitors may exist in PV patients. This is consistent with previous cytogenetic studies, although it is also possible that some malignant clones may include both chromosomally normal and abnormal components. Evidence in favor of such a possibility has in fact recently been obtained in CML (77).

All of the above three markers have their drawbacks. G6PD heterozygotes with PV are rare. Only two such females have been identified to date. PV patients with cytogenetic changes are more common but still represent only approximately 10% of the total, and the application of this methodology to the assessment of colonies, although now feasible (78), is still very labor-intensive. Use of extended chromosome analysis may increase the number of patients found to have cytogenetic changes, but use of this procedure will also increase the amount of labor required. Progenitors with an altered EPO responsiveness are relatively easily detected and appear to be present in all patients with PV, but this approach suffers from the fact that not all members of the abnormal clone are identified.

Clearly, it would be extremely helpful to have new markers. One possibility is the production of monoclonal antibodies to unique surface antigens (79). Another is based on the expectation that cells of the malignant clone may be found to have alterations in their DNA not detectable as karyotypic changes but demonstrable using appropriate probes. Hopefully, these will help to unravel the mechanisms that determine karyotype instability, clonal dominance, expression of EPO independence, the unbalanced production of mature blood cells, and how these different abnormalities combine to give the various types of myeloproliferative disorders commonly recognized.

IX. ACKNOWLEDGMENTS

Supported in part by the National Cancer Institute of Canada and the British Columbia Medical Services Foundation (Vancouver Foundation), with core support from the British Columbia Cancer Foundation and the Cancer Control Agency of B.C. Dr A. Eaves is a Research Scholar of the B.C. Health Care Research Foundation. Dr C. Eaves is a Research Associate of the National Cancer Institute of Canada.

IX. REFERENCES

1. Vaquez, H. M. (1892). 'Sur une forme speciale de cyanose s'accompagnant d'hyperglobulie excessive et persistante', *C.R. Soc. Biol. (Paris)*, **44**, 384.
2. Osler, W. (1903). 'Chronic cyanosis with polycythemia and enlarged spleen: A new clinical entity', *Am. J. Med. Sci.*, **126**, 187–201.
3. Türk, W. (1904). 'Beiträge zur Kenntnis des Symptomenbildes Polycythämie mit Milztumor und Zyanose', *Wien, Klin. Wochenschr.*, **17**, 153–189.
4. Hutchinson, R., and Miller, C. H. (1906). 'A case of splenomegalic polycythaemia, with report of post-mortem examination', *Lancet*, **i**, 744–746.
5. Dameshek, W. (1951). 'Some speculations on the myeloproliferative syndromes', *Blood*, **6**, 372–375.
6. Till, J. E., and McCulloch, E. A. (1961). 'A direct measurement of the radiation sensitivity of normal mouse bone marrow cells', *Radiat. Res.*, **14**, 213–222.
7. Nowell, P. C., and Hungerford, D. A. (1960). 'A minute chromosome in human chronic granulocytic leukemia', *Science*, **132**, 1497.
8. Fialkow, P. J. (1980). 'Clonal and stem cell origin of blood cell neoplasms', in *Contemporary Hematology/Oncology*, (Eds. R. Silber, A. S. Gordon, J. LoBue, and F. M. Muggia), Plenum Medical, New York, vol. 1, pp. 1–46.
9. Krantz, S. B. (1968). 'Response of polycythemia vera marrow to erythropoietin *in vitro*', *J. Lab. Clin. Med.*, **71**, 999–1012.
10. Prchal, J. F., and Axelrad, A. A. (1974). 'Bone marrow responses in polycythemia vera', *N. Engl. J. Med.*, **290**, 1382.
11. Metcalf, D. (1977). 'Hemopoietic colonies. *In vitro* cloning of normal and leukemic cells', in *Recent Results in Cancer Research*, Springer-Verlag, Berlin/Heidelberg, vol. 61.
12. Hara, H., and Ogawa, M. (1978). 'Murine hemopoietic colonies in culture containing normoblasts, macrophages, and megakaryocytes', *Am. J. Hemat.*, **4**, 23–34.
13. Johnson, G. R., and Metcalf, D. (1977). 'Pure and mixed erythroid colony formation *in vitro* stimulated by spleen conditioned medium with no detectable erythropoietin', *Proc. Natl. Acad. Sci., USA*, **74**, 3879–3882.
14. Humphries, R. K., Eaves, A. C., and Eaves, C. J. (1979). 'Characterization of a primitive erythropoietic progenitor found in mouse marrow before and after several weeks in culture', *Blood*, **53**, 746–763.
15. Fauser, A. A., and Messner, H. A. (1978). 'Granuloerythropoietic colonies in human bone marrow, peripheral blood, and cord blood', *Blood*, **52**, 1243–1248.
16. Fauser, A. A., and Messner, H. A. (1979). 'Identification of megakaryocytes, macrophages, and eosinophils in colonies of human bone marrow containing neutrophilic granulocytes and erythroblasts', *Blood*, **53**, 1023–1027.

17. Humphries, R. K., Jacky, P. B., Dill, F. J., Eaves, A. C., and Eaves, C. J. (1979). 'CFU-S in individual erythroid colonies derived *in vitro* from adult mouse marrow', *Nature*, **279**, 718–720.
18. Humphries, R. K., Eaves, A. C., and Eaves, C. J. (1981). 'Self-renewal of hemopoietic stem cells during mixed colony formation *in vitro*', *Proc. Natl. Acad. Sci., USA*, **78**, 3629–3633.
19. Messner, H. A., and Fauser, A. A. (1980). 'Culture studies of human pluripotent hemopoietic progenitors', *Blut*, **41**, 327–333.
20. Ash, R. C., Detrick, R. A., and Zanjani, E. D. (1981). 'Studies of human pluripotential hemopoietic stem cells (CFU-GEMM) *in vitro*', *Blood*, **58**, 309–316.
21. Eaves, C. J., Humphries, R. K., amd Eaves, A. C. (1979). '*In vitro* characterization of erythroid precursor cells and the erythropoietic differentiation process', in *Cellular and Molecular Regulation of Hemoglobin Switching* (Eds. G. Stamatoyannopoulos and A. W. Nienhuis), Grune and Stratton, New York, pp. 251–273.
22. Robinson, J., Sieff, C., Delia, D., Edwards, P. A. W., and Greaves, M. (1981). 'Expression of cell-surface HLA-DR, HLA-ABC, and glycophorin during erythroid differentiation', *Nature*, **289**, 68–71.
23. Iscove, N. N. (1978). 'Erythropoietin-independent stimulation of early erythropoiesis in adult marrow cultures by conditioned media from lectin-stimulated mouse spleen cells', in *Hematopoietic Cell Differentiation* (Eds. D. W. Golde, M. J. Cline, D. Metcalf, and C. F. Fox), Academic Press, New York, pp. 37–52.
24. Axelrad, A. A., McLeod, D. L., Suzuki, S., and Shreeve, M. M. (1978). 'Regulation of population size of erythropoietic progenitor cells', in *Differentiation of Normal and Neoplastic Hematopoietic Cells* (Eds. B. Clarkson, P. Marks, and J. E. Till), Cold Spring Harbor Laboratory, pp. 155–163.
25. Wagemaker, G. (1978). 'Cellular and soluble factors influencing the differentiation of primitive erythroid progenitor cells (BFU-e) *in vitro*', in *In Vitro Aspects of Erythropoiesis* (Ed. M. J. Murphy, Jr.), Springer-Verlag, New York, pp. 44–57.
26. Aye, M. T. (1977). 'Erythroid colony formation in cultures of human marrow: Effect of leukocyte conditioned medium', *J. Cell Physiol.*, **91**, 69–79.
27. Gregory, C. J., and Eaves, A. C. (1977). 'Human marrow cells capable of erythropoietic differentiation *in vitro*: Definition of three erythroid colony responses', *Blood*, **49**, 855–864.
28. Iscove, N. N., and Sieber, F. (1975). 'Erythroid progenitors in mouse bone marrow detected by macroscopic colony formation in culture', *Exp. Hemat.*, **3**, 32–43.
29. Eaves, C. J., Humphries, R. K., Krystal, G., and Eaves, A. C. (1981). 'Erythropoietin action: Models, data, and speculation', in *Hemoglobins in Development and Differentiation* (Eds. G. Stamatoyannopoulos and A. W. Nienhuis), Alan R. Liss, Inc., New York, pp. 63–72.
30. Eaves, C. J., and Eaves, A. C. (1979). 'Erythroid progenitor cell numbers in human marrow—Implications for regulation', *Exp. Hemat.*, **7 (Suppl. 5)**, 54–64.
31. Ogawa, M., Grush, O. C., O'Dell, R. F., Hara, H., and MacEachern, M. D. (1977). 'Circulating erythropoietic precursors assessed in culture: Characterization in normal men and patients with hemoglobinopathies', *Blood*, **50**, 1081–1092.
32. Clarke, B. J., and Housman, D. (1977). 'Characterization of an erythroid precursor cell of high proliferative activity in normal human peripheral blood', *Proc. Natl. Acad. Sci., USA.*, **74**, 1105–1109.
33. Eaves, A. C., Henkelman, D., and Eaves, C. J. (1980). 'Abnormal erythropoiesis

in the myeloproliferative disorders: An analysis of underlying cellular and humoral mechanisms', *Exp. Hemat., 8* (**Supl. 8**), 235–247.

34. Grilli, G., Carbonell, F., and Fliedner, T. M. (1980). 'Variations in erythroid and myeloid progenitor cell numbers in normal human peripheral blood', *Br. J. Haemat., 44*, 679–681.
35. Chervenick, P. A. (1973). 'Increase in circulating stem cells in patients with myelofibrosis', *Blood, 41*, 67–71.
36. Öhl, S., Carsten, A. L., Chanana, A. D., Chikkappa, G., and Cronkite, E. P. (1976). 'Increased erythrocytic and neutrophilic progenitors in myelofibrosis with myeloid metaplastia', *Europ. J. Cancer, 12*, 131–135.
37. Eaves, A. C., and Eaves, C. J. (1979). 'Abnormalities in the erythroid progenitor compartments in patients with chronic myelogenous leukemia (CML)', *Exp. Hemat., 7* (**Suppl. 5**), 65–75.
38. Paran, M., Sachs, L., Barak, Y., and Resnitzky, P. (1970). '*In vitro* induction of granulocyte differentiation in hematopoietic cells from leukemic and non-leukemic patients', *Proc. Natl. Acad. Sci., USA, 67*, 1542–1545.
39. Moore, M. A. S. (1977). '*In vitro* culture studies in chronic granulocytic leukaemia', *Clinics in Haemat., 6*, 97–112.
40. Goldman, J. M., Th'ng, K. H., and Lowenthal, R. M. (1974). '*In vitro* colony forming cells and colony stimulating factor in chronic granulocytic leukaemia', *Br. J. Cancer, 30*, 1–12.
41. Goldman, J. M., Shiota, F., Th'ng, K. H., and Orchard, K. H. (1980). 'Circulating granulocytic and erythroid progenitor cells in chronic granulocytic leukaemia', *Br. J. Haemat., 46*, 7–13.
42. Hara, H., Kai, S., Fushimi, M., Taniwaki, S., Ifuku, H., Okamoto, T., Ohe, Y., Fujita, S., Noguchi, K., Kanamaru, A., Nagai, K., and Inada, E. (1981). 'Pluripotent, erythrocytic and granulocytic hemopoietic precursors in chronic granulocytic leukemia', *Exp. Hemat., 9*, 871–877.
43. Prchal, J. F., Adamson, J. W., Murphy, S., Steinmann, L., and Fialkow, P. J. (1978). 'Polycythemia vera: The *in vitro* response of normal and abnormal stem cell lines to erythropoietin', *J. Clin. Invest., 61*, 1044–1047.
44. Adamson, J. W., Singer, J. W., Catalano, P., Murphy, S., Lin, N., Steinmann, L., Ernst, C., and Fialkow, P. J. (1980). 'Polycythemia vera: Further *in vitro* studies of hematopoietic regulation', *J. Clin. Invest., 66*, 1363–1368.
45. Becker, A. J., McCulloch, E. A., Siminovitch, L., and Till, J. E. (1965). 'The effect of differing demands for blood cell production on DNA synthesis by haemopoietic colony-forming cells of mice', *Blood, 26*, 296–308.
46. Byron, J. W. (1972). 'Comparison of the action of ^{3}H-thymidine and hydroxyurea on testosterone-treated hemopoietic stem cells', *Blood, 40*, 198–203.
47. Fauser, A. A., and Messner, H. A. (1979). 'Proliferative state of human pluripotent hemopoietic progenitors (CFU-GEMM) in normal individuals and under regenerative conditions after bone marrow transplantation', *Blood, 54*, 1197–1200.
48. Rubin, S. H., and Cowan, D. H. (1973). 'Assay of granulocytic progenitor cells in human peripheral blood', *Exp. Hemat., 1*, 127–131.
49. Fauser, A. A., and Messner, H. A. (1981). 'Pluripotent hemopoietic progenitors (CFU-GEMM) in polycythemia vera: Analysis of erythropoietin requirement and proliferative activity', *Blood, 58*, 1224–1227.
50. Suzuki, S., and Axelrad, A. A. (1980). '*Fv-2* locus controls the proportion of erythropoietic progenitor cells (BFU-E) synthesizing DNA in normal mice', *Cell, 19*, 225–236.

51. Axelrad, A. A., Croizat, H., and Eskinazi, D. (1981). 'Gene control of progenitor cell proliferation during erythropoietic differentiation', in *Hemoglobins in Development and Differentiation* (Eds. G. Stamatoyannopoulos and A. W. Nienhuis), Alan R. Liss, Inc., New York, pp. 45–55.
52. Barach, A. L., and McAlpin, K. R. (1933). 'Negative results of oxygen therapy in polycythemia vera', *Am. J. Med. Sci.*, **185**, 178–181.
53. Lawrence, J. H., Elmlinger, P. J., and Fulton, G. (1952). 'Oxygen and the control of cell production in primary and secondary polycythemia: Effects on the iron turnover patterns with Fe[59] as tracer', *Cardiologia*, **21**, 337–346.
54. Stohlman, F., Jr. (1966). 'Pathogenesis of erythrocytosis', *Semin. Hemat.*, **3**, 181–192.
55. Koeffler, H. P., and Goldwasser, E. (1981). 'Erythropoietin radioimmunoassay in evaluating patients with polycythemia', *Ann. Intern. Med.*, **94**, 44–47.
56. de Klerk, G., Rosengarten, P. C. J., Vet, R. J. W. M., and Goudsmit, R. (1981). 'Serum erythropoietin (ESF) titers in polycythemia', *Blood*, **58**, 1171–1174.
57. Adamson, J. W. (1968). 'The erythropoietin/hematocrit relationship in normal and polycythemic man: Implications of marrow regulation', *Blood*, **32**, 597–609.
58. Popovic, W. J., and Adamson, J. W. (1979). 'Erythropoietin assay: Present status of methods, pitfalls, and results in polycythemic disorders', *Crit. Rev. Clin. Lab. Sci.*, **9**, 57–87.
59. Krystal, G., Eaves, A. C., and Eaves, C. J. (1981). 'Determination of normal human serum erythropoietin levels, using mouse bone marrow', *J. Lab. Clin. Med.*, **97**, 158–169.
60. Krantz, S. B. (1968). 'Application of the *in vitro* erythropoietin system to the study of human bone marrow disease: Polycythemia vera', *Ann. N.Y. Acad. Sci.*, **149**, 430–436.
61. Golde, D. W., Bersch, N., and Cline, M. J. (1977). 'Polycythemia vera: Hormonal modulation of erythropoiesis *in vitro*', *Blood*, **49**, 399–405.
62. Adamson, J. W., Fialkow, P. J., Murphy, S., Prchal, J. F., and Steinmann, L. (1976). 'Polycythemia vera: Stem-cell and probable clonal origin of the disease', *N. Engl. J. Med.*, **295**, 913–916.
63. Eaves, C. J., and Eaves, A. C. (1978). Erythropoietin (Ep) dose–response curves for three classes of erythroid progenitors in normal human marrow and in patients with polycythemia vera', *Blood*, **52**, 1196–1210.
64. Lacombe, C., Casadevall, N., and Varet, B. (1980). 'Polycythemia vera: *In vitro* studies of circulating erythroid progenitors', *Br. J. Haemat.*, **44**, 189–199.
65. Zanjani, E. D., Lutton, J. D., Hoffman, R., and Wasserman, L. R. (1977). 'Erythroid colony formation by polycythemia vera bone marrow *in vitro*', *J. Clin. Invest.*, **59**, 841–848.
66. Eaves, A. C., Henkelman, D. H., and Eaves, C. J. 'Polycythemia vera: Diagnosis by *in vitro* erythroid colony assay', (in preparation).
67. Cashman, J., Henkelman, D., Eaves, C., and Eaves, A. 'Polycythemia vera: Heterogeneity in the proportion of phenotypically abnormal CFU-E derived from individual BFU-E'. (in preparation).
68. MacDonald, M. E., Johnson, G. R., and Bernstein, A. (1981). 'Different pseudotypes of Friend spleen focus-forming virus induce polycythemia and erythropoietin-independent colony formation in serum-free medium', *J. Virol.*, **110**, 231–236.
69. Miyake, T., Kung, C. K. H., and Goldwasser, E. (1977). 'The purification of human erythropoietin', *J. Biol. Chem.*, **252**, 5558–5564.
70. Casadevall, N., Vainchenker, W., Lacombe, C., Vinci, G., Chapman, J., Breton-Gorius, J., and Varet, B. (1982). 'Erythroid progenitors in polycythemia

vera: Demonstration of their hypersensitivity to erythropoietin using serum free cultures', *Blood,* **59**, 447–451.
71. Singer, J. W., Fialkow, P. J., Adamson, J. W., Steinmann, L., Ernst, C., Murphy, S., and Kopecky, K. J. (1979). 'Increased expression of normal committed granulocytic stem cells *in vitro* after exposure of marrow to tritiated thymidine', *J. Clin. Invest.,* **64**, 1320–1324.
72. Berlin, N. I. (1975). 'Diagnosis and classification of the polycythemias', *Semin. Hemat.,* **12**, 339–351.
73. Lutton, J. D., and Levere, R. D. (1979). 'Endogenous erythroid colony formation by peripheral blood mononuclear cells from patients with myelofibrosis and polycythemia vera', *Acta Haemat.,* **62**, 94–99.
74. Prchal, J. F., Axelrad, A. A., and Crookston, J. H. (1974). 'Erythroid colony formation in plasma culture from cells of peripheral blood in myeloproliferative disorders', *Blood,* **44**, 912 (abstract).
75. Wurster-Hill, D. H., and McIntyre, O. R. (1978). 'Chromosome studies in polycythemia vera', *Virchows Arch. B. Cell Path.,* **29**, 39–44.
76. Testa, J. R. (1980). 'Cytogenetic patterns in polycythemia vera', *Cancer Genet. Cytogenet.,* **1**, 207–215.
77. Fialkow, P. J., Martin, P. J., Najfeld, V., Penfold, G. K., Jacobson, R. J., and Hansen, J. A. (1981). 'Evidence for a multistep pathogenesis of chronic myelogenous leukemia', *Blood,* **58**, 158–163.
78. Dubé, I. D., Eaves, C. J., Kalousek, D. K., and Eaves, A. C. (1981). 'A method for obtaining high quality chromosome preparations from single hemopoietic colonies on a routine basis', *Cancer Genet. Cytogenet.,* **4**, 157–168.
79. Köhler, G., and Milstein, C. (1975). 'Continuous cultures of fused cells secreting antibody of predefined specificity', *Nature,* **256**, 495–497.

Current Concepts in Erythropoiesis
Edited by C. D. R. Dunn
© 1983 John Wiley & Sons Ltd.

CHAPTER 8

Mechanism of the anemia of chronic renal failure

JAMES W. FISHER*, HEINZ W. RADTKE† and ARVIND B. REGE*

*Department of Pharmacology
Tulane University School of Medicine
New Orleans, Louisiana

Contents

I. INTRODUCTION

The primary site of production of erythropoietin (EPO) has been known for several years to be the kidney (1,2,3). Patients with chronic renal failure usually suffer from a hypoproliferative bone marrow and a normocytic

†Department of Nephrology, University Hospital, Frankfurt, West Germany

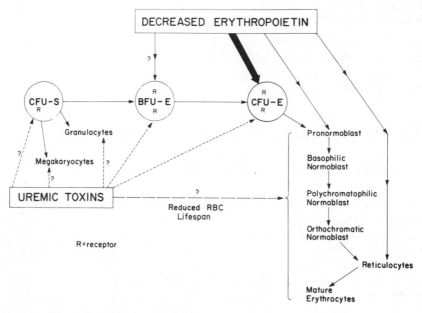

Figure 1. Model for mechanism of anemia of renal disease

normochromic anemia (4,5,6). Inadequte EPO production to sustain erythro-poiesis is probably the primary case of the anemia of chronic renal failure (CRF). Uremic toxins are increased in plasma and other biological fluids, thus, exposing the blood forming organs to high levels of these toxic substances to add further to this anemia. As renal insufficiency becomes more severe, the accumulation in body fluids of toxic materials causes the anemia to become progressively worse, because of the failure of the kidney to produce sufficient amounts of EPO to meet the increased demand for new red blood cells (RBC) caused by the uremic inhibitors (7) and factors which produce a reduction in the normal RBC lifespan (6,8–11). Shreiner and Maher (12) in 1961 and Bergstrom and Bittar (13) in 1969 outlined very clearly most substances which were known to be accumulated in body fluids, some of which produce suppression of erythropoiesis in patients with renal insufficiency. Jebsen *et al* (14) have reported that prolonged dialysis of patients with anemia and uremia of CRF can reverse the peripheral neuropathy independent of changes in BUN and creatinine. However, anemia of CRF, even though slightly improved, usually persists in the dialyzed patient primarily because of the failure of the erythropoietic function of the kidney.

II. MODEL FOR THE MECHANISM OF ANEMIA OF RENAL FAILURE

Our model for the mechanism of the anemia of renal disease is shown in Figure 1. EPO deficiency is probably the first and primary etiological factor in the anemia of renal disease. The kidney is unable to produce sufficient amounts of EPO to meet the increased demands for new RBC created by the shortened RBC lifespan, blood loss especially through the dialyzer unit, and/or inhibitors of erythropoiesis. The second major cause of the anemia is inhibitors of erythropoiesis which apparently include inhibitors of heme synthesis (15–23) and of the erythrocytic progenitor cell compartment (CFU-E, BFU-E) (24–30). It is quite possible that the decrease in heme synthesis is a late *sequelae* which reflects the inhibitory effects of uremic toxins on erythrocytic progenitor cells (EPO responsive cells, BFU-E, CFU-E) which ultimately give rise to the heme synthesizing nucleated erythrocytic cells (24–29). Uremic toxins may also act directly to suppress the pluripotential stem cell (CFU-S) compartment thus leading to a depletion of the erythrocytic progenitor cells (BFU-E, CFU-E). On the other hand, it is quite possible that inhibitors of erythropoiesis in uremia may inhibit the cycling and differentiation of BFU-E and CFU-E. High concentrations of uremic toxins may also lead to a direct suppression of the heme synthesizing nucleated erythrocytic cell compartment. The third major cause of the anemia of renal failure is shortened RBC lifespan due to retained uremic toxin(s) (6,8–11).

III. INHIBITORS OF HEME SYNTHESIS

Several investigators (16–23) have reported inhibition of heme synthesis with plasma and sera from anemic uremic patients with renal disease. Moriyama and co-workers (20,21,31) and Lindemann *et al* (19) have reported low molecular weight serum (20,21) and urinary (19) inhibitors of heme synthesis—generally assessed by the incorporation of ^{59}Fe. Wallner *et al* (23,28,32) have also more recently reported an inhibitor of heme synthesis in sera from patients with anemia of CRF. These investigators did not find a significant difference in the serum iron values between normal and uremic rabbits or normal and uremic patients (23,28,32) studied indicating that a change in the cold iron pool did not influence their results.

IV. INHIBITORS OF ERYTHROCYTIC PROGENITOR CELLS (CFU-E AND BFU-E)

Moriyama and Fisher (21) and Ohno and Fisher (26) have reported an inhibitor of CFU-E (erythrocytic colony-forming progenitor cell) in the sera of uremic rabbits using a nephrectomy CRF model and an inhibitor of both CFU-E and BFU-E (erythrocytic burst-forming unit) in the sera of patients with anemia of CRF (27). This inhibitor was partially removed by hemodialysis (27). In addition, Freedman and Saunders (33) have reported an inhibitor of CFU-E in plasma of anemic uremic children. Even though further work is necessary to completely characterize this inhibitor of the erythrocytic

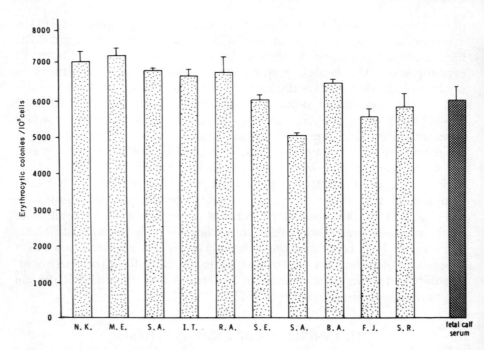

Figure 2. Effects of ten normal human sera at a concentration of 15% compared to fetal calf serum only (30%) on erythrocytic colony formation. Bars indicate s.e.m. of three replicates

progenitor cell compartment and to further determine whether the inhibitors reported for heme synthesis are the same as those which have been reported for CFU-E and BFU-E; our recent work (30) strongly implicates the polyamines as important uremic toxins as a causal agent in the anemia of CRF. Parathyroid hormone has also been postulated to be a uremic toxin which may contribute to and worsen the anemia of CRF (34) in that a significant increase in the hemoglobin levels occurred in four dialysis patients after parathyroidectomy (35). This improvement in hemoglobin levels after parathyroidectomy has been suggested not to be due to an inhibitor of erythropoiesis but rather to a change in the oxygen dissociation curve (9).

In order to evaluate the influence of normal human serum on erythrocytic colony formation in the fetal liver cell cultures as a control over our uremic human sera studies, ten normal human sera at a concentration of 15% were tested. This serum concentration was obtained by replacing 50% of the usual fetal calf serum supplement. These sera allowed the formation of 5080–7250 colonies/plate with a mean of 6435 ± 680, which was in the same range as 30% fetal calf serum (Figure 2). Since the variation in erythrocytic colony formation did not exceed the limits of accuracy of the assay, no indication for a

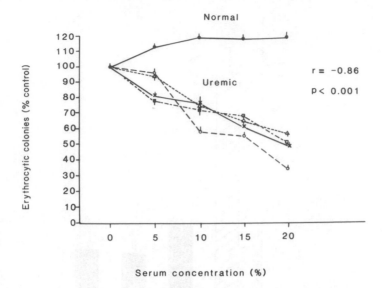

Figure 3. Effects of increasing concentrations of sera from normal human subjects (pooled sample of ten sera) and four azotemic patients on erythroid colony formation in fetal mouse liver cultures. Bars indicate s.e.m. of three replicates

heterogeneous effect of the normal sera on colony formation was seen. Therefore, pooled human sera derived from our normal human volunteers served as a control for comparison with the sera from CRF patients.

In the next experimental series the influence of sera from anemic azotemic patients prior to regular hemodialysis treatment was investigated. Representative sera from four patients were added to the fetal mouse liver cell cultures at concentrations of 0, 5, 10, 15, and 20% and compared to the effects of the pooled normal sera tested at the same concentrations. As shown in Figure 3, the predialysis sera inhibited erythrocytic colony (CFU-E type) formation in a dose-dependent manner. There was a significant negative correlation ($r = -0.86$, $p < 0.001$) between the concentration of all four sera from the CRF patients and the number of erythrocytic colonies formed. At the same time, the pooled normal human sera produced a slight but not significant enhancement in erythrocytic colony formation. To evaluate the significance of this inhibitor effect on CFU-E formation three uremic sera were also tested in normal human bone marrow CFU-E cultures. As illustrated in Figure 4, the serum of each of three uremic patients when included in the serum fraction of the culture media resulted in a marked inhibition of normal human bone marrow erythrocytic colony growth. As was seen in fetal mouse liver cell CFU-E cultures, inhibition of human CFU-E formation was also dose related (Figure 5).

As shown in Table 1, each of the 15 sera from the anemic azotemic patients prior to regular hemodialysis treatment (predialysis sera) markedly inhibited

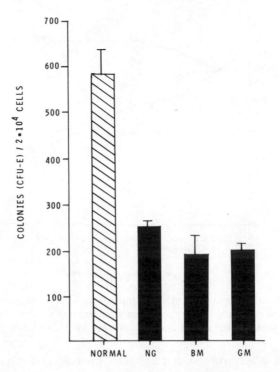

Figure 4. The effects of sera from three uremic patients and one normal human subject on erythrocytic colony formation in normal human bone marrow cultures. Uremic serum constituted two-thirds of the serum fraction in each culture. Bars indicate s.e.m. of three replicates

erythrocytic colony formation. They were 39–65% of the normal control values with a mean of 52 ± 8.8 (s.d.)%. When directly compared in the same assay, erythrocytic colony formation was restored to 83 ± 7.6 (s.d.)% of the control values following 48 hr *in vitro* dialysis (molecular weight 3500D) of 15 predialysis sera. Sera from eight of these patients were tested in culture again after 16–20 weeks of regular hemodialysis therapy (postdialysis sera) and a significant reduction in the inhibitory effects of the sera on erythrocytic colony formation was seen (Figure 6). When these post-dialysis sera were tested in the same fetal mouse liver cell culture as the original predialysis sera, erythrocytic colony formation was 61–92% of the normal human sera controls with a mean of 82 ± 3.58 (s.d.) %, which was significantly (*p* < 0.01) higher than the mean of the respective eight predialysis sera (49.5 ± 2.98). Thus, both *in vivo* and *in vitro* dialysis caused a significant reduction in the level of the inhibitor in the sera of azotemic patients. There was no statistically significant difference between the effects of *in vitro* dialysis and *in vivo* hemodialysis in their ability to remove the inhibitor from the sera. As further noted in Figure 6 a moderate

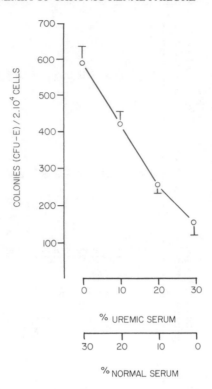

Figure 5. The effect of increasing dilution of serum from a uremic patient on human erythrocytic colony formation. Bars indicate s.e.m. of three replicates

elevation in hematocrit occurred in four and no change in two of the patients from their predialysis hematocrit values after 16–20 weeks (4–6 hr, three days a week) of regular hemodialysis.

In a previous study, where a larger group of 42 patients was followed over a longer period of 3–27 months on regular hemodialysis, the mean hematocrit increased from 21.7% to 28.6% which was highly significant ($p < 0.001$) (36). Since during this period there was neither a decrease in blood loss nor an increase in EPO production (36), this observation indicates the improvement in erythropoiesis following hemodialysis and lends strong support to the hypothesis that dialysis is effective in removing an inhibitor of erythropoiesis.

The Amicon stirred cell was used to separate two molecular weight fractions, above and below 500D from the uremic serum dialysate. When tested for colony inhibition the activity was found to be in the less than 500D molecular weight fraction (Figure 7). This ultrafiltrate produced a dose-related inhibition of fetal liver erythrocytic colony formation. No inhibition was seen in the molecular weight fractions above 500D. Neither the high nor the low molecular

Table 1 Clinical data on 15 anemic uremic pre- and postdialysis patients. Mean of three replicates of erythrocytic colony formation in the fetal mouse liver cell culture presented as percent of normal control. Predialysis sera, in vitro dialyzed predialysis sera, and postdialysis sera were tested at a concentration of 15% in the culture

Patient	Sex	Age	Diagnosis	BUN mg/10 ml	Creatinine mg/100 ml	Hct predialysis	Erythrocytic colonies (CFU-E) % of control	
							Predialysis	In vitro dialyzed predialysis sera
1 B.M.	F	16	Pyelonephritis	160	20.0	15	63	88
2 E.S.	M	46	Mal. nephrosclerosis	218	38.6	17	45	93
3 P.L.	M	67	Glomerulonephritis	67	8.9	17	51	87
4 T.I.	M	73	Pyelonephritis	130	9.5	19	45	85
5 BY.M.	F	65	Mal. nephrosclerosis	162	23.5	21	50	90
6 C.A.	M	55	Mal. nephrosclerosis	141	28.2	16	44	80
7 P.J.	M	40	Mal. nephrosclerosis	129	24.0	20	49	78
8 M.G.	F	28	Mal. nephrosclerosis	148	24.8	19	39	74
9 C.B.	M	33	Glomerulonephritis	198	27.4	16	62	86
10 L.J.	M	42	Glomerulonephritis	225	36.6	11	65	75
11 A.M.	F	54	Pyelonephritis	180	21.0	17	62	86
12 T.S.	F	58	Glomerulonephritis	197	24.3	14	60	85
13 M.A.	F	62	Glomerulonephritis	207	26.4	18	44	68
14 C.M.	F	54	Multiple myeloma	160	24.0	16	41	69
15 W.R.	M	18	Rejection post-transplant	104	7.4	23	51	91
N				15	15	15	15	15
mean		47.4		162	23.0	17.3	52.1	83.3
s.D. (±)		17		43	8.7	2.8	8.8	7.6
							$p < 0.001$	

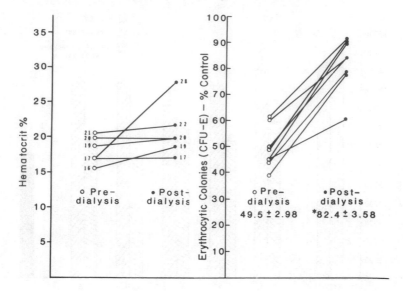

Figure 6. The effects of hemodialysis (16–20 weeks, 4–6 hr, three days/week) on hematocrit and serum levels of inhibitors of erythrocytic colony (CFU-E) formation. ± = s.e.m.

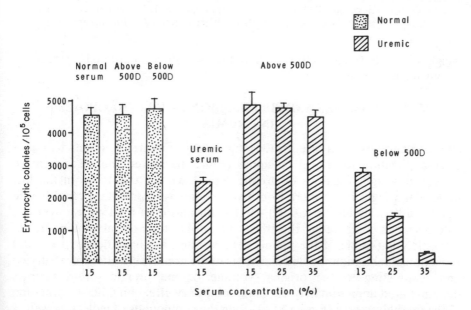

Figure 7. Effects of normal and uermic serum dialysate fractions above and below 500 D and crude normal and uremic sera on erythrocytic colony formation. Bars indicate s.e.m. of three replicates

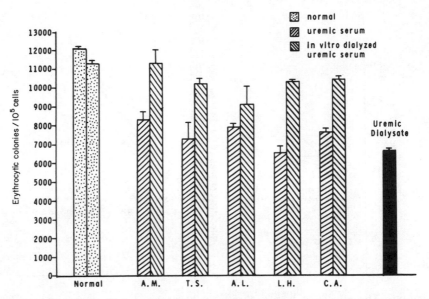

Figure 8. The effects of normal and uremic human sera before and after *in vitro* dialysis and the uremic dialysate itself (solid bar) on erythrocytic colony formation (CFU-E) in fetal mouse liver cultures containing 100 mu EPO/ml. The uremic sera produced significantly ($p < 0.01$) less inhibition of erythrocytic colony formation after *in vitro* dialysis. Bars indicate s.e.m. of three replicates of 15% human serum plus 15% fetal calf serum. Reproduced with permission from *J. Clin. Invest.* (30)

weight dialysate fractions from normal human subjects inhibited erythrocytic colony formation (Figure 7).

V. POLYAMINES AND SUPPRESSION OF ERYTHROPOIESIS IN UREMIA

We have demonstrated recently (30) that inhibitor in uremic serum dialysates after application to Biogel columns, (which permitted the assessment of molecular weight fractions of uremic sera down to 100D) was in the low molecular weight range. Sera from five patients with end-stage renal failure significantly inhibited ($p < 0.01$) CFU-E formation in fetal mouse liver cell cultures when compared to the effect of a pool of ten normal human sera. *In vitro* dialysis (48 hr) of the uremic sera resulted in a significant ($p < 0.01$) reduction of inhibition. Pooled dialysates of the uremic sera after freeze-drying and readjusting to the original volume of the uremic serum samples demonstrated approximately the same inhibitory effect on CFU-E formation as the predialysis sera (Figure 8). Among the compounds of molecular weight ∼ 200D found to be significantly elevated in the serum of uremic patients (37) the polyamines were selected for further study, since they have been reported

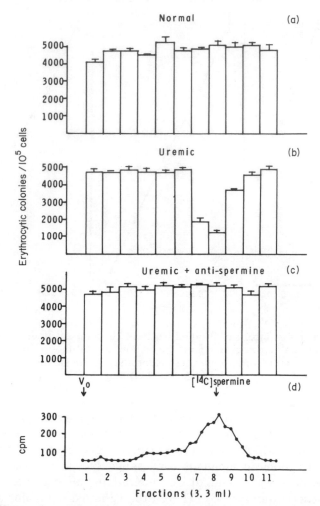

Figure 9. Effects of uremic serum dialysate fractions derived from gel filtration chromatogrphy (Bio-Gel P–2) on erythrocytic colony formation (a) to (c). Enumeration of the fractions (3.3 ml) begins with the void volume (V_0). (a) illustrates the effects of Bio-Gel fractions from a normal serum dialysate, (b) is a serum dialysate from an azotemic patient, and (c) a serum dialysate from an azotemic patient, which was preincubated with spermine antiserum, (d) shows the radioactivity (cpm) of 1.1 ml fractions, when ^{14}C-spermine tetrahydrochloide was added to a uremic serum dialysate prior to fractionation. Bars indicate s.e.m. of three replicates. Reproduced with permission from *J. Clin. Invest.* (30)

previously to suppress cell proliferation (38). In addition, the inhibitor of erythropoiesis was found to elute with the same polyacrylamide gel fractions as did radiolabeled spermine added prior to separation (Figure 9).

Disturbances in polyamine metabolism have been described in patients with

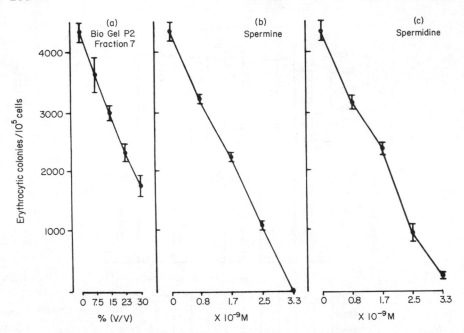

Figure 10. Inhibitory effects of Bio-Gel fraction 7 in comparison to that of spermine and spermidine on erythrocytic colony formation in fetal mouse liver cell cultures. Bars indicate s.e.m. of three replicates. Reproduced with permission from *J. Clin. Invest.* (30)

different stages of renal insufficiency (39,40). Polyamines have also been found to suppress the activity of such crucial endogenous enzymes as adenylate cyclase (41) and Na-K-ATPase (42). Furthermore, because of the high avidity of these polycationic compounds for anionic sites, the surface charge of erythrocytic cells was found to be reduced in the presence of elevated polyamine concentrations (43). Therefore, we tested the major endogenous mammalian polyamines, spermine and spermidine, in the fetal mouse liver culture to determine whether they might elicit an inhibitory effect on erythrocytic colony formation. As indicated in our present studies (9), both spermine and spermidine produced a dose-related inhibition of erythrocytic colony formation in fetal mouse liver (Figure 10) and spermine also inhibited human bone marrow cultures (Figure 11).

In an attempt to prove that spermine molecules present in sera from azotemic patients were the only inhibitors of erythrocytic colony formation, specific spermine antiserum was added to the *in vitro* test system. As shown in Figure 12, spermine antiserum completely neutralized the inhibitory activity of each of eight different uremic sera. For comparison, when added to a normal human serum, spermine antiserum did not influence CFU-E formation in the

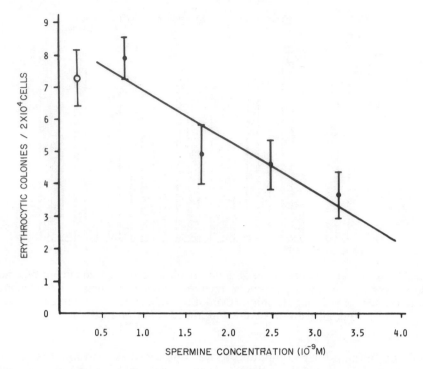

Figure 11. Inhibitory effects of spermine added to normal sera on human erythrocytic colony (CFU-E) formation in normal human bone marrow cultures containing 200 mu EPO. (0) = 200 mu EPO alone in normal human sera. (N = 4). Reproduced with permission from *J. Clin. Invest.* (30)

fetal mouse liver cell culture. The same observation was made when spermine antiserum was added to the uremic serum dialysate 5 hr before passing it through a polyacrylamide gel column. As shown in Figure 9, there was no inhibition of CFU-E formation by any of the Bio-Gel fractions of uremic serum following the addition of spermine antiserum. The addition of normal rabbit serum did not interfere with the inhibitory effects of uremic serum on erythrocytic colony formation.

These observations provide suggestive evidence that spermine may be responsible for the inhibition of the erythrocytic progenitor cell (CFU-E) compartment in the bone marrow of patients with anemia of chronic renal failure. Our studies do not completely discount the possibility of other inhibitors of erythropoiesis as yet unidentified; however, if other substances are involved in the inhibition of erythropoiesis in uremia, their effects on the CFU-E compartment would appear to be minimal, i.e., below the level of inhibition detectable in our fetal mouse liver cell culture assay system.

Four criteria were recently proposed by Bergstrom and Furst (37) which

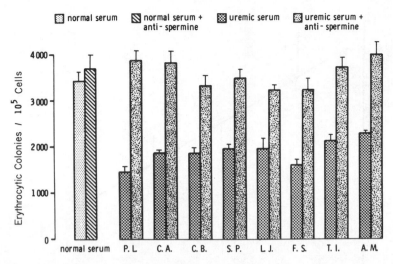

Figure 12. Effects of preincubation of eight uremic sera and a normal control serum with and without spermine antiserum on erythrocytic colony formation in fetal mouse liver cell cultures containing 100 mu EPO/ml. Bars indicate s.e.m. of three replicates. Reproduced with permission from *J. Clin. Invest.* (30)

should be fulfilled for a compound to be considered as a uremic toxin. Our present data provide evidence that spermine meets all four of these criteria for an inhibitor of erythropoiesis in chronic renal failure; (a) spermine has been chemically identified in uremic sera and can be measured quantitatively in biological fluids (39,40); (b) the serum concentrations of spermine in uremic patients have been shown to be elevated above normal controls (39); (c) inhibitory effects of spermine on *in vitro* erythrocytic colony growth can clearly be demonstrated at concentrations in the range of serum polyamine levels found in uremic patients; and (d) high polyamine concentrations have been shown to be associated with anemia of CRF, dysfunction of cellular immunity, and uremic neuropathy (39). Furthermore, there is suggestive evidence that serum concentrations of a heretofore unknown inhibitor of erythropoiesis are directly correlated with the severity of anemia of CRF. This is derived from the observation that anemia of uremia progresses relentlessly in the course of renal insufficiency up to the point where hemodialysis support is essential (44), and that anemia improves after several weeks of adequate dialysis therapy, in spite of a significant drop in the patients' serum EPO concentration (36,44). Thus, it is highly likely that it is an inhibitory factor which accumulates in uremia and is removed, at least in part, by dialysis, that correlates with the degree of anemia. It is of interest that continuous ambulatory peritoneal dialysis (CAPD) produces a more marked increase in hemoglobin levels in CRF patients with anemia than hemodialysis (45). Further studies are necessary to determine whether CAPD is more effective than hemodialysis in removing the polyamines spermine and spermidine. The inhibitor of erythropoiesis that we have previously shown to be removable from predialysis sera of azotemic patients by both *in vivo* and *in vitro* dialysis (46) may, indeed, be spermine, since the inhibitory effect of uremic sera could be mimicked by increasing concentrations of pure spermine added to normal sera. In addition, the effect of the uremic sera on erythrocytic colony formation could be completely abolished by the addition of specific spermine antiserum. On the other hand, systematic studies to determine an inverse correlation between the patients' hematocrit values and serum spermine or spermidine concentrations have not yet been performed in patients with end-stage renal failure.

VI. ERYTHROPOIETIN DEFICIENCY IN THE ANEMIA OF CHRONIC RENAL FAILURE

EPO deficiency is probably the most important factor causing the anemia of renal insufficiency. The nephric CRF patient can probably produce elevated levels of EPO but not of a sufficient titer to meet the increased demand for new RBC. On the other hand, the anephric CRF patient depends upon extrarenal EPO production which is more resistant to anemic hypoxic stimulation. Therefore, the completely anephric subject usually suffers a more severe degree of anemia than the nephric CRF patient. EPO titers in plasma of patients with anemia of CRF have been reported to be increased (44,47–52), unchanged (44,47) or undetectable (53) utilizing various bioassays and immunoassays for EPO. An important factor in determining the level of EPO is the residual renal erythropoietic mass and the sensitivity of extra-renal sites for EPO production. It is well known that extra-renal EPO production, perhaps from the liver, is more resistant to suppression by transfusion (54) and is probably more resistant to hypoxic stimulation (55,56). Utilizing an immunoassay for EPO most investigators (44,47–52) have reported elevated titers of immunologically reactive EPO in patients with anemia of CRF. However, Garcia *et al* (57) attributed the increase in immunoreactive erythrocytic activity in sera of patients with anemia of CRF to impure antigen used in his RIA since when pure EPO was used as the antigen no increase in serum EPO levels above normal were seen. In addition, Caro *et al* (47) have recently measured EPO levels in plasma of CRF patients using biological (polycythemic mouse assay) and immunological assays for EPO as well as a special concentration method for plasma. Nephric uremic patients were demonstrated to fall into two groups, one group having EPO titers in the range of normal non-uremic individuals and a second group with EPO titres higher than normal. Decreased but detectable levels of EPO were found in anemic anephric patients (46,58). Radtke *et al* (44) using a fetal mouse liver assay for EPO have also recently reported the results of an assay of 135 nephric uremic patients at various stages of CRF and found that most EPO titers were at a normal range or elevated. Sherwood and Goldwasser (52) and Lertora *et al* (51) using radioimmunoassays for EPO also reported that serum levels of EPO were higher in uremic anemic patients than that of normal human sera.

Recent animal models (59,60) have demonstrated that the anemia of renal failure can be partially corrected by administering EPO. It has been demonstrated (60) that a decrease in renal function, produced by subtotal nephrectomy, not severe enough to require dialysis, results in an anemia which is correctable by the administration of EPO. However, it seems clear that a more marked reduction in renal function produces uremia due to the retention of uremic toxins requiring dialysis and causes a suppression of erythropoiesis and a shortened RBC lifespan. In addition, it is not known whether these anemic non-uremic animal models are comparable to the anemia of CRF in man. The work of Essers *et al* (61) in the human subject may indicate that when uremia is superimposed upon the compromised erythropoietic function of the kidney, higher doses of EPO are required to correct the anemia because of the suppression of erythropoiesis by the retained uremic toxins.

VII. THE ROLE OF SHORTENED RED BLOOD CELL LIFESPAN IN THE ANEMIA OF CHRONIC RENAL FAILURE

Shortened RBC lifespan plays a variable role in the anemia of renal disease (8,11). Even though the primary cause of anemia of renal insufficiency is a failure of erythropoiesis which is due, at least in part, to inadequate production of EPO by the diseased kidney, another important factor contributing to the anemia is shortened RBC lifespan (6,8–11). The hemolysis in the anemia of renal disease appears to be due to an extracorpuscular hemolytic factor and not to any abnormality in the RBC itself, because RBC from patients with renal disease have been transfused into healthy recipients and appear to have a normal lifespan. However, when normal RBC have been transfused into uremic recipients their lifespan has been found to be shortened. The hemolysis is usually mild or may not be present at all until the terminal stages of renal disease. Circulating RBC in uremia usually are markedly distorted and fragmented with bizarre shapes; triangular, helmet-like, egg shell, burr cells, very small, and hyperpigmented spherocytes (6,9,10). Giovannetti *et al* (62–65) have demonstrated that guanidine derivatives, especially methylguanidine (MG) which has been demonstrated to be elevated in the serum of uremic patients, may be the cause of the hemolysis seen in chronic uremia. These investigators (66) have found that MG dialyzes quite differently to urea and creatinine and have postulated a role for MG in the shortened RBC lifespan in chronic uremia (63).

VIII. SUMMARY AND CONCLUSIONS

It seems clear from our model that the primary mechanism of the anemia of chronic renal failure in man is an insufficient production of EPO, because of the compromised erythropoietic function of the kidney, to sustain normal erythropoiesis and to meet the increased demand for new RBC formation created by the uremic toxins which inhibit erythropoiesis and shorten RBC lifespan. In that the primary cause of the anemia of CRF is a relative EPO deficiency, it seems important to attempt to provide large amounts of purified EPO to treat this anemia. Our present work strongly implicates the polyamines spermine and spermidine as important uremic toxins and inhibitors of erythropoiesis. Thus, it should be determined whether the reason that CAPD is more effective than hemodialysis in improving the anemia of CRF is due to the more effective removal of polyamines. Therefore, proper maintenance dialysis, especially intermittent peritoneal dialysis and CAPD, combined with the administration of purified EPO would seem to be the most effective therapy in the treatment of anemia of renal failure in man.

IX. ACKNOWLEDGMENTS

Supported by USPHS Grant No. AM–13211

X. REFERENCES

1. Jacobson, L. O., Goldwasser, E., Fried, W., and Plzak, L. (1957). 'Role of the kidney in erythropoiesis', *Nature (Lond.)*, **179**, 633–534.
2. Fisher, J. W., and Birdwell, B. J. (1961). 'The production of an erythropoietic factor by the *in situ* perfused kidney', *Acta Haemat.,* **26**, 224–232.
3. Kuratowska, Z., Lewartowski, B., and Michalak, E. (1961). 'Studies on the production of erythropoietin by isolated perfused organs', *Blood,* **18**, 527–634.
4. Callen, J. R., and Limarzi, L. R. (1950). 'Blood and bone marrow studies in renal disease', *Am. J. Clin. Path.,* **20**, 3–23.
5. Kaye, M. (1957). 'The anemia associated with renal disease', *J. Lab. Clin. Med.,* **52**, 83–100.
6. Loge, J. R., Lange, R. D., and Moore, C. V. (1958). 'Characterization of the anemia associated with chronic renal insufficiency', *Am. J. Med.* **24**, 4–18.
7. Fisher, J. W. (1980). 'Mechanism of the anemia of chronic renal failure', (Edit. Rev.), *Nephron,* **25**, 106–111.
8. Castaldi, P. A., Rozenberg, M. D., and Stewart, J. H. (1966). 'The bleeding disorder of uremia. A qualitative platelet defect', *Lancet,* ii, 66–69.
9. Connelly, T. J., Caro, J., and Erslev, A. J. (1979). 'Prevention of the anemia of partially nephrectomized rats by a low phosphate diet', *Clin. Res.* **27**, 291A.
10. Joske, R. A., McAlister, J. M., and Prankerd, T. A. J. (1956). 'Isotope investigations of red cell production and destruction in chronic renal disease', *Clin. Sci.,* **15**, 511–522.

11. Shaw, A. B. (1967). 'Haemolysis in chronic renal failure', *Br. Med. J.,* **ii**, 213–216.
12. Schreiner, G. E., and Maher, J. (1961). *Uremia.* Thomas, Springfield.
13. Bergstrom, J., and Bittar, E. E. (1969). 'The basis of uremic toxicity', in *The Biological Basis of Medicine* (Eds. A. Bittar and E. E. Bittar), Academic Press, New York, vol. 6, p. 495.
14. Jebsen, R. H., Tenckhoff, H., and Hoult, J. C. (1967). 'Natural history of uremic polyneuropathy and the effects of dialysis', *New Engl. J. Med.,* **277**, 327–333.
15. Erslev, A. J., McKenna, P. J., Capelli, J. P., Hamburger, R. J., Cohn, H. E. and Clark, J. E. (1968). 'Rate of red cell production in two nephrectomized patients', *Arch. Intern. Med.,* **122**, 230–235.
16. Fisher, J. W., Hatch, F. E., Roh, B. L., Allen, R. C. and Kelley, B. J. (1968). 'Erythropoietin inhibitor in kidney extracts and plasma from anemic uremic human subjects', *Blood,* **31**, 440–452.
17. Fisher, J. W., Lertora, J. J. L., Lindholm, D. D., Tornyos, K. and Moriyama, Y. (1973). 'Erythropoietin production and inhibitors in serum in the anemia of uremia', *Proc. Clin. Dialysis Transplant Forum.,* **III**, 22–23.
18. Fisher, J. W., Ohno, Y., Barona, J., Martinez, M., and Rege, A. (1978). 'The role of erythropoietin and inhibitors of erythropoiesis in the mechanism of the anemia of renal insufficiency', in *Heintz Symposium of Uremic Toxins,* pp. 21–23, McGraw-Hill, New York.
19. Lindemann, R. (1971). 'Erythropoiesis inhibitory factor (EIF). I. Fractionation and demonstration of urinary EIF', *Br. J. Haemat.,* **21**, 623–631.
20. Moriyama, Y., Saito, H., and Kinoshita, Y. (1970). 'Erythropoietin inhibitor in plasma from patients with chronic renal failure', *Haematologica,* **4**, 15–20.
21. Moriyama, Y., and Fisher, J. W. (1975). 'Effects of erythropoietin on erythroid colony formation in uremic rabbit bone marrow cultures', *Blood,* **45**, 659–664.
22. Stuckey, W. J., Fisher, J. W., Lindholm, D., Beltran, G., and Lertora, J. J. L. (1972). 'The study of anemia in patients with renal disease', 5th Ann. Contractors Conf. Artif. Kidney Program. USPHS-NIAMDD, Bethesda, MD., pp. 157–158.
23. Wallner, S., Kurnick, J., Ward, H., Vautrin, R., and Alfrey, A. C. (1976). 'The anemia of chronic renal failure and chronic diseases. *In vitro* studies of erythropoiesis', *Blood,* **47**, 561–569.
24. Fisher, J. W., Ohno, Y., Barona, J., Martinez, M., and Rege, A. B. (1978). 'Role of erythropoietin and inhibitors of erythropoiesis in the anemia of renal insufficiency', *Dialysis Transplant,* **7**, 472–481.
25. Fisher, J. W., Ohno, Y., Barona, J., Martinez, M., and Rege, A. B. (1978). 'The role of serum inhibitors of erythroid colony forming cells in the mechanism of the anemia of renal insufficiency', in *In Vitro Aspects by Erythropoiesis,* (Ed. M. J. Murphy) Capri, Springer, New York, pp. 181–191.
26. Ohno, Y., and Fisher, J. W. (1977). 'Inhibition of bone marrow erythroid colony forming cells (CFU-E) by serum from chronic anemic uremic rabbits', *Proc. Soc. Exp. Biol. Med.,* **156**, 56–59.
27. Ohno, Y., Rege, A. B., Fisher, J. W., and Barona, J. (1978). 'Inhibitors of erythroid colony forming cells (CFU-E and BFU-E) in sera of azotemic patients with anemia of renal disease', *J. Lab. Clin. Med.,* **92**, 916–923.
28. Wallner, S. F., and Vautrin, R. M. (1978). 'The anemia of chronic renal failure: Studies of the effect of organic solvent extraction of serum', *J. Lab. Clin. Med.,* **92**, 363–369.
29. Fisher, J. W., Modder, B. H., Foley, J. E., Ohno, Y., and Rege, A. B., (1977). 'The role of erythropoietin and inhibitors of erythropoiesis in the mechanism of the anemia of renal insufficiency', in *Kidney Hormones* (Ed. J. W. Fisher), Academic Press, London, vol. II, pp. 551–570.

30. Radtke, H. W., Rege, A. B., LaMarche, M. B., Bartos, D., Bartos, F., Campbell, R. A., and Fisher, J. W. (1981). 'Identification of spermine as an inhibitor of erythropoiesis in patients with chronic renal failure', *J. Clin. Invest.*, **67**, 1623–1629.
31. Moriyama, Y., Rege, A., and Fisher, J. W. (1975). 'Studies on an inhibitor of erythropoiesis. II. Inhibitor effects of serum from uremic rabbits on heme synthesis in rabbit bone marrow cultures', *Proc. Soc. Exp. Biol. Med.*, **148**, 94–97.
32. Wallner, S. F., Ward, H. P., Vautrin, R., Alfrey, A. C., and Mishell, J. (1975). 'The anemia of chronic renal failure. *In vitro* response of bone marrow to erythropoietin', *Proc. Soc. Exp. Biol. Med.*, **149**, 939–944.
33. Freedman, M. H., and Saunders, E. F. (1976). 'Erythroid stem cell studies in chronic renal failure', *Proc. 16th Int. Congr. Hemat., Kyoto*, 6 (abstract).
34. Massry, S. F. (1977). 'Parathyroid hormone; A uremic toxin?', *Nephron*, **19**, 125–130.
35. Better, O. S., Shasha, S. M., Windver, J., and Chaimovitz, C. (1976). 'Improvement in the anemia of hemodialysis patients following parathyroidectomy (PTX)', *Proc. Am. Soc. Nephrol.*, **9**, 1.
36. Radtke, H. W., Frei, U., Erbes, P. M., Schoeppe, W., and Koch, K. M. (1980). 'Improving anemia by hemodialysis: Effect on serum erythropoietin', *Kidney Int.*, **17**, 382–387.
37. Bergstrom, J., and Furst, P. (1978). 'Uremic toxins', *Kidney Int. Supl.*, **8**, S9–S12.
38. Grahl, W. A., Changus, J. W., and Pitot, H. C. (1976). 'The effect of spermine and spermidine on proliferation *in vitro* of fibroblasts from normal and cystic fibrosis patients', *Pediatr. Res.*, **12**, 531–535.
39. Campbell, R., Talwalker, Y., Bartos, D., Bartos, F., Musgrave, J., Harner, M., Puri, H., Grettie, D., Dolney, A. M., and Logan, B. (1978). 'Polyamines, uremia, and hemodialysis', in *Polyamines* (Ed. R. A. Campbell) Raven Press, New York, vol. 2, pp. 319–344.
40. Swendseid, M., Panaque, M., and Kopple, J. D. (1980). 'Polyamine concentrations in red cells and urine of patients with chronic renal failure', *Life Sci.*, **26**, 533–539.
41. Atmar, V. J., and Kuehn, G. D. (1977). 'Effects of polyamines on adenylate cyclase activity and acidic nuclear protein phosphorylation in physarum polydephalum', *Fed. Proc.*, **36**, 686.
42. Quarforth, G., and Ahmed, K. (1977). 'Sites of action of polyamines on Na,K-ATPase', *Fed. Proc.*, **36**, 360.
43. Chun, P. W., Rennart, O. M., Paffen, E. E., and Taylor, W. J. (1976). 'Effects of polyamines on the electrokinetic properties of red blood cells', *Biochem. Biophys. Res. Commun.*, **69**, 1095–1101.
44. Radtke, H. W., Claussner, A., Erbes, P. M., Scheuermann, E. H., Schoeppe, W., and Koch, K. M. (1979). 'Serum erythropoietin concentration in chronic renal failure: Relationship to degree of anemia and excretory renal function', *Blood*, **54**, 877–884.
45. Gokal, R., McHugh, M., Fryer, R., Ward, M. K., and Kerr, D. N. S. (1980). 'Continuous ambulatory peritoneal dialysis: One year's experience in a UK dialysis unit', *Br. Med. J.*, **281**, 474–477.
46. Radtke, H. W., Rege, A. B., LaMarche, M. B., and Fisher, J. W. (1979). 'Characterization of erythroid inhibiting factors (EIF) in patients with chronic renal failure', *Proc. Clin. Dialysis Transplant Forum.*, **9**, 179–183.
47. Caro, J., Brown, S., Miller, O., Murray, T., and Erslev, A. J. (1979). 'Erythropoietin levels in uremic nephric and anephric patients', *J. Lab. Clin. Med.*, **93**, 449–458.
48. Kozura, M., and Noda, Y. (1976). 'Immunochemical studies on the serum

erythropoietin by use of the anti-human erythropoietin', *Proc. 16th Int. Congr. Hemat., Kyoto,* 18 (abstract).

49. Lange, R. D., McDonald, T. P., Jordan, T. A., Trobaugh, F. E., Jr., Kretchmar, A. L., and Chernoff, A. I. (1970). 'The hemagglutination-inhibition assay for erythropoietin: A progress report', in *Hemopoietic Cellular Proliferation* (Ed. F. Stohlman, Jr.), Grune and Stratton, New York, pp. 122–132.
50. Lange, R. D. and Ichiki, A. T. (1977). 'Immunological studies of erythropoietin', in *Kidney Hormones* (Ed. J. W. Fisher), Academic Press, London, vol. II, pp. 111–149.
51. Lertora, J. J. L., Dargon, P. A., Rege, A. B., and Fisher, J. W. (1975). 'Studies on a radioimmunoassay for human erythropoietin, *J. Lab. Clin. Med.,* **86**, 140–151.
52. Sherwood, J. W., and Goldwasser, E. (1979). 'A radioimmunoassay for erythropoietin', *Blood,* **54**, 885–893.
53. Krugers-Dagneaux, P. G. L. C., Goudsmit, R., and Krijnen, H. W. (1968). 'Investigations on an immunoassay of erythropoietin', *Ann. N.Y. Acad. Sci.,* **149**, 294–297.
54. Lucarelli, G., Porcellini, A., Carvevali, C., and Stohlman, F., Jr. (1968). 'Fetal and neonatal erythropoiesis', *Ann. N.Y. Acad. Sci.,* **149**, 544–559.
55. Anagnostou, A., Vercellotti, G., Barone, J., and Fried, W. (1976). 'Factors which affect erythropoiesis in partially nephrectomized and sham-operated rats', *Blood,* **48**, 425–433.
56. Fried, W., and Anagnostou, A. (1977). 'Extrarenal erythropoietin production', in *Kidney Hormones* (Ed. J. W. Fisher), Academic Press, London, vol. II, pp. 231–244.
57. Garcia, J. F., Sherwood, J. W., and Goldwasser, E. (1979). 'Radioimunoassay for erythropoietin', *Blood Cells,* **5**, 405–419.
58. Rege, A. B., Brookins, J., and Fisher, J. W. (1981). 'A radioimmunoassay for erythropoietin: Serum levels in normal subjects and patients with some hemopoietic disorders', *J. Lab. Clin. Med.,* (submitted).
59. Van Stone, J. C., and Max, P. (1979). 'Effect of erythropoietin on anemia of peritoneally dialyzed anephric rats', *Kidney Int.,* **15**, 370–375.
60. Mladenovic, J., Eschbach, J. W., Garcia, J., and Adamson, J. W. (1981). 'Anemia of chronic renal failure (CRF) in the sheep: Response to erythropoietin (Ep) *in vivo* and *in vitro*', *Blood,* **58**, (**Suppl. 1**), 99a (abstract).
61. Essers, V., Muller, W., and Brunner, E. (1974). 'Further studies on the effectiveness of erythropoietin in renal failure', *Dt. Med. Wschr.,* **99**, 1618–1624.
62. Giovannetti, S., Balestri, P. L., and Cioni, L. (1965). 'Spontaneous *in vitro* autohaemolysis of blood from chronic uraemic patients', *Clin. Sci.,* **29**, 407–416.
63. Giovannetti, S., Giagnono, P., Balestri, P. L., and Cioni, L. (1966). 'Red cell survival in chronic uraemia. Its relationship with the spontaneous *in vitro* autohaemolysis and with the degree of anaemia', *Experientia,* **22**, 739.
64. Giovannetti, S., Cioni, L., Balestri, L., and Baigini, M. (1968). 'Evidence that guanidines and some related compounds cause haemolysis in chronic uraemia', *Clin. Sci.,* **34**, 141–148.
65. Giovannetti, S., Balestri, P. L., and Barsotti, G. (1973). 'Methylguanidine in uremia', *Arch. Intern. Med.,* **131**, 709–713.
66. Giovannetti, S., and Barsotti, G. (1974). 'Dialysis of methylguanidine', *Kidney Int.,* **6**, 177–183.

Current Concepts in Erythropoiesis
Edited by C. D. R. Dunn
© 1983 John Wiley & Sons Ltd.

CHAPTER 9

The anemia of chronic disorders: Clinical and pathological features

S. F. WALLNER

Medical Services Department
Veterans Administration Medical Center
Denver, Colorado

Contents

I. INTRODUCTION

Anemia of mild to moderate degree is seen complicating the disease course of patients with a wide variety of chronic infectious, inflammatory, and malignant conditions. Despite the wide variation in diseases causing this anemia, its features are remarkably constant from patient to patient. While a variety of names have been proposed, for the want of better terminology, it is simply called, 'the anemia of chronic disorders' (ACD).

In the preface to Chapter 13 of his book, *A Text-Atlas of Hematology*, Mathew Block states that 'the single most important and common problem in hematology, and the one to which the least attention is paid, is the reason sick people form red blood cells at a decreased rate' (1). While this might be somewhat of an overstatement, it is the purpose of this chapter to examine some of the clinical and pathophysiologic features of the ACD.

A good definition of the ACD is given by Cartwright and Lee (2) as 'that anaemia usually mild in degree, not progressive in severity, which is characterized by decreased plasma iron, decreased total iron-binding capacity of the plasma, decreased saturation of the transferrin with iron, decreased bone marrow sideroblasts, and normal or increased reticuloendothelial iron'. Data to be reviewed show that the pathophysiologic events leading to anemia are a mild degree of hemolysis with inadequate marrow compensation.

A wide variety of illnesses associated with anemia are lumped under this category. However, here we will discuss only that anemia seen with the commonly accepted infectious, inflammatory and malignant diseases. Specifically to be excluded will be the anemias seen in patients with malaria or schistosomiasis; in patients with hematologic malignancy such as lymphoma or myeloma since the mechanism producing anemia may be somewhat different; in patients who have extensive involvement of the bone marrow with either myelofibrosis or metastatic malignant diseases; in patients who have been burned.

II. CLINICAL FEATURES

A. Review

Complete review of the clinical findings of the ACD is beyond the scope of this work and has been the subject of recent reviews (2–4). The interesting feature is the constancy of the hematologic abnormalities despite the wide diversity of underlying diseases.

Anemia begins to develop shortly after the acquisition of the chronic process and generally becomes relatively stable by four to six weeks (Figure 1). It remains constant throughout the duration of the illness and improves when therapy directed at the underlying disease is begun. The majority of patients have a hematocrit between 30% and 40% with an average of about 35%, while

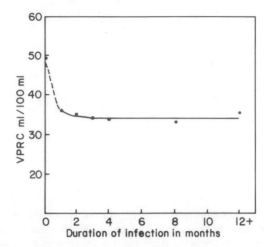

Figure 1. The relationship between the degree of anemia, (VPRC) and the duration of disease in 50 patients with chronic infections. Reproduced by permission from Cartwright, *Semin Hemat.,* 1966, **3**, 351–375

levels as low as 25% are encountered. Values under this are not usually found and another process must be suspected although some severely anemic patients fulfill all the criteria for the ACD and no other cause can be determined (3).

Ordinarily, red blood cell (RBC) indices are within the normocytic and normochromic ranges, however, in a significant number of cases, the RBC are microcytic and hypochromic (5). Reticulocytosis is uncommon; the reticulocyte count is usually normal to slightly elevated.

The diagnosis can be made clinically with assurance by the unique set of iron findings. The serum iron and transferrin (iron-binding capacity) are low. The percentage transferrin saturation is also reduced, although not to the degree seen in patients with iron deficiency anemia. Paradoxically, the bone marrow reticuloendothelial system (RES) iron stores are normal or increased while a decrease in sideroblasts is found. Usually 30% to 50% of marrow erythroblasts have fine iron granules, but in the ACD it is between 5% and 20% (3,4). This pattern is typical and diagnostic of the ACD and is not seen in any other process. Not infrequently, the ACD will coexist with iron deficiency and present some diagnostic problem. This can be resolved by measuring serum ferritin which is usually low in iron deficiency or by looking at marrow iron stores. The typical pattern seen in the ACD will emerge when these patients are treated with iron. The remainder of the bone marrow morphology is generally normal unless it has been modified by the underlying disease process.

B. Is the ACD an 'anemia'?

It has been proposed previously that the ACD may be 'physiologic' or adaptive

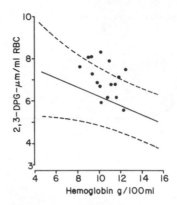

Figure 2. The relationship between red cell 2,3-DPG and hemoglobin concentration in 16 patients with ACD. The regression line and 95% confidence limits are those of 56 non-uremic subjects with anemia. Reproduced by permission from Douglas and Adamson, *Blood*, 1975, **45**, 55–65

in the sense that the low hematocrit reflects a decrease in tissue oxygen requirements in these chronically ill patients. This has been suggested in patients with panhypopituitarism or growth hormone deficiency in whom no change in RBC 2,3-diphosphoglycerate(2,3-DPG) occurs (6). In most anemic patients there is an increase in levels of 2,3-DPG and an increase in whole blood P_{50} thus resulting in an improvement in tissue oxygen delivery. Douglas and Adamson have found that patients with the ACD do increase 2,3-DPG levels and P_{50} (7) and this has been confirmed by Wallner *et al* (8) (Figure 2). Neither of these studies presents a complete analysis of oxygen delivery with simultaneous measurement of arterial and venous pH. However, the available data suggest that the ACD is not adaptive and shows that these patients have a normal reponse to anemia by attempting to shift oxygen delivery in favor of the tissues.

III. ANIMAL MODELS

A number of animal models have been developed in an attempt to duplicate the ACD of humans. These models have been used in many studies and inferences have been drawn concerning the pathophysiology of the human condition. It is critical to realize that there may be and often are important differences between these models and the human situation and this may bear upon the interpretation of experimental results and their applicability to understanding the human condition. The principal models will be reviewed briefly.

A. Turpentine abscess model

Perhaps the most frequently used model is that in which sterile abscesses are induced by intramuscular injection of turpentine in dogs or rodents. After injection a chronic sterile abscess forms associated with the development of anemia and hypoferremia (9,10). Mild to moderate reticulocytosis is seen (11). Thus, an anemia occurs which is due to a mild degree of hemolysis plus inadequate marrow compensation. These features simulate the ACD of humans. However, normal or elevated transferrin levels are seen in some of these animals (12) and the anemia is often microcytic (11), unlike the majority of patients the ACD who have normocytic RBC and low transferrin levels.

In addition, particularly in rodents, major changes in hematopoiesis occur in the spleen (13), a situation not seen in the human. Some have attempted to compensate for this by performing studies on splenectomized animals (13) and this does appear to be somewhat closer to the human situation. However, inferences concerning the pathophysiology of the ACD in humans which are drawn from an animal which has been splenectomized and whose iron status does not simulate that of human ACD must be made somewhat tentatively.

B. Adjuvant disease model

Another model which simulates the anemia of inflammation is the adjuvant induced immunologic injury in the rat in which Freund's complete adjuvant is injected into the heel pads of the animals. This process induces a generalized inflammatory reaction which is regarded as a type of delayed hypersensitivity to the mycobacterial antigen. Several weeks later the rats develop a mild and stable anemia which shares many of the morphologic and kinetic features of the ACD in humans (14,15,16). Mild shortening of RBC survival has been shown to occur in this animal and the anemia is presumed to result from incomplete marrow compensation for the mild hemolytic process. However, the spleen contributes significantly to hematopoiesis in rodents and splenomegaly with an fincrease in splenic erythropoiesis occurs in these animals (14,15,16). In addition, while serum iron levels fall, the level of transferrin does not change early (15) but falls late in the process (14). The anemia is usually hypochromic and microcytic (14).

C. Erhlich's ascites carcinoma

The Erhlich's ascites carcinoma can be transmitted in mice as either an ascitic or solid tumor. In the latter, the cells are injected intramuscularly and a discrete solid tumor develops without marrow involvement (17,18,19). Chromium studies show a modest decrease in RBC survival, and reticulocyte counts are low, analogous to the human situation. However, the anemia is progressive and increases until the time of the animal's death. Importantly, neutrophilia occurs with counts rising to two or three times baseline value. A significant but slight decrease in serum iron occurs, but transferrin rises.

Ferrokinetic studies show that an impressive wave of erythropoiesis occurs in the spleen.

D. Mycoplasma Arthritidis Arthritis

Mycoplasma Arthritidis is pathogenic for mice. After the intravenous injection of this organism an acute arthritis develops. This is followed by more chronic changes and after three weeks changes in the joints are characterized by synovial proliferation, mononuclear cell infiltration, and pannous formation. These features are similar to those seen in rheumatoid arthritis. A mild anemia develops and is accompanied by neutrophilia. The serum iron is low but transferrin rises significantly. Reticuloendothelial iron stores are abundant (20).

E. Walker 256 Carcinosarcoma

This model is that of a malignancy maintained in rats. As in the Ehrlich's ascites carcinoma model, anemia develops but is progressive and is associated with neutrophilia. Chromium survival studies show a modest decrease in RBC survival with an inadequate marrow response as judged by reticulocyte count. However, ferrokinetic studies show that there is a marked splenic compensation in animals with this condition (21).

F. Hepatoma 7777

The hepatoma 7777 is a model in rats. After implantation of tumor cells a progressive anemia develops which becomes severe. Leucocytosis occurs and there is a shift of erythropoiesis to the spleen. The anemia is microcytic and hypochromic and is characterized by a mild decrease in RBC survival. The serum iron level falls but the transferrin is elevated (22).

In summary, the anemias which occur in a variety of animal models have been proposed to parallel some of the features of the ACD of humans. Most of these successfully simulate the two major pathophysiologic events, a mild hemolytic process with an incomplete bone marrow erythrocytic response. However, all suffer from some differences from the human situation including a tendency for transferrin to be elevated rather than reduced, a marked increase in splenic erythropoiesis, microcytosis, and leucocytosis. None is a perfect model of the ACD. Considerable caution must be exercised in transposing data obtained in experimental animals to the human situation.

IV. PATHOPHYSIOLOGY

A. Overview

Abundant data, both from human and animal studies of the ACD indicate that the processes resulting in anemia are mild hemolysis due to an extracorpuscular event(s) with an inadequate marrow compensation. In this section we will review the available information which attempts to explain the nature of the hemolytic defect and the mechanisms leading up to the inadequate erythro-poietic response.

B. Hemolysis

A modestly reduced RBC survival was an early finding in patients with chronic diseases (23,24). This has been confirmed in numerous studies as reviewed by Cartwright (3) and is present in most of the animal models. Cross transfusion studies have shown that this process is extracorpuscular (24,25). The nature of the hemolytic abnormality has eluded detection and is difficult to study since, as pointed out by Erslev (4), it would take only minor changes in the RBC to bring about the mild hemolysis seen. The diversity of conditions leading to the ACD makes it difficult to suggest a common denominator which may account for the hemolysis. One feature may be tissue damage, whether this be from infection, inflammation or malignancy. It is possible that a substance is released as a result of tissue damage which in some way alters RBC shortening their survival. Another possible mechanism is that RBC are somehow injured when they pass through the diseased tissues. Finally, the reticuloendothelial system (RES) is in a state of some hyperactivity in patients with chronic diseases and it has been suggested that RES cells are sequestering more RBC than they do normally (26). The role of the RES in iron storage will be described below.

Studies in the hepatoma 7777 model show that RBC taken from the tumor-bearing animals have an increased osmotic fragility and examination of these cells with scanning electronmicroscopy shows echinocytic changes (22). This may account for some of the shortening of RBC survival in this model, however, changes in osmotic or mechanical fragility are not characteristic of cells taken from patients with the ACD (23), but it may be that changes are so subtle that they cannot be detected by these tests. Recall that the anemia in the hepatoma model is much more profound than in the human situation.

C. Marrow failure

1. Failure of marrow to compensate for hemolysis

Considerably more data exist to permit hypotheses concerning the failure of the marrow to compensate for the mild hemolytic process. A variety of conditions could conceivably result in a reduction in bone marrow RBC production and these will be considered in detail. Among the questions to be addressed are;

1. Is there an abnormality of iron metabolism?

2. What is the role of erythropoietin (EPO)?
3. Is there an inhibitor of EPO or erythropoiesis?
4. Are the erythrocytic cells normally responsive to EPO?
5. Are the numbers of stem cells normal?
6. Is the hematopoietic microenvironment normal?

2. Iron kinetics

The unique iron findings seen in the ACD early suggested that an abnormality of iron metabolism may be in part responsible for this condition. Initial attention was paid to the finding of the low serum iron and transferrin. Early studies in the rat showed that hypoferremia developed rapidly following induction of inflammation (turpentine abscess) and that this was accompanied by a fall in transferrin (27). Others showed that there was a decrease in iron absorption in patients with the ACD (28). While it was attractive to ascribe the hypoferremia to inadequate iron absorption, the finding of an increase in RES storage iron made it unlikely that the low serum iron was due to inadequate iron absorption or that iron absorption played any role at all in the development of the ACD.

Freireich *et al* studied dogs with turpentine abscesses which were given ^{59}Fe-labeled non-viable RBC or [^{59}Fe]transferrin (29). Such labeled RBC are handled in the RES and the reappearance of the labeled iron was followed in new RBC. A significant delay was found compared to control animals while the utilization of transferrin iron for hemoglobin synthesis was normal. These investigations suggested that impaired iron release from the RES led to a form of 'iron deficient erythropoiesis' despite the fact that more than adequate storage iron was present. Using an identical technique, Weinstein (30) and Noyes *et al* (31) described similar findings in patients with the ACD as did Haurani *et al* who used [^{59}Fe]hemoglobin as the tracer (32). The concept of an 'RES block' of iron release was suggested. This held that reduced flow of iron from the RES accounted for the low serum iron, the decreased marrow sideroblasts, the anemia and the increased iron stores (Figure 3). The concept that an RES block was entirely responsible for the ACD was first challenged by studies which showed that treatment of animals with models of the ACD with cobalt (33) or EPO (12) would result in partial correction of the anemia, a finding subsequently confirmed.

A number of more recent studies have addressed the issue of the RE block. Beamish *et al* used [^{59}Fe]transferrin and [^{59}Fe]dextran to study patients with the ACD. They found normal use of the transferrin iron, but reduced release of the dextran iron from RES cells in some patients (34). This confirmed the earlier work suggesting a block in RES iron release. Kumar studied patients with chronic infections and evaluated normal subjects and subjects with iron deficiency as controls (35). Using ^{59}FeCl$_3$ as the tracer he

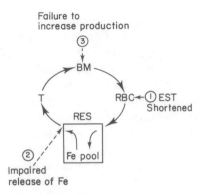

Figure 3. Representation of the defects involved in the pathogenesis of the anemia of chronic disorders. T, transferrin; BM, bone marrow; RBC, red blood cells; RES, reticuloendothelial system; EST, erythrocyte survival time. Reproduced by permission from Cartwright, *Semin Hemat.*, 1966, **3**, 351–375

found a normal RBC iron utilization and RBC iron turnover in all of his groups of patients. Plasma iron clearance, RBC iron utilization, and RBC iron turnover were also studied and no significant differences were found. It was concluded that studies with iron chloride did not indicate the true state of erythropoiesis in these patients and was suggested that the results would be heavily influenced by other factors, for example, the size of labile (storage) iron pool. Bennett *et al* also studied the uptake, release and use of RES iron with [^{59}Fe]dextran in patients with rheumatoid arthritis and found a decrease in iron release at 14 days accompanied by a decrease in hepatic mobilization of iron, and a decrease in the splenic uptake of iron. They concluded that the data showed ineffective RES iron elease (36). At variance, Williams *et al* used labeled iron dextran to measure RES iron uptake and release in patients with rheumatoid arthritis and were unable to detect a block of iron release (37).

The ferrokinetic studies of Douglas and Adamson confirmed that marrow failure occurred in the ACD. They found that the majority of erythropoiesis was effective and suggested that supply of iron to the bone marrow was the limiting factor in erythropoiesis (7). Cavill *et al* introduced a technique in which the patients own transferrin was labeled with iron and studied patients with chronic inflammatory diseases and iron deficiency. There was no increase in ineffective erythropoiesis in the ACD but they found a significant increase in iron deficiency. It was concluded that the ACD was not due to 'iron deficient erythropoiesis' since it was totally unlike the picture seen in pure iron deficiency anemia from the ferrokinetic standpoint (38). However, using the same method, Dinant and deMaat found an increase in ineffective erythropoiesis (39).

Although results of studies in animal models have been presented it must be recalled in the outset that no animal model completely simulates the ACD of humans. This is especially important when iron metabolism is studied since no change or an increase rather than a decrease in transferrin is seen in some models. However, some important data are available. Haurani and O'Brien recorded the effect of thorium dioxide, an RES blocking agent on erythro-poiesis in normal dogs, and showed a stimulatory effect which could not be attributed to release of EPO, thyroid hormone or corticosteroids (40). They concluded that the thorium dioxide caused release of iron from the RES and that this stimulated erythropoiesis and proposed that this was the reverse of the situation seen in the ACD in which RES iron release was 'blocked' and erythropoiesis was inhibited. In another acute experiment, Hershko *et al* evaluated iron kinetics in rats with turpentine abscesses. A fall of serum iron and transferrin occurred within the first 24 hr following the induction of injury. Iron turnover was measured with labeled heat-damaged RBC and labeled transferrin. The RES release of iron was reduced as was the hepatic parenchymal cell release of iron. Ferritin stores were shown to be increased in hepatocytes and it was concluded that accumulation of tissue iron occurred in these animals with an impaired release of RES iron, confirming previous data (27).

In a study producing contradictory results, Zarrabi *et al* studied iron kinetics in rats with Walker 256 carcinosarcoma. Unlike several previous studies, the animals were studied three weeks after engraftment of the tumor when a chronic anemia had been established. The utilization of iron-labeled heat-damaged RBC and the sequestration of this iron in organs was studied. Iron re-utilization in the tumor-bearing *versus* the control group was not significantly different. No excessive iron sequestration in liver or spleen was observed in their work. EPO levels were evaluated appropriately to the degree of anemia. They concluded that in the presence of sufficient EPO there were no significant changes in iron kinetics in this animal model (41).

Thus, the data concerning iron kinetics in humans and animals with ACD are in conflict. Significant methodological considerations must be taken into account when evaluating these studies. In an attempt to reconcile the contra-dictions, Zarrabi *et al* carefully reviewed previous studies and pointed out that in early studies of RES function the amount of non-viable RBC adminis-tered was often far in excess of what would occur physiologically. Perhaps more would be deposited in RES cells and dilution of the tracer by the large amount of storage iron could give the appearance of delayed release. Studies using labeled hemoglobin are flawed by the fact that this material is largely handled by liver parenchymal cells and not by RES cells (42). Additional studies have confirmed that the size of labile iron pool is extremely important when evaluating ferrokinetics. The large amount of storage iron typically seen in the ACD may effect the studies by dilution of the tracer by 'cold iron'.

In summary, the data available are not reconcilable. Early studies may have suffered from methodological problems which make interpretation difficult. Recent studies utilizing improved techniques suggest that there is

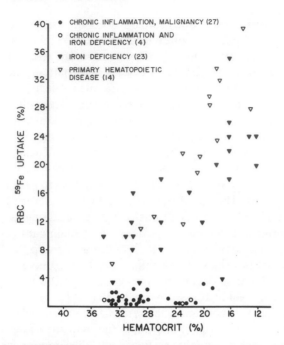

Figure 4. Levels of EPO hematocrit in subjects with the anemia of chronic disorders and in those with primary hematopoietic disease, primarily iron deficiency. Levels of EPO are expressed as ^{59}Fe incorporation into red blood cells of ex-hypoxemic mice. Patients with the ACD do not elevate levels of EPO compared to those patients with primary hematopoietic disorders. Reproduced from *The Journal of Clinical Investigation*, 1971, **50**, 332–335 by copyright permission of The American Society for Clinical Investigation

not an intrinsic abnormality of iron metabolism by RES cells, but further study is needed to clarify these issues.

3. The role of erythropoietin

(a) Human Work. Studies in this area have yielded more consistent data than the work in the area of iron metabolism. Using the ex-hypoxic mouse bioassay technique for measuring EPO, Ward *et al* described that serum levels in patients with rheumatoid arthritis were less than those which would be expected when these patients were compared to a group of iron deficient subjects whose EPO levels were felt to be appropriately elevated (43). This work was extended to include patients with a variety of infectious and inflammatory diseases and a group with lymphomas and other carcinomas, (Figure 4) (44). Some of the patients with malignancies had a significant elevation of serum EPO when compared to normal levels, but in few cases did this reach the levels seen in the group of patients with iron deficiency anemia

and similar hematocrit. Firat and Banzon used the starved mouse bioassay technique and studied patients with lymphomas, leukemias, and solid tumors and found that the majority of their patients had serum levels of EPO less than those of control subjects (45). Only an occasional patient had a level in the normal range and this occurred in the least anemic subjects. The lowest levels were seen in those subjects who were most anemic. These initial three studies led to the concept that EPO levels were reduced relative to the degree of anemia in most patients with chronic infectious, inflammatory, and malignant states. Somewhat contradictory data appeared when Zucker *et al* reported that serum EPO levels in patients with malignancy were often elevated appropriately for the degree of anemia when compared to patients with iron or folate deficiency (46). They confirmed that EPO levels were low in patients with infectious and inflammatory diseases. Likewise, Douglas and Adamson found that a significant number of patients with malignant diseases had an increase in the urinary excretion of EPO (7) but as a group the ACD subjects had lesser amounts of urinary EPO than would be expected on the basis of hematocrit. Additional studies of serum and urine EPO have also indicated that these are usually not increased in the ACD (8,47).

It appears remarkably constant that serum and urine EPO are inappropriately low relative to the degree of anemia in the majority of patients, certainly those with infectious or inflammatory disorders. The situation is somewhat less clear for the anemia seen in patients with malignant disorders, some patients with solid tumors having an increased level of EPO as can also be seen in leukemias and lymphomas. As previously mentioned, the mechanisms controlling RBC production in patients with a primary hematologic malignancy may be somewhat different than those with solid tumors. Thus, it is suggested that there is a subset of patients with solid tumor and anemia in whom EPO levels are appropriately elevated. Considering the widely diverse nature of the conditions producing the ACD it seems hardly surprising that some variations in pathophysiologic mechanisms would be found.

(b) Animal Studies. Work in this field has been somewhat limited, partly because of the relatively large amount of serum needed to measure EPO activity when the ex-hypoxic mouse assay technique is used. Lukens found that the serum EPO levels of rats with Freund's adjuvant arthritis were somewhat less though not statistically so compared to levels in normal rats (48). One might argue that such levels are, in fact, significantly low when one takes into account the fact that the animals were anemic. The hematocrit response to hypoxia was uniformly less in the Freund's adjuvant rats compared to normal rats although some elevation did occur. This suggested that there was some abnormality of EPO elaboration in these animals. Low EPO levels have also been found in rats with turpentine abscesses (11) and in mice with the solid phase Erhlich ascites carcinoma (19). In distinction, levels in rats with Walker

256 malignancy were significantly and appropriately elevated (21,24). These data are roughly parallel to results seen in humans. Animals with anemia due to inflammatory processes and some animals with malignant disease have low levels of serum EPO while other animals with malignancy have elevated levels.

(c) Why is EPO Reduced? The reason for the depressed level of EPO is not totally clear but has been the subject of some study. Three mechanisms could account for this phenomenon. First, the absolute amount of EPO synthesized could be reduced; second, an abnormal EPO molecule could be produced; and third, an inhibitor to the action of EPO may be present. That the first mechanism is correct, is suggested but not proved in studies which show that animals with the ACD will respond normally to cobalt (33), hypoxia (12), or exogenous EPO (12,48). No data exist to test the second hypothesis although it is difficult to conceive why these diverse processes should be associated with he synthesis of a biologically non-functioning protein. A number of studies have addressed the issue of an inhibitor. These studies have primarily used an *in vitro* neutralization test in which serum from patients with the ACD is mixed with EPO solutions which are incubated and subsequently checked for erythropoietic activity. In two studies, Ward *et al* were unable to find evidence of inactivation of EPO with ACD serum (43,44). Firat and Banzon approached the problem slightly differently by injecting ACD serum simultaneously with EPO into their test mice and found no alteration in response to EPO (45), but it is certainly possible that the intact mouse excreted or metabolized an inhibitor. Zucker *et al* incubated EPO with human ACD serum and subsequently studied its ability to stimulate heme synthesis in suspension cultures of erythroblasts, finding no loss of activity (11). Thus, while EPO inhibitors are known to exist in a variety of tissues (49), there is no evidence at present that such substances are responsible for the low levels of EPO activity seen in the ACD.

Lack of appropriate production of EPO appears to be an important event in the ACD and several studies have attempted to find a mechanism for this phenomenon. Kurnick *et al* studied albumin, transferrin, and EPO levels in a group of patients with chronic diseases and found significant correlations between hematocrit and albumin and between hematocrit and transferrin levels (50). It was proposed that the low level of EPO reflected a generalized hyposynthetic state in which proteins were synthesized at a rate not commensurate with breakdown. Direct data on EPO synthesis rates have not appeared, however.

Indirect evidence that starvation with decreased protein intake is implicated in a reduction of EPO production comes from use of the starved rat as an EPO assay system. Starvation is known to alter the rate at which thyroxine (T4) is converted to the more metabolically active tri-iodothyronine (T3) (51). It is felt that a large fraction of thyroid hormone action is a result of this peripheral conversion of T4 to T3. It has been shown that in starvation this conversion is reduced and/or in fact may proceed in the direction of the metabolically inactive 'reverse' T3. Caro *et al* recently confirmed that EPO production in starved rats was low and that the EPO response to hypoxia was blunted. This abnormal response was corrected when the animals were given glucose. T3 and T4 levels were also reduced in these animals. Thyroid hormones have a stimulatory effect on erythropoiesis *in vitro* and on EPO production in response to hypoxia, thus it appears possible that alterations in EPO seen in starved animals are due to changes which occur in thyroid hormone balance (52). Patients suffering from chronic diseases also have a depression in level of T3 and an increase in the inactive 'reverse' T3 (53). These are the same patients who tend to have low levels of EPO and anemia. One can speculate that alterations in thyroid hormone metabolism induced by chronic illnesses and/or starvation are responsible in part for the reduced levels of EPO seen in these patients.

4. Is there an inhibitor of erythropoiesis in the ACD?

Studies reviewed above suggest that the low level of EPO seen in patients with the ACD is the result of failure to synthesize adequate amounts of EPO and not the result of reduction of activity by an inhibitory substance. A substance directly inhibitory to erythrocytic cells might account, in part, for the inadequate marrow response and several studies have addressed this issue. The work cited in which plasma from patients with the ACD was studied *in vitro* would not distinguish between an inhibitor of EPO or of erythropoiesis, but the failure to find inhibition of heme synthesis in suspension culture argues against any inhibitor being present in the plasma (46).

Wallner *et al* (54) studied serum from patients with the anemia of chronic renal failure and the ACD in a similar suspension culture system measuring labeled iron heme synthesis by normal dog marrow as end point. Inhibition was found in cultures prepared with serum from patients with uremia but no statistically significant difference was noted between heme synthesis in plates prepared with normal and the ACD sera. However, in each experiment the amount of heme synthesized in the presence of ACD serum was somewhat less than the normal serum control plates, raising the possibility that a larger number of experiments might have demonstrated some inhibition.

Lukens showed that rats with adjuvant disease responded to EPO normally compared to control animals (Figure 5) (48), but, the response was never quite the same as that seen in the normal animals. A larger series might have detected a significant difference in response suggesting that an inhibitor was present. In unpublished observations on the *Mycoplasma arthriditis* model in

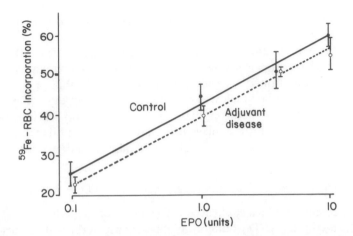

Figure 5. The effect of Freund's adjuvant disease on the erythropoietic response of hypertransfused rats to sheep EPO. Points and bars identify means and s.e.m.s for groups of rats. Reproduced by permission from Lukens. *Blood*, 1973, **41**, 37–44

the mouse, our results were similar. The hematocrit response to daily serially administered exogenous EPO in the anemic animals was not statistically different than in controls but on each day after EPO treatment the increase was less. The results of these studies leave open the possibility that there is an inhibitory substance present in the ACD. One would anticipate that the level of inhibitor activity would be low since it has not been easy to detect with currently available methods but inhibition may still play some role in the production of the ACD as has been suggested in uremia (55).

The normal, or near normal, responses of animals to EPO suggest that, when properly stimulated, erythrocytic cells are able to extract iron from RE cells in amounts sufficient to support a normal rate of erythropoiesis and tend to argue against the hypothesis that a block of RE release of iron is the sole limiting factor in RBC formation in the ACD. Recent studies of iron laden macrophages *in vitro* show that EPO does not cause release of iron directly (56) and it must be proposed that iron release is related to activity of the cells.

In some distinction, Zucker *et al* have proposed that serum of rats with the Walker 256 malignancy contains a lipoprotein inhibitor of erythropoiesis (57,58). In additional studies with this model, they showed that the presence of cancer cells would inhibit either the amount of heme synthesized in suspension culture or the number of erythrocytic colonies formed when marrow was cultured using the semi-solid methylcellulose technique. This did not appear to be due to cell contact since immobilization of the malignant cells in an agar underlayer also resulted in a reduction in erythrocytic colony formation, suggesting that the cancer cells were releasing some substance capable of inhibiting erythrocytic tissue (59). With the exception of this model, evidence to suggest that inhibitors of erythropoiesis play a role in the ACD is sketchy.

If inhibitors exist in humans their nature is entirely unknown. It is perhaps noteworthy that Herman *et al* have recently described that when tissue culture medium was 'conditioned' *in vitro* by human neutrophils a material was released into the media which was capable of inhibiting erythrocytic colony growth (60). Certainly, neutrophilia is part of a variety of infectious and inflammatory states and it is conceivable that the neutrophils themselves are releasing some substance which results in mild inhibition of erythropoiesis.

5. Are the erythrocytic cells normally responsive to EPO in the ACD?

Another mechanism which could account, in part, for the failure of the marrow to compensate in the ACD would be an abnormality in the cellular response to EPO. Several studies have appeared directed at this issue. Bone marrow erythrocytic cells taken from rats with turpentine abscesses had a normal response to EPO when studied in suspension culture with labeled iron heme synthesis measured as the endpoint (11). Bone marrow from humans with the ACD have also been studied in suspension culture and cells taken from patients with infectious or inflammatory processes responded to EPO similarly to controls. However, some reduction in heme synthesis was noted when the cells were taken from patients with malignant diseases. (Figure 6) (46). Further studies confirmed that the response to EPO was reduced when cells from patients who had bone marrow involvement were studied (61). Finally, a decrease in heme synthesis has been found when bone marrow cells of rats with the Walker 256 carcinosarcoma were cultured (32).

These studies indicate that the erythrocytic tissue appears to be normally responsive to EPO in tissue culture when the cells were from animals or humans with infectious or inflammatory processes. There is some reduction in heme synthesis when cells from either patients or animals with malignant diseases are studied. The previously cited work suggests that the cancer cells may elaborate some substance which inhibits erythropoiesis, therefore, this work does not necessarily imply that an abnormality intrinsic to erythrocytic cells has occurred. It is possible that some inhibitory substance may be elaborated which alters EPO responsiveness. This issue requires further study.

6. Are the number of stem cells altered in the ACD?

Several studies directed at this issue have used animal models. DeGowin and Gibson studied erythropoiesis in mice with the solid phase Ehrlich ascites tumor (18). Anemia developed after implantation of the tumor and using ^{59}Fe as a tracer a marked decrease in iron incorporation into the bone marrow was noted with a compensatory increase in iron incorporation in the spleen.

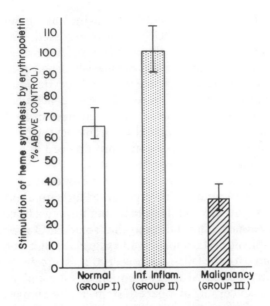

Figure 6. The effect of EPO (0.2 or 0.6 units/ml on ^{59}Fe incorporation into heme) in marrow cultures from normal subjects, from those with inflammatory or infectious diseases and from those with malignant conditions. Stimulation of heme synthesis is recorded as percentages above saline controls. Results include the mean ± the s.e.m. of each group. Reproduced from *The Journal of Clinical Investigation*, 1974, **53**, 1132–1138 by copyright permission of The American Society for Clinical Investigation

Differential counts of bone marrow cells showed that erythrocytic and lymphocytic tissue had been largely replaced by an intense granulocytosis, granulocytic tissue increasing from 50% to approximately 90% of marrow cells whereas erythrocytic cells fell from 20% to 6%.

This affect was partially ablated when the spleen had been removed previously; the number of marrow erythroblasts remained higher in the post-splenectomy tumor-bearing animals. Essentially similar results were obtained when the same group studied mice with turpentine abscesses (16).

Reissmann and Udupa extended this work by studying numbers of stem cells in mice with turpentine abscesses (13). They measured the number of splenic colony-forming units (the CFU-S) using the lethally-irradiated mouse method and numbers of primitive erythrocytic precursors (erythrocytic burst forming units, the BFU-E) and later erythrocytic precursors (erythrocytic colony forming units, the CFU-E) in addition to white blood cell colony-forming units (the CFU-C) in methylcellulose culture. After injection of the turpentine and during the development of the anemia, a marked fall in femoral marrow CFU-E was noted (Figure 7), accompanied by a rise in CFU-C. It appeared that a wave of granulopoiesis occurred in the marrow as a response to inflammation. This was compensated for by an increase in numbers of CFU-E in the spleen. Splenic CFU-S and CFU-C also increased. Data paralleling the colony-forming unit results were found when differential counts of hemato-poietic cells were done. Further studies in mice which had been splenectomized confirmed that a lesser decrease in marrow erythrocytic tissue occurred in the splenectomized abscess-bearing mice. It was concluded that unknown mediators of inflammation resulted in major changes in the bone marrow by permitting the accelerated production of granulocytes perhaps altering the environment so that erythropoiesis could not proceed at a normal rate. This effect could be partially ablated by splenectomy.

These studies suggested that a reduction in the amount of erythrocytic tissue occurred in marrow of animals in response to inflammation or malignancy. Some compensation occurred in the spleen, but this must be considered partial since anemia developed. This indicated that some EPO is produced, at least enough to drive splenic erythropoiesis, and suggested that a process other than EPO lack accounted for the fall in marrow erythrocytic cells, perhaps mediated by some substance(s) released as a consequence of the underlying process. No data are available concerning numbers of stem cells in humans.

7. Is there an abnormality of the hematopoietic microenvironment in patients with the ACD?

Changes in the marrow microenvironment may have important influences on modifying hematopoiesis. For example, studies in mice have indicated that the defects in erythropoiesis noted in aged mice are not intrinsic to stem cells themselves (62) and the abnormalities are not corrected by engraftment of normal marrow from younger animals (63). These findings suggest that abnormalities of the microenvironment occur in ageing. Results reviewed above would be consistent with some change in the microenvironment such that granulopoiesis was favored at the expense of erythropoiesis. Studies in the turpentine abscess-bearing mouse model and in the solid phase Ehrlich ascites carcinoma have been done using a technique in which colonies of marrow derived fibroblasts, felt to represent marrow stomal cells (MSC), were cultured.

The cells for culture were obtained by flushing the medullary cavities. Studies in both models showed that MSC were reduced in the anemic animals (16,18). Somewhat less of a decrease in MSC occurred in animals which had been splenectomized and this parallels the lesser decrease in erythrocytic cells noted in the marrow. This work suggested that changes in the hematopoietic microenvironment occur and that this may correlate with the reduced rate of erythropoiesis. Support for the concept that adherence of cellular elements to microenvironmental cells is important comes from studies of erythropoiesis and granulopoiesis in long-term bone marrow cell cultures in which differential adhesion of granulocytic and/or erythrocytic precursors to fat cells and/or macrophages has important modifying features on the rates of production of granulocytes or erythrocytes (64). It is conceivable that some humoral event produced by the chronic disorder modifies the number of stromal cells in the bone marrow resulting in a reduced rate of RBC production and allowing granulopoiesis to proceed at an accelerated rate. Recent work has shown that MSC elaborate prostaglandin E and this may have important effects on hematopoietic proliferation (65).

8. Is something missing from serum in patients with the ACD?

For completeness, a final possibility which may account for the reduced rate of erythropoiesis in the ACD would be the absence of some material from plasma of these patients which is required for erythropoiesis to proceed at a normal rate. Certainly EPO and iron levels are low. However, iron levels do not appear to be a limiting feature since erythropoiesis can proceed at a normal rate when exogenous EPO is given. Studies of other vitamins have failed to detect deficiencies in the ACD. Thus, while this mechanism remains a possibility, no data have been advanced for lack of any material other than EPO in these patients.

V. SUMMARY

This review has focused primarily on the pathophysiology of the ACD. The primary events are a mild hemolytic process produced by an extra corpuscular process and an inadequate bone marrow compensation for this hemolysis. The nature of the event inducing hemolysis is unknown. A variety of events have been postulated to account for the failure of the erythrocytic compartment to repair the mild hemolysis. Early studies focused on an apparent block of iron release by RE cells. Recent studies suggest that alterations in iron metabolism, while present, are not as important an etiologic feature as felt previously. This statement must be qualified by pointing out that great controversy exists concerning methodology. Much work has focused on the lack of EPO which is seen in both humans and animals with the ACD. Indeed, many authorities suggest that a central event in the ACD is lack of production of sufficient EPO, although there are exceptions particularly in patients and animals with malignant diseases. No evidence has been presented in support of an inhibitor of EPO in the ACD or that the EPO molecule is abnormal. The reason for reduced level of EPO seems to be an inadequate rate of synthesis of hormone and that this may be related to a general protein hyposynthetic state or to alterations in thyroid hormone metabolism. With the exception of studies in patients with malignancy and in some animal models of malignancy, no evidence of an inhibitor of erythropoiesis *per se* has been presented in this

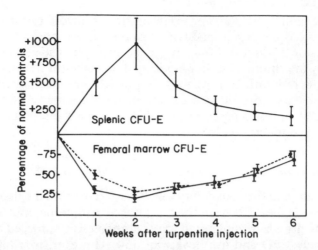

Figure 7. The effect of turpentine-induced abscess (day 0) on CFU-E in femoral marrow and spleen. The dashed line represents femoral CFU-E in mice splenectomized two weeks before turpentine injection. Mean and s.e.m. of ten mice in each group. Reproduced from Reissmann and Udupa. Effect of inflammation on erythroid precursors (BFU-E and CFU-E) in bone marrow and spleen of mice. *J. Lab. Clin. Med.*, 1978, **92**, 22–29

condition and the erythrocytic cells of most patients with ACD appear to respond normally to EPO *in vitro*. Preliminary studies of stem cells in experimental animals have suggested that important changes occur in the bone marrow and spleens of these animals. Further studies have suggested that this may be due to changes in the hematopoietic microenvironment.

Considerable progress has been made in our understanding of the events leading to the ACD. Methodologic improvements are needed to clarify the alterations in iron metabolism which occur in the ACD. Additional studies of hematopoetic stem cells and regulatory factors will continue to elucidate their role in the ACD.

VI. REFERENCES

1. Block, M. H. (1976). *A Text-Atlas of Hematology*, Lea and Febriger, Philadelphia, p. 607.
2. Cartwright, G. E., and Lee, G. R. (1971). 'The anaemia of chronic disorders', *Br. J. Haemat.*, **21**, 147–151.
3. Cartwright, G. E. (1966). 'The anemia of chronic disorders', *Semin. Hemat.*, **3**, 351–375.
4. Erslev, A. J. (1977). 'Anemia of chronic disorders', in *Hematology*, (Eds. W. J. Williams, E. Beutler, A. J. Erslev and R. W. Rundles), McGraw-Hill Book Company, New York, pp. 434–442.
5. Chernow, B., and Wallner, S. F. (1978). 'Is the anemia of chronic disorders normochromic-normocytic?', *Mil. Med.*, **143**, 345–346.

6. Rodriguez, J. M., and Shahidi, N. T. (1971). 'Erythrocyte 2,3-diphosphoglycerate in adaptive red-cell volume deficiency', *N. Engl. J. Med.*, **285**, 479–482.
7. Douglas, S. W., and Adamson, J. W. (1975). 'The anemia of chronic disorders. Studies of marrow regulation and iron metabolism', *Blood*, **45**, 58–65.
8. Wallner, S. F., Kurnick J. E., Vautrin, R. M., White, M. J., Chapman, R. G., and Ward, H. P. (1977). 'Levels of erythropoietin in patients with the anemia of chronic diseases and liver failure', *Am. J. Hemat.*, **3**, 37–44.
9. Yuile, C. L., Bly, C. G., Steward, W. B., Izzo, A. J., Wells, J. C., and Whipple, G. H. (1949). 'Plasma and red cell radioiron following intravenous injection. Turpentine abscesses in normal and anemic dogs', *J. Exp. Med.*, **90**, 273–282.
10. Rigby, P. G., Strasser, H., Emerson, C. P., Betts, A., and Friedell, G. H. (1962). 'Studies in the anemia of inflammatory states. 1. Erythrocyte survival in dogs with acute and chronic turpentine abscess', *J. Lab. Clin. Med.*, **59**, 244–248.
11. Zucker, S., and Lysek, R. (1974). 'Bone marrow erythropoiesis in anemia of inflammation', *J. Lab. Clin. Med.*, **84**, 620–631.
12. Gutnisky, A., and Van Dyke, D. (1963). 'Normal response to erythropoietin or hypoxia in rats made anemic with turpentine abscess', *Proc. Soc. Exp. Biol. Med.*, **112**, 75–78.
13. Reissmann, K. R., and Udupa, K. B. (1978). 'Effect of inflammation on erythroid precursors (BFU-E and CFU-E) in bone marrow and spleen of mice', *J. Lab. Clin Med.*, **92**, 22–29.
14. Lukens, J. N., Cartwright, G. E., and Wintrobe, M. M. (1967). 'Anemia of adjuvant induced inflammation in rats', *Proc. Soc. Exp. Biol. Med.*, **126**, 346–349.
15. Mikolajew, M., Kurantniska, Z., Kossakowska, M., Plachecka, M., and Kopec, M. (1969). 'Haematological changes in adjuvant disease in the rat', *Ann. Rheum. Dis.*, **28**, 172–179.
16. Werts, E. D., Gibson, D. P., and DeGowin, R. L. (1979). 'Chronic inflammation suppresses bone marrow stromal cells and medullary erythropoiesis', *J. Lab. Clin. Med.*, **93**, 995–1003.
17. DeGowin, R. L., Grund, F. M., and Gibson, D. P. (1978). 'Erythropoietic insufficiency in mice with extramedullary tumor', *Blood*, **51**, 33–43.
18. DeGowin, R. L., and Gibson, D. P. (1978). 'Suppressive effects of an extramedullary tumor on bone marrow erythropoiesis and stroma', *Exp. Hemat.*, **6**, 568–575.
19. DeGowin, R. L., and Gibson, D. P. (1979). 'Erythropoietin and the anemia of mice bearing extramedullary tumors', *J. Lab. Clin. Med.*, **94**, 303–311.
20. Edwards, C. O., Deiss, A., Cole, B. C., and Ward, J. R. (1975). Hematologic changes in chronic arthritis of mice induced by mycoplasma arthritides', *Proc. Soc. Exp. Biol. Med.*, **150**, 664–668.
21. Zucker, S., Lysik, R. M., and DiStefano, J. (1977). 'Pathogenesis of anemia in rats with Walker 256 carcinosarcoma', *J. Lab. Clin. Med.*, **90**, 502–511.
22. Lamar, C., Green, A. S., and Green, W. B. (1979). 'Host-tumor interactions: Basis for the anemia in rats bearing the hepatoma 7777', *Am. J. Hemat.*, **7**, 127–135.
23. Hyman, G. A. (1954). 'Studies on anemia of disseminated malignant neoplastic disease. I. The hemolytic factor', *Blood*, **9**, 911–919.
24. Hyman, G. A., Gellhorn, A., and Harvey, J. L. (1956). 'Studies on the anemia of disseminated malignant neoplastic disease. II. Study of the life span of the erythrocyte', *Blood*, **11**, 618–631.
25. Alexander, W. R. M., Richmond, J., Roy, L. M. H., and Duthie, J. J. R. (1956). 'Nature of anaemia in rheumatoid arthritis. II. Survival of transfused erythrocytes in patients with rheumatoid arthritis', *Ann. Rheum. Dis.*, **15**, 12–20.

26. O'Shea, M. J., Kershenolich, D., and Tavill, A. S. (1973). 'Effects of inflammation on iron and transferrin metabolism', *Brit. J. Haemat.*, **25**, 707–714.
27. Hershko, C., Cook, J. D., and Finch, C. A. (1974). 'Storage iron kinetics. VI. The effect of inflammation on iron exchange in the rat', *Brit. J. Haemat.*, **28**, 67–75.
28. Haurani, F. I., Green, D., and Yound, K. (1965). 'Iron absorption in hyporferremia', *Am. J. Med. Sci.*, **249**, 537–547.
29. Freireich, E. J., Miller, A., Emerson, C. P., and Ross, J. F. (1957). 'The effect of inflammation on the utilization of erythrocyte and transferrin bound radioiron for red cell production', *Blood*, **12**, 972–983.
30. Weinstein, I. M. (1959). 'A correlative study of the erythrokinetics and disturbances in iron metabolism associated with the anemia of rheumatoid arthritis', *Blood*, **14**, 950–966.
31. Noyes, W. D., Bothwell, T. M., and Finch, C. A. (1960). 'The role of the reticuloendothelial cell in iron metabolism', *Brit. J. Haemat.*, **6**, 43–55.
32. Haurani, F. I., Burke, W., and Martinez, E. J. (1965). 'Effective reutilization of iron in the anemia of inflammation', *J. Lab. Clin. Med.*, **65**, 560–570.
33. Wintrobe, M. M., Grinstein, M., Dubash, J. J., Humphreys, S. R., Ashenbrucker, H., and Worth, W. (1947). 'The anemia of infection. VI. The influence of cobalt on the anemia associated with inflammation', *Blood*, **2**, 323–331.
34. Beamish, M. R., Davies, A. G., Eakins, J. D., Jacobs, A., and Trevett, D. (1971). 'The measurement of reticuloendothelial iron release using iron-dextran', *Brit. J. Haemat.*, **21**, 617–622.
35. Kumar, R. (1974). 'Ferrokinetic studies. Red cell iron utilization and red cell iron turnover in the anaemia of chronic infection', *Indian J. Med. Res.*, **62**, 53–64.
36. Bennett, R. M., Holt, P. J. L., and Leurs, S. M. (1974). 'Role of the reticuloendothelial system in the anaemia of rheumatoid arthritis', *Ann. Rheum. Dis.*, **33**, 147–152.
37. Williams, P., Cavill, I., and Kanakakorn, K. (1974). 'Iron kinetics and the anaemia of rhematoid arthritis', *Rheumatol. Rehab.*, **13**, 17–20.
38. Cavill, I., Ricketts, C., and Napier, J. A. F. (1977). 'Erythropoiesis in the anaemia of chronic disease', *Scand. J. Haemat.*, **19**, 509–512.
39. Dinant, H. J., and deMaat, C. E. M. (1978). 'Erythropoiesis and mean red cell lifespan in normal subjects and in patients with the anaemia of active rheumatoid arthritis', *Brit. J. Haemat.*, **39**, 437–444.
40. Haurani, F. I., and O'Brien, R. (1973). 'The erythropoietic effect of a reticuloendothelial blocking agent', *J. Reticuloendothelial. Soc.*, **13**, 126–133.
41. Zarabi, M. H., Lysik, R., DiStefano, J., and Zucker, S. (1977). 'The anaemia of chronic disorders: studies of iron reutilization in the anaemia of experimental malignancy and chronic inflammation', *Brit. J. Haemat.*, **35**, 647–658.
42. Sanchez-Mandel, L., Duarte, L., and Labardini, J. (1970). 'Hemolysis and erythropoiesis. VI. A comparative study of the utilization of hemoglobin iron and transferrin iron by the erythropoietic tissue', *Blood*, **35**, 721–726.
43. Ward, H. P., Gordon, B., and Pickett, J. C. (1969). 'Serum levels of erythropoietin in rheumatoid arthritis', *J. Lab. Clin. Med.*, **74**, 93–97.
44. Ward, H. P., Kurnick, J. E., and Pisaczyk, M. J. (1971). 'Serum level of erythropoietin in anemias associated with chronic infection, malignancy, and primary hematopoietic disease', *J. Clin. Invest.*, **50**, 332–335.
45. Firat, D., and Banzon, J. (1971). 'Erythropoietic effect of plasma from patients with advanced cancer', *Cancer Res.*, **32**, 1353–1359.
46. Zucker, S., Freidman, S., and Lysik, R. M. (1974). 'Bone marrow erythropoiesis in the anemia of infection, inflammation, and malignancy', *J. Clin. Invest.*, **53**, 1132–1138.

47. Mahmood, T., Robinson, W. A., Kurnick, J. E., and Vautrin, R. (1977). 'Granulopoietic and erythropoietic activity in patients with anemias of iron deficiency and chronic disease', *Blood,* **50**, 449–455.
48. Lukens, J. N. (1973). 'Control of erythropoiesis in rats with adjuvant induced chronic inflammation', *Blood,* **41**, 37–44.
49. Kazal, L. A., Erslev, A. J., Miller, O. P., and Abardoo, K. J. R. (1972). 'Inhibition of erythropoietin by lipid extracts of kidney and other tissues', *Ann. Clin. Lab. Sci.,* **2**, 209–216.
50. Kurnick, J. E., Ward, H. P., and Pickett, J. C. (1972). 'Mechanism of the anemia of chronic disorders', *Arch. Int. Med.,* **130**, 323–326.
51. Balsam, A., and Ingbar, S. H. (1979). 'Observations on the factors that control the generation of triodothyronine from thyroxine in rat liver and the nature of the defect induced by fasting', *J. Clin. Invest.,* **63**, 1145–1156.
52. Caro, J., Silver, R., Erslev, A. J., Miller, O. P., and Birgegard, G. (1981). 'Erythropoietin production in fasted rats. Effects of thyroid hormones and glucose supplementation', *J. Lab. Clin. Med.,* **98**, 860–868.
53. Chopra, I. J., Solomon, D., Hepner, G. W., and Morgenstein, A. (1979). 'Misleading low free thyroxine index and usefulness of reverse triiodothyronine measurements in nonthyroidal illness', *Ann. Intern. Med.,* **90**, 905–912.
54. Wallner, S. F., Kurnick, J. E., Ward, H. P., Vautrin, R., and Alfrey, A. C. (1976). 'The anemia of chronic renal failure and chronic diseases: *in vitro* studies of erythropoiesis', *Blood,* **47**, 561–569.
55. Wallner, S. F., and Vautrin, R. M. (1981). 'Evidence that inhibition of erythropoiesis is important in the anemia of chronic renal failure', *J. Lab. Clin. Med.,* **97**, 170–178.
56. Reeves, W. B., Fairman, R. M., and Maurani, F. I. (1981). 'Influence of hormones on the release of iron by macrophages', *J. Reticuloendothelial. Soc.,* **29**, 173–179.
57. Zucker, S., Michael, M. S., Lysik, R. M., Glucksman, M. J., Reese, J., Rudin, A., and DiStefano, J. (1979). 'Lipoprotein inhibitor of bone marrow cells in tumor-bearing rats', *Cell Tissue Kinet.,* **12**, 393–404.
58. Zucker, S., Lysik, R. M., Chikkappa, G., Glucksman, M. J., Gomez-Reino, J., and DiStefano, J. F. (1980). 'Very low density lipoprotein hematopoiesis inhibitor from rat plasma', *Exp. Hemat.,* **8**, 895–905.
59. Zucker, S., Lysik, R. M., and DiStefano, J. F. (1980). 'Cancer cell inhibition of erythropoiesis'. *J. Lab. Clin. Med.,* **96**, 770–782.
60. Herman, S. P., Golde, D. W., and Cline, M. J. (1978). 'Neutrophil products that inhibit cell proliferation: relation to granulocytic "Chalone" ', *Blood,* **51**, 207–219.
61. Zucker, S., Lysik, R., and Friedman, S. (1976). 'Diminished bone marrow responsiveness to erythropoietin in myelophthisic anemia', *Cancer,* **37**, 1308–1315.
62. Hotta, T., Hirabayashi, N., Utsumi, M., Murate, T., and Yamada, H. (1980). 'Age-related changes in the function of hemopoietic stroma in mice', *Exp. Hemat.,* **8**, 933–936.
63. Harrison, D. E. (1975). 'Defective erythropoietic responses of aged mice not improved by young marrow', *J. Geront.,* **30**, 286–288.
64. Dexter, T. M., Testa, N. G., Allen, T. D., Rutherford, T., and Scolnick, E. (1981). 'Molecular and cell biologic aspects of erythropoiesis in long-term bone marrow cultures', *Blood,* **58**, 699–707.
65. Gibson, D. T., DeGowin, R. L., and Knapp, S. A. (1982). 'Effect of X-irradiation on release of prostaglandin E from marrow stromal cells in culture', *Radiat. Res.,* **89**, 537–545.

Current Concepts in Erythropoiesis
Edited by C. D. R. Dunn
© 1983 John Wiley & Sons Ltd.

CHAPTER 10

The role of protein and other nutritional factors in the regulation of erythropoiesis

WALTER FRIED* and ATHANASIUS ANAGNOSTOU†
*Michael Reese Hospital and Medical Center, Chicago, Illinois
†University of Illinois at the Medical Center, Chicago, Illinois

CONTENTS

I. INTRODUCTION

Synthesis of the numerous essential proteins required for the various specialized function of human organ systems requires a constant ingestion of

233

complete proteins capable of supplying an adequate amount of all of the essential amino acids. Decrease of total protein intake or ingestion of qualitatively inferior proteins with resultant deficiency in one or more essential amino acids can lead to impairment of synthesis of specific proteins that in turn result in impairment of various organ systems. Several investigators have proposed that the various proteins are assigned priorities by the organism (1,2) and therefore their vulnerability to the affects of protein deprivation differ. Stated differently, when the supply of one or more amino acids is insufficient, these will be diverted preferentially towards synthesis of high priority proteins at the expense of others. The hematopoietic system is predictably sensitive to the consequences of protein deprivation since the constant turnover of hematopoietic cells requires continuous cell proliferation, differentiation, and maturation as well as production of the regulating polypeptide hormone, erythropoietin (EPO).

Protein deprivation is a common occurrence in underdeveloped countries, among refugee populations, and among prisoners whose access to quantitatively and qualitatively adequate sources of protein is limited. It may also be prevalent among persons with chronic illnesses (particularly neoplasms) who are anorexic, yet have an increased demand for proteins to satisfy the appetites of tumors and also the needs of the host defense mechanisms. Hematologic abnormalities, particularly anemia, are common in these populations.

However, the exact causative role of protein deprivation is usually difficult to dissect out since infections, various other nutritional deficiencies, and hormonal deficiencies, also contribute to the pathogenesis of the anemia.

In this chapter we review the current state of knowledge regarding the effects of protein deprivation on erythropoiesis.

II. CHARACTERISTICS OF THE ANEMIA OF PROTEIN DEFICIENCY

Anemia has been recognized as a consistent occurrence in patients with Kwashiorkor (3–7). Although protein deprivation contributes to this anemia, as evidenced by improvement after high protein feedings, other nutritional deficiencies (i.e., carbohydrates, vitamins, and minerals) may also contribute. Accordingly, the characteristics of pure protein deprivation anemia in humans are not clearly definable. A study in rhesus monkeys deprived selectively of proteins (8) suggests that the anemia is normocytic, normochronic, and non-regnerative. The anemia in these studies was associated with a low serum iron and TIBC, a low total protein (with a low serum albumin but high γ globulin fraction), and a reduced rate of ^{59}Fe absorption. The percentage saturation of transferrin is usually normal or high as is the serum iron in protein depleted humans. In rats (9,10), protein deprivation causes decreases in the plasma iron turnover; in the rate of ^{59}Fe incorporation into the red blood cells

(RBC); and in the red cell mass (RCM). The reticulocyte count is lower than expected for a normal response to anemia but increases in response to hypoxic stimulation. Bone marrow erythrocytic hypoplasia has been described in children both during protein deprivation and transiently during protein repletion (5,11).

III. PATHOGENESIS

A. Regulation of erythropoiesis

According to current concepts on the regulation of erythropoiesis (12,13; see also Chapter 1) the primary factor is the circulating titer of EPO, a glycoprotein produced primarily by the kidneys of adult animals. In fetal and neonatal life, the liver is the principal site of EPO production. The liver retains the capability of producing EPO into adulthood. However, it does so at only a fraction of that of the kidneys; it is unclear whether any EPO is being regularly produced by the liver of adult animals in the presence of functioning kidneys.

EPO production is regulated primarily by the demands of the producing cells for O_2 relative to the rate at which O_2 is supplied. Other factors also modulate this function, but will not be discussed here.

The principal targets for the action of EPO are the EPO-responsive cells—committed erythrocytic precursor cells found in the bone marrow of humans, and in both marrow and spleen of rodents. EPO triggers these cells to complete the maturation process into mature erythrocytes. This involves both DNA synthesis with consequent cell division and production of the protein which is essential for the erythrocytes' prime function of O_2 storage and delivery: i.e., hemoglobin. The rate of erythropoiesis, accordingly, is determined by the plasma titer of EPO and by the number and functional integrity of the precursor cells in the marrow.

The provision of an adequate number of 'late' precursor cells (CFU-E) depends on the existence of an adequate supply of hematopoietic precursors and of the various humoral and microenvironmental factors required for them to both proliferate and differentiate. Since the CFU-E compartment consists of cells incapable of significant self-replication, it is probably not capable of maintaining itself for prolonged periods of time, particularly when there are frequent demands for expansion of the compartment or increased pressures for maturation. The precursor cells capable of maturing into CFU-E and therefore responsible for feeding new cells into the CFU-E compartment are called BFU-E (burst-forming unit), a name descriptive of its tissue culture characteristics. The BFU-E compartment consists of erythrocytic committed progenitors, a smaller percentage of which are in cell cycle at any given time; which are relatively insensitive to EPO; and which may enter the circulation, where they are found as well as in the bone marrow. The forces which influence maturation of BFU-E to CFU-E are not clearly understood but this process is dependent on factors other than EPO, including substances secreted by monocytes and T-lymphocytes. The characteristics of the more mature BFU-E approach more and more those of CFU-E with regard to responsiveness to EPO, increased cell density, increased proliferative fraction, and decreased ability to traverse the marrow sinusoids and enter the circulating blood. The properties of the more primitive populations of BFU-E, on the other hand, approach those of the pluripotential stem cells, the CFU-S (colony-forming units—spleen; a name based on their ability to produce discrete, hematopoietic colonies in the spleens of irradiated mice), which are more buoyant, contain a very small proliferative fraction, are unresponsive to EPO, are found in the bloodstream as well as in hematopoietic tissues, and are capable of differentiating into erythrocytic progenitors (to become primitive BFU-E) but also into progenitor cells of the granulocyte–macrophage series or of the megakaryocytes. Proliferation and differentiation of CFU-S depends on interactions with cells in the hematopoietic microenvironment and on the structural and functional integrity of fixed stromal elements in hematopoietic sites.

Maturation of CFU-E into erythrocytes is dependent, not only on EPO but also on an adequate supply of B_{12} and folate to permit cell division and of iron for hemoglobin synthesis.

The normally constructed erythrocyte survives approximately 110–120 days in a healthy human circulatory system. Abnormalities in the lipid and protein components of the erythrocyte membrane, the enzymes necessary to prevent oxidation of erythrocyte proteins and to generate energy for its metabolic process, or of the hemoglobin, can shorten the survival of the erythrocyte. Also abnormalities in the chemical composition of the plasma, or of the vessels and organs through which blood flows, can traumatize the erythrocytes and shorten their survival. Protein deprivation affects all of the various processes involved in the production of erythrocytes and their normal survival.

B. Effect of protein deprivation on erythropoietin production

Bethard et al (14) showed that the rate of ^{59}Fe incorporation declines in protein deprived rats, and Fried et al (15) demonstrated that moderately starved rats have an increased sensitivity to exogenous EPO, although this sensitivity declines as the period of starvation becomes more prolonged. Fried et al (15) concluded, on this basis, that an early response to starvation is a decline in the rate of EPO production and speculated that this is caused by a reduction in the rats' rate of O_2 utilization. Reissmann in a classic series of experiments showed that rats fed a diet deficient only in protein have a decrease in their rate of erythropoiesis (9), and produce less EPO in response to hypoxia than rats fed a normal diet. However, rats responded normally to exogenous EPO (16), even after prolonged protein deprivation (10). Reissmann concluded that protein deprivation results in a decrease in EPO production, whereas hemoglobin synthesis is unaffected in the presence of adequate EPO. This conclusion is in accord with the concept of Whipple *et al* (1) that protein caloric deprivation results in a decrease in the production of some proteins while the synthesis rate of other essential proteins is preserved on a priority basis. High priority is given to hemoglobin synthesis, whereas the synthesis of albumin and transferrin is given lower priority. The studies by Reissmann showed that the synthesis of EPO is also lower in the priority scale of rats.

In humans, there is also compelling evidence that EPO synthesis declines in response to protein deprivation. The sensitivity of the synthetic rate of EPO to changes in the amount of protein ingested was shown in three normal individuals fed for eight days a diet containing 17% of the recommended daily protein requirements (17). At the end of this short period, the 24-hr urinary EPO excretion and the reticulocyte response to phlebotomy were significantly depressed. Since a small decrease in total caloric intake also occurred, one cannot ascertain that the erythrocytic depression was due only to protein deprivation *per se* and not to the moderate restriction in total caloric intake. The changes observed were not large enough to be of clinical importance in healthy individuals, but they may acquire special significance in patients with already compromised erythropoiesis.

Anagnostou *et al* (18–20) reported on the results of a series of studies designed to further characterize the manner in which protein deprivation effects EPO production in rats and demonstrated the exquisite dependence of EPO production in rats on a continuous supply of dietary proteins. Rats fed diets, containing as much as 60% of the recommended amount of protein produced significantly less EPO in response to hypoxia than did those fed normal diets; and those fed protein-free diets for only one day prior to hypoxic exposure produced less EPO than did normally fed controls. Additionally, rats fed a protein-free diet for six days produced as much EPO as normally fed ones if they received a single bolus protein feeding immediately prior to being exposed to hypoxia for 7 hr. Even if they were given the protein 4 hr after initiating the hypoxic stimulus, they produced significantly more EPO during the subsequent 3 hr of hypoxia than did controls which received saline rather than the protein feeding. Although the rate of O_2 consumption declined significantly in protein-deprived rats and again returned to normal on refeeding proteins, these changes did not occur nearly as rapidly as did the changes in EPO production (18). Accordingly, the effect of protein deprivation on EPO production seemed independent of its effects on O_2 utilization and is more likely due to the dependence of EPO synthesis on amino acids derived from dietary sources of protein. Anagnostou *et al* (19) also demonstrated that feeding protein-deprived rats with suspensions containing single amino acids, partially corrected their inability to synthesize EPO in response to hypoxia. Most effective were the amino acids methionine and cystine. The significance of this observation is presently unclear. Another interesting observation regarding the effect of protein deprivation on EPO production is that of Lucarelli *et al* (21) that EPO production in neonatal rats is not influenced by protein deprivation. Since EPO production in these animals is predominantly of extra-renal origin, this suggested that extra-renal sites of EPO production are not as directly dependent on amino acids derived from dietary protein intake as are the kidneys. This suggestion was confirmed by Anagnostou *et al* (19), who showed that EPO production in anephric rats is not decreased by protein deprivation. This is not surprising in view of the special role of the liver in amino acid metabolism.

In concluding this discussion of the effects of protein deprivation on EPO synthesis, we must re-emphasize that EPO synthesis is only relatively suppressed and not irreversibly shut off by even severe protein deprivation. Increase in the intensity of the hypoxic stimulus (16), or the administration of cobaltous chloride (22) and/or androgens (23), (substances known to enhance endogenous EPO production) have been shown to increase EPO production and/or erythropoiesis in experimental animals and also in children with Kwashiorkor (23). This emphasizes the probability that the priority assigned by the organism for sparing the synthesis of specific essential proteins during protein-deprived states is a dynamic one and is influenced by increased demands for that protein (2).

C. Effects of protein deprivation on hematopoietic progenitor cells and the marrow microenvironment

Fried *et al* (15) observed that the response of starved rats to EPO decreases as the period of starvation is prolonged. Naets and Wittek (24) reported that starved polycythemic rats are less responsive to EPO than are normally fed polycythemic ones. There are, however, conflicting data on the responsiveness of protein-deprived rats to EPO. Whereas Reissmann *et al* (16) found this to be unimpaired, Giglio *et al* (25) and Alippi *et al* (26) reported it to be markedly decreased, although not as severely so as in starved rats. Fondu *et al* (27) also reported that in humans with protein-energy malnutrition the responsiveness of the bone marrow to EPO was impaired.

Furthermore, Alippi *et al* (26) showed that the ability of rats to respond to EPO is dependent not only on the quantity of ingested protein but also on its quality. When the dietary protein consisted of casein or egg yolk, less was required to enable a maximum responsiveness to EPO than when it consisted of wheat gluten or corn protein. The effects of feeding diets deficient in only one or more essential amino acids on erythropoiesis, and the effects of feeding single amino acids on the erythrocytic response of protein-deprived animals to hypoxic stimuli or to anemia has been extensively studied by Whipple and his co-workers (1) and also by Aschkenasy (28). These numerous studies and their conclusions cannot be individually decribed here. In summary, however, they indicate that some individual amino acids can ameliorate the erythrocytic defect caused by protein deprivation to a greater or lesser extent. However, complete restoration of erythrocytic function requires ingestion of adequate amounts of all of the essential amino acids. Fried et al (29) have shown that prolonged feeding of diets with little or no protein content to mice resulted in a decrease in the platelet and lymphocyte count as well as the hematocrit, suggesting that protein deprivation may affect the pluripotential hematopoietic stem cells or CFU-S.

These authors showed that the number of pluripotential hematopoietic stem cells (CFU-S) in the protein-depleted mouse spleens decline shortly after initiating the deficient diet, whereas CFU-S in the bone marrow declined only after prolonged and severe protein deprivation. Bell et al (30) reported similar results in newborn mice. Also, the rate of regeneration of CFU-S following irradiation-induced damage is slower in protein-depleted mice than in those on a complete diet (29). These findings may help to explain the clinical observation that patients undergoing chemotherapy for neoplasms have less severe and less prolonged hematopoietic suppression if their protein intake is maintained by parenteral hyperalimentation.

Pololi-Anagnostou et al (31) showed that mice fed a protein-free diet for six days have a decreased number of CFU-E and of BFU-E in their femoral marrow. The decreased number of CFU-E could be secondary to the decrease in EPO titers of protein-deprived animals, since the size of this cell population is correlated with and dependent upon the plasma EPO titer. However, BFU-E are relatively independent of plasma EPO titers and consequently the decrease in the numbers of these cells is more likely to reflect a direct effect of protein deprivation. It is interesting that the BFU-E decline occurred at a time when there was no decrease of the CFU-S concentration.

Although no definitive evidence exists to demonstrate a protein-related defect in the hematopoietic microenvironment which is essential to promote maximum proliferation and differentiation of hematopoietic progenitors, morphologic studies suggest that such functional changes may exist. About 50% of the volume of the marrow in normal individuals is occupied by fat cells (32). The general opinion about its function is that it is a passive space filler expanding in times of depressed hematopoiesis and shrinking when hematopoiesis is enhanced (33,34). Early studies in starved experimental animals concluded that marrow fat is storage fat, and thus its absolute quantity decreases during starvation (35). After 25 days of complete starvation the marrow of rabbits is replaced by a gelatinous mass (36). Cohen and Gardner (37) made a distinction between the distal or yellow marrow fat and the proximal or red marrow fat. Whereas the first was unaffected in starvation, the second was mobilized in a similar way to the extramedullary fat. Tavassoli (38) found no mobilization of the distal marrow fat in acute starvation and raised the speculation that it has a different function from the extramedullary fat which has an active role in the regulation of hematopoiesis. A recent study in rabbits (39) starved for two weeks concluded that despite a severe decrease in body weight there was no change in the volume, the number, or the esterification capacity of the marrow fat cells. The hypothesis that marrow fat does not follow changes in the animal total body energy requirements, but has an active role in the control of hematopoiesis, has recently received additional support from the finding that in long term *in vitro* cultures of marrow cells, fat cells constitute an essential part of the microenvironment supporting the hematopoietic process (40).

D. Effect of protein deprivation on red blood cell survival

RBC survival is decreased in protein-depleted rats (41) and in children with Kwashiorkor (42). This phenomenon has been ascribed to alterations in the RBC membrane lipids (43), lowering of intracellular ATP levels (44), or extracorpuscular factors (42,45). Lanzkowsky *et al* (42) found the RBC survival to be considerably reduced in children with protein malnutrition and ascribed it to both corpuscular and extra-corpuscular factors. An improvement in half-life of RBC was seen following protein feeding, leading the authors to speculate that protein deficiency was the main factor responsible for the shortened RBC survival. Hemolysis becomes apparent only as protein deprivation is prolonged in experimental animals. This has been associated with an increase in the rate of erythropoiesis in spite of a continued slow decline in the RCM. The increase in erythropoiesis associated with hemolysis in rats on protein-depleted diets for prolonged periods of time may be due to the increased availability of amino acids from the increased turnover of hemoglobin; or to the direct effects of hemolysates on erythropoiesis or EPO production. In humans and experimental animals, the hemolysis which occurs in association with protein depletion is probably not of primary importance in the etiology of the anemia.

E. Other changes secondary to protein deprivation which impact on erythropoiesis

With severe and prolonged protein deprivation, the rate of iron absorption from the intestine declines. The exact cause of this defect is unclear but may be attributed to the lack of amino acids which enhance iron absorption from the intestinal lumen (46), to a deficiency of apoferritin in the intestinal wall, or to a decline in the serum transferrin level (1,47). This decrease in iron absorption is rarely severe and not likely to contribute significantly to the anemia of patients, since the serum iron level of protein-deprived humans is usually high or normal as is the storage iron level. Changes in the plasma volume occur frequently in patients with severe protein deprivation (6). This is probably related to diffusion of plasma into the extravascular space and consequent contraction of the plasma volume which is associated with hypoalbuminemia. With protein refeeding, a rapid rise in the serum albumin may cause an early expansion of the plasma volume which may mask the increase in the RCM (10,48).

IV. THE ROLE OF CARBOHYDRATES

Patients with anorexia nervosa primarily develop deficiency of carbohydrates and calories. The serum albumin, an early indicator of protein deficiency, usually remains near the normal level. Despite the strong interest of western medicine in this peculiar clinical entity, little has been written about hematological abnormalities in this condition, a fact indicative perhaps of the infrequency of such abnormalities. Only few of the patients have a mild or moderate anemia (49,50) and a hypoplastic bone marrow in which the fat has been replaced by a gelatinous ground substance, probably acid mucopolysaccharide (49,51). A more distinctive feature is the frequent finding in the peripheral blood smear of numerous acanthocytes (52) related perhaps to low levels of β-lipoproteins.

Caro *et al* (53) reported recently that rats fasted for 48 hr have decreased post-hypoxic renal and extra-renal EPO levels with recovery of the EPO titers to normal levels when the fasted animals were given 25% glucose in drinking water. These authors concluded that;
1. A caloric deficiency was the cause of the decreased plasma EPO levels, and
2. This effect was mediated by a decreased serum T3 level and decreased responsiveness of EPO production to T3.

In our own studies in much younger and only protein-deprived rats, a single feeding of glucose produced only a small increase in renal EPO production (18). The discrepancies between these experimental results may be explained by differences in the effects of total nutritional deprivation as compared to selective protein deprivation. These observations warrant further study.

V. WATER DEPRIVATION AND ERYTHROPOIESIS

It has long been known that water deprivation depresses erythropoiesis (54,55). In fact, one of the earlier bioassays for the measurement of EPO utilized dehydrated rats as assay animals (54). The underlying mechanism for the observed depression of erythropoiesis was thought to be a decrease in endogenous EPO production (55). Later studies concluded that water deprivation is invariably associated with decreased food intake (25,26) and thus the response of dehydrated rats to a stimulus for endogenous EPO production or to the administration of exogenous EPO is indistinguishable from that of starved animals, i.e., is diminished. Similarly, both late (CFU-E) and early (BFU-E) erythrocytic precursor cells are decreased in the marrow and spleen of dehydrated mice (56), an effect also thought to be due mainly to reduced protein intake. However, further experiments are required to ascertain whether dehydration *per se* influences erythropoiesis.

VI. CORRECTION OF PROTEIN DEFICIENCY

Although the correction of all hematopoietic abnormalities caused by protein deprivation is best achieved by feeding adequate amounts of high quality proteins (animal proteins with a complete amino acid content), amelioration of the anemia can also be accomplished by administration of substances such as thyroxine (53), androgenic steroids (23), and cobaltous chloride (22), which increase endogenous EPO production.

VII. REFERENCES

1. Whipple, G. H. (1956). *The Dynamic Equilibrium of Body Proteins*, Charles C. Thomas, Springfield, Ill.
2. Waterlow, J. C. (1968). 'Observations on the mechanism of adaptation to low protein intakes', *Lancet,* **ii**, 1091–1097.
3. Altmann, A., and Murray, J. F. (1948). 'The anaemia of malignant malnutrition (infantile pellagra, Kwashiorkor): Protein deficiency as a possible aetological factor', *S. African J. Med. Sci.,* **13**, 91.
4. Walt, F., Taylor, J. E. D., and Robertson, L. (1961). 'The anaemias in Kwashiorkor', *Med. Proc.,* **7**, 47.
5. Neame, P. B., and Simson, J. C., (1964). 'Acute transitory erythroblastopenia in Kwashiorkor', *S. African J. Lab. Clin. Med.,* **10**, 27.
6. Adams, E. B. (1970). 'Anemia associated with protein deficiency', *Semin. Hemat.,* **7**, 55–66.
7. Finch, C. A. (1975). 'Erythropoiesis in protein-caloric malnutrition', in *Protein-Caloric Malnutrition*, Little, Brown & Co., Boston, pp. 247–256.
8. Sood, S. K., Deo, M. G., and Ramalingaswami, V. (1965). 'Experimental protein deficiency: Pathological features in the rhesus monkey', *Arch. Path. (Chicago)*, **80**, 14–23.
9. Reissmann, K. R. (1964). 'Protein metabolism and erythropoiesis. I. The anemia of protein deprivation', *Blood,* **23**, 137–145.
10. Ito, K., and Reissmann, K. R. (1966). 'Quantitative and qualitative aspects of steady state erythropoiesis induced in protein-starved rats by long-term erythropoietin injection', *Blood,* **27**, 343–351.
11. Allen, D. M., and Dean, R. F. A. (1965). 'The anaemia of Kwashiorkor in Uganda', *Trans. Royal Soc. Trsp. Med. Hyg.,* **59**, 326–341.
12. Zanjani, E. D., and Kaplan, M. E. (1979). 'Cell-cell interactions in erythropoiesis', in *Progress in Hematology*, (Ed. E. Brown), Grune and Stratton, New York, pp. 173–191.
13. Peschle, C. (1980). 'Erythropoiesis', *Ann. Rev. Med.,* **31**, 303–314.

14. Bethard, W. F., Wissler, R. W., Thompson, J. S., Schroeder, M. A., and Robson, M. J. (1958). 'The effect of acute protein deprivation upon erythropoiesis in rats', *Blood*, **13**, 216–225.

15. Fried, W., Plzak, L. F., Jacobson, L. O., and Goldwasser, E. (1957). 'Studies on erythropoiesis. III. Factors controlling erythropoietin production', *Proc. Soc. Exp. Biol. Med.*, **94**, 237–241.

16. Reissmann, K. R. (1964). 'Protein metabolism and erythropoiesis. II. Erythropoietin formation and erythroid responsiveness in protein deprived rats', *Blood*, **23**, 146–153.

17. Catchatourian, R., Eckerling, G., and Fried, W. (1980). 'Effect of short-term protein deprivation on hemopoietic functions of healthy volunteers', *Blood*, **55**, 625–628.

18. Anagnostou, A., Schade, S., Ashkinaz, M., Barone, J., and Fried, W. (1977). 'Effect of protein deprivation on erythropoiesis', *Blood*, **50**, 1093–1097.

19. Anagnostou, A., Schade, S., Barone, J., and Fried, W. (1978). 'Effect of protein deprivation on extrarenal erythropoietin production', *Blood*, **51**, 549–553.

20. Anagnostou, A., Schade, S., and Fried, W. (1978). 'Stimulation of erythropoietin secretion by single amino acids', *Proc. Soc. Exp. Biol. Med.*, **159**, 139–141.

21. Lucarelli, G., Porcellini, A., Carnevali, C., Carmena, A., and Stohlman, F., Jr. (1968). 'Fetal and neonatal erythropoiesis', *Ann. N.Y. Acad. Sci.*, **149**, 544–559.

22. Orten, J. M., and Orten, A. U. (1945). 'The production of polycythemia in rats made anemic by a diet low in protein', *Am. J. Physiol.*, **144**, 464–467.

23. Aschkenasy, A. (1963). 'Etudes sur la production d'erythropoietine cher le rat carence en proteines', *Rev. Fr. Etud. Clin. Biol.*, **8**, 985–999.

24. Naets, J. P., and Wittek, M. (1974). 'Effect of starvation on the response to erythropoietin in the rat', *Acta Haemat.*, **52**, 141–150.

25. Giglio, J. M., Alippi, R. M., Barcelo, A. C., and Bozzini, C. E. (1979). 'Mechanism of the decreased erythropoiesis in the water deprived rat', *Brit. J. Haemat.*, **42**, 93–100.

26. Alippi, R. M., Giglio, J. M., Barcelo, A. C., Bozzini, C. E., Farina, R., and Rio, M. E. (1979). 'Influence of dietary protein concentration and quality on response to erythropoietin in the polycythemic rat', *Brit. J. Haemat.*, **43**, 451–456.

27. Fondu, P., Haga, P., and Halvorsen, S. (1978). 'The regulation of erythropoiesis in protein-energy malnutrition', *Brit. J. Haemat.*, **38**, 29–36.

28. Aschkenasy, A. (1962). 'Inhibition precoce de l'erythropoiese apres privation de divers aeides amines essential cher le rat male', *C.R. Soc. Biol.*, **156**, 1971–1976.

29. Fried, W., Shapiro, S., Barone, J., and Anagnostou, A. (1978). 'Effect of protein deprivation on hematopoietic stem cells and on peripheral blood counts', *J. Lab. Clin. Med.*, **92**, 303–310.

30. Bell, R. G., Hazell, L. A., and Sheridan, J. W. (1976). 'The influence of dietary deficiency on hematopoietic cells in the mouse', *Cell Tissue Kinet.*, **9**, 305–311.

31. Pololi-Anagnostou, A., Schade, S., and Anagnostou, A. (1981). 'The effect of protein deprivation on erythroid stem cell growth', *Int. J. Vitamin and Nutr. Res.*, **51**, 59–63.

32. Rohr, K. (1960). *Das Menschliche Knochenmark*, Georg Thieme Verlag, Stuttgart, pp. 29–43.

33. Ascenzi, A. (1976). 'Physiological relationships and pathological inferences between bone, tissue and marrow', *Biochem. Physiol. of Bone*, **4**, 403–444.

34. Erslev, A. J. (1967). 'Medullary and extramedullary blood formation', *Clin. Orthoped.*, **52**, 25–36.

35. Newlin, H. E., and McCay, C. M. (1948). 'Bone marrow for fat storage in rabbits', *Arch. Biochem.*, **17**, 125–128.

36. Dietz, A. A., and Steinberg, B. (1953). 'Chemistry of bone marrow; VII. Composition of rabbit bone marrow in inanition', *Arch. Biochem.*, **45**, 10–20.
37. Cohen, P., and Gardner, F. H. (1965). 'Effect of massive triamcinolone administration in blunting the erythropoietic response to phenylhydrazine', *J. Lab. Clin. Med.*, **65**, 88–101.
38. Tavassoli, M. (1974). 'Differential response of bone marrow and extramedullary adipose cells to starvation', *Experientia*, **30**, 424–425.
39. Bathija, A., Davis, S., and Trubowitz, S. (1979). 'Bone marrow adipose tissue: Response to acute starvation', *Am. J. Hemat.*, **6**, 191–198.
40. Dexter, T. M. (1979). 'Cell interactions *in vitro*', *Clinics in Hematology*, **8**, 453–468.
41. Delmonte, L., Aschkenasy, A., and Eyquem, A. (1964). 'Studies on the hemolytic nature of protein-deficiency anemia in the rat', *Blood*, **24**, 49–68.
42. Lanzkowsky, P., McKenzie, D., Katz, S., Hoffenberg, R., Friedman, R., and Black, E. (1967). 'Erythrocyte abnormality induced by protein malnutrition', *Brit. J. Haemat.*, **13**, 639–649.
43. Coward, W. A. (1971). 'The erythrocyte membrane in Kwashiorkor', *Brit. J. Nutr.*, **25**, 145–151.
44. Aschkenasy, A., Gajdos-Torok, U., Spach, C., and Gajdos, A. (1969). 'Etude de la privation de proteines alimentaires sur les teneurs erythrocytaires en ATP cher le rat', *C.R. Soc. Biol.*, **163**, 1275.
45. Aschkenasy, A. (1967). 'Nouvelles etudes sur la duree de ire des erythrocytes dans la carence prolongee en proteines. II. Demonstration d'une intervention de facteurs extra-erythrocytaires, dans l'hemolyse *in vivo* chez des rats carences en proteines', *C.R. Soc. Biol.*, **161**, 1925–1928.
46. Kroe, D., Kinney, T. D., Kaufman, N., and Klavins, J. V. (1963). 'The influence of amino acids on iron absorption', *Blood*, **21**, 546–552.
47. Cartwright, G. E., and Wintrobe, M. M. (1948). 'Studies on free erythrocyte protoporphyrin, plasma copper and plasma iron in protein-deficient and iron-deficient swine', *J. Biol. Chem.*, **176**, 571–583.
48. Leonard, P. J., MacWilliams, K. M., and Jones, K. W. (1965). 'The relationship between change in plasma volume, plasma proteins, and hemoglobin concentration during treatment of Kwashiorkor', *Trans. Royal Soc. Trsp. Med. Hyg.*, **59**, 582.
49. Mant, M. J., and Faragher, B. S. (1972). 'The hematology of anorexia nervosa', *Brit. J. Haemat.*, **23**, 737–749.
50. Lampert, F., and Lau, B. (1976). 'Bone marrow hypoplasia in anorexia nervosa', *Eur. J. Pediat.*, **124**, 65–71.
51. Pearson, H. A. (1967). 'Marrow hypoplasia in anorexia nervosa', *J. Pediat.*, **71**, 211–215.
52. Amrein, P. C., Friedman, R., Kosinski, K., and Ellman, L. (1979). 'Hematologic changes in anorexia nervosa', *J. Am. Med. Assoc.*, **24**, 2190–2191.
53. Caro, J., Silver, R., Erslev, A. J., Miller, O. P., and Biregegard, G. (1981). 'Erythropoietin production in fasted rats. Effects of thyroid hormones and glucose supplementation', *J. Lab. Clin. Med.*, **98**, 860–868.
54. Keighley, G., Lowy, P. H., Borsook, H., Goldwasser, E., Gordon, A. S., Prentice, T. C., Rambach, W. A., Stohlman, F., Jr., and Van Dyke, D. C. (1960). 'A cooperative assay of a sample with erythropoietic stimulating activity', *Blood*, **16**, 1424–1432.
55. Kilbridge, T. M., Fried, W., and Heller, P. (1969). 'The mechanisms by which plethora suppresses erythropoiesis', *Blood*, **33**, 104–113.
56. Dunn, C. D. R., and Smith, L. N. (1980). 'The effect of dehydration on erythroid progenitor cells in mice', *Exp. Hemat.*, **8**, 620–625.

Current Concepts in Erythropoiesis
Edited by C. D. R. Dunn

CHAPTER 11

The effect of physical exercise on plasma volume and red blood cell mass

L. Röcker, M. Laniado, and K. Kirsch
Institute of Physiology, Free University of Berlin

CONTENTS

I. INTRODUCTION

Until the sixties, exercise physiology was a field which attracted only a few physiologists and some cardiologists. Their main aim was to explore the ultimate biological limitations of the human body and to help the athletes to improve their performance. However, in the last two decades the interest in physical fitness has increased leading to a greater participation in all sports. Moreover the medical community has become increasingly aware of the fact that some kinds of exercise can be used for medical purposes. To improve the muscular strength during the rehabilitation of the disabled, aerobic and anaerobic short-term exercises are applied. For the prevention of cardiovascular diseases long-term exercise has become very popular (jogging). In the last decade especially, the latter fact has stimulated research in this field of exercise and the hematological studies attracted many investigators. In the course of this kind of research many new facts could be elaborated. It is, however, for a clinician, who is not particularly experienced in this field of physiology, hard to take advantage of all the knowledge which has emerged from the many sometimes very specialized studies. This chapter aims to bring together what we think is the most usable information for clinicians working in the field of hematology. We will concentrate on the effects of short-term and repeatedly performed long-term (endurance) exercise on the blood constituents. Special emphasis will be placed on the differentiation of the various forms of exercise with respect to their effects on the plasma volume (PV) as well as the red blood cell mass (RCM).

The reader must, however, keep in mind that the exercise stimulus not only has effects on the blood constituents. Nearly every system in the organism is involved, especially the thermoregulatory, cardiovascular, and respiratory systems. Blood indeed is an important link within all the above mentioned systems but the changes must always be seen to serve the purposes of the other systems as well.

II. CHANGES OF BLOOD VOLUME IN RESPONSE TO ACUTE PHYSICAL EXERCISE

In contrast to some animals (e.g., dog, cat) (1), humans have no reserve of preformed red blood cells (RBC) which can suddenly be emptied into the intravascular space. Therefore, the RCM cannot change rapidly under acute physical exercise. This observation has been reported by several groups of investigators using chromium-51 labeled autologous RBC to measure RCM (2–8). However, blood volume (BV) is known to change under certain exercise conditions. Because of pores (of an average size of 4 nm) in the capillary membrane, plasma water and small molecules can rapidly be shifted into or out of the intravascular space. Based on the early studies of Starling (9), Landis and Pappenheimer (10) showed that the extracellular fluid distribution depends on the difference of the hydrostatic pressure in the capillaries (P_c) and in the interstitial space (P_i) as well as on the difference of the colloidal osmotic pressure in the capillaries (π_c) and in the interstitial space (π_i). The following equation was given to explain the capillary fluid shift (F) between the intravascular space and the interstitium;

$$F = k(P_c - P_i + \pi_i - \pi_c),$$

where k represents the filtration coefficient. If the value of F is positive, fluid is filtrated and the PV decreases, if it is negative, fluid is absorbed and PV increases.

Under resting conditions filtration and absorption are in an equilibrium resulting in a constant PV. However, this equilibrium can be shifted to a new steady state by exercise.

A. Plasma volume changes after short-term physical exercise (less than 10 min)

To our knowledge no studies have been performed to compare the effect of short-term physical exercise on PV in trained versus untrained subjects. Therefore, the hematological changes in response to acute exercise will be discussed in general.

It is well documented that the PV is diminished 200–600 ml after short-term exercise (2,5,7,11–25). Even a change from the supine to the upright position is associated with a decrease of PV (26–28). However, it has been confirmed that physical exercise itself produces a significant reduction of PV (12,14,17,18,29–31). Due to an augmentation of the capillary pressure and an enlargement of the filtration surface area, fluid is shifted from the intravascular to the interstitial space (32–36). Another factor which is believed to account for the fluid shift is the accumulation of osmotic substances from the anerobic working muscles, e.g., lactic acid, that temporarily might withhold water in the interstitial space (37–39). The augmentation of the capillary pressure is mediated by the increased blood flow through maximally dilated vessels (33). The vasodilatation mainly occurs in the precapillary sphincters and is supposed to be operated by local chemical factors of a hypoxic or metabolic nature, and only to a smaller degree by the activation of the sympathetic nervous system (40). The dilatation of precapillary sphincters increases the distribution of blood flow to previously unperfused capillaries. Thereby the filtration surface expands. Folkow et al (41) demonstrated that the mean muscular venous pressure is lowered during exercise in the upright posture even during situations with maximal blood flow. Most likely this is due to the action of the muscle pump. The capillary pressure rise during exercise appears to be limited effectively by this phenomenon. The tissue hyperosmolality is due to the accumulation of metabolic substances in the working muscles (39). In addition, during exercise blood is diverted to the working muscles. Whereas usually only 15–20% of the cardiac output is diverted to the muscle compartment, this relative distribution may change to 85% during exercise (42). At the same time the cardiac output can increase considerably compared to the resting state which enhances the effectiveness of the above described mechanisms, i.e., transcapillary fluid shifts. These mechanisms overcome the water binding capacity of the intravascular protein mass. However, after normalization of the capillary pressure and after the decrease of the filtration surface area following the cessation of muscular exercise, the colloidal osmotic capacity of the intravascular protein mass is able to bind corresponding amounts of fluid. Thereby the PV returns to pre-exercise values within 30 min (43).

It has been mentioned above that there is no reserve of RBC in the human. On the other hand no noteworthy intravascular hemolysis occurs during short-term exercise. Therefore, the total number of circulating erythrocytes can be considered constant and BV changes are totally due to changes of PV. Since PV is generally diminished a hemoconcentration is usually observed.

Depending on the intensity and duration of exertion, RBC concentration increases have been found. A large rise of the RBC count (24.8%) was found after a sprint of 100 yards, whereas a small increase (8.8%) occurred after a run of two miles (44). These changes as well as those in hematocrit (Hct) and hemoglobin (Hb) concentration are a reflection of the fluid shift from the intravascular space to the interstitium with the resulting PV decrease.

B. Plasma volume changes after long-term physical exercise (more than 1 hr)

Since long-term physical exercise can only be performed by physically active subjects, no data are available for untrained subjects. Whereas in all investigations of short-term exercise a decrease in PV was found, conflicting results have been reported following long-term physical exercise (6,15,21,45–52). Differences in the methodologies may be at least partly responsible for this discrepancy. Due to the complexity of mechanisms involved in the fluid shifts during long-term physical exercise, the environmental temperature and the fluid uptake, for example, have to be considered as parameters greatly influencing the PV. Åstrand and Saltin (6) determined PV (Evans Blue space) on six well-trained subjects before and 1 hr after an 85 km race in cross-country skiing. The PV was increased 11% after exercise. In their study the outdoor temperature was below or just around 0 °C and the athletes ingested in average 2.0 kg of water.

Refsum et al (53) studied Hb concentration, Hct, and a series of serum and blood parameters related to RBC turnover in highly-trained athletes taking part in long-distance cross-country ski races (70 km and 90 km). The subjects were allowed to drink freely during the exercise. However, no information has been given concerning the environmental temperature. The races led to a parallel fall in Hb and Hct. Immediately after exercise Hb concentration was 14.92 g/100 ml whereas the pre-race value was 15.73 g/100 ml ($p < 0.001$). Measurements of serum haptoglobin, iron, and bilirubin as well as total iron binding capacity revealed that exercise-induced intravascular hemolysis was only partly responsible for the significant reduction in Hb concentration. Therefore, this phenomenon was probably due to a PV expansion after prolonged heavy exercise. However, the observations of Refsum et al (53) did not give a true measure of the extent of PV expansion and the possibility discussed in their paper was that the Hb concentration also may have been influenced by transitory changes of the relationship between peripheral and whole-body Hct.

An unchanged PV after long-term exercise has been reported by several investigators (25,48,54). Exercise with low intensity (2 hr walking in the desert) as well as 1 hr of submaximal exercise (67% $\dot{V}_{O_2}$ max) on a bicycle ergometer was not accompanied by a change in PV.

However, in most of the studies dealing with long-term physical exercise a decrease of PV was found (15,25,45,47–52,54). In these investigations no fluid was taken during or immediately after exercise. The PV decreased 5–18%.

From studies in our own laboratory (43) with 13 highly trained endurance athletes the PV decrease amounted to 5.8% immediately after a 32 km race. The decrease, however, was much less than after short-term exercise; 90 min after the end of the exercise period the PV returned to the pre-exercise level. As mentioned above, no fluid was taken during and after the race.

As discussed above, PV changes in short-term exercise are totally due to fluid shifts from the intravascular space to the interstitial space. In contrary more mechanisms are involved in PV changes during long-term exercise; sweat loss, intracellular water liberation due to glycogen combustion, increase in intravascular protein mass, to mention probably the most important. There is some evidence that immediate losses of PV are rapidly made up and often lead to an 'overshoot' several hours after cessation of exercise.

The relationship between these mechanisms is not completely understood. However, some considerations are possible. A well-trained endurance athlete, weighing 70 kg, may store up to 800 g of glycogen in the muscle cells (55). About 2.4 l of intracellular water are bound by 800 g glycogen. Due to the combustion of glycogen during long-term exercise this amount of water leaves the intracellular space (55,56). By osmosis and filtration a considerable amount of plasma water is lost to the active muscles. Simultaneously the interstitial fluid pressure in the working muscles begins to increase and most likely opposes the outward flux of fluid (57). As an effect of work-induced arterial hyperosmolality and reflex adrenergic mechanisms, this fluid loss is partly balanced by the simultaneous absorption of extravascular fluid from the

250 CURRENT CONCEPTS IN ERYTHROPOIESIS

inactive tissues (22). On the other hand, and in contrast to short-term exercise, the homeostatic demand requires sweat production for the temperature regulation. As a result, the BV as an important link in the O_2-transporting system remains relatively constant. The importance of the intravascular protein mass in the regulation of PV has already been noted. The intravascular protein mass undoubtedly contributes to the recovery of PV several hours after exercise. Senay (58) and Senay and Kok (59) were one of the first to suggest that during exercise proteins enter the intravascular space *via* the lymphatics resulting in a fluid uptake into the vascular bed. The importance of plasma proteins for the size of PV was further described by Scatchard *et al* (60) who showed that 1 g of protein is able to bind 14 ml of fluid in the intravascular space. Consistent with the above information, studies in our own laboratory have shown that the intravascular protein mass was increased 90 min after exercise (43). On the basis of the findings of Scatchard *et al* (60) an increased colloidal osmotic force into the intravascular space could be assumed. It seems that a redistribution of some proteins occurs in the vascular bed in response to long-lasting exercise increasing the intravascular protein mass. Due to the water binding capacity of the intravascular protein mass, the intravascular space increases. This mechanism seems to be an important factor for the homeostasis of PV during and after physical exercise and would tend to produce an increase in PV. This mechanism is also an important prerequisite for the neuro-humoral control of PV (Figure 1). According to this concept, described by Gauer and Henry (61), a change of BV is sensed by cardiovascular stretch receptors which transmit this information to the central nervous system. From here two main routes are involved, the ADH mechanism for the control of water, and the sympathetic renin–angiotensin–aldosterone system for the control of sodium. The validity of Gauer's hypothesis has been confirmed under several different physiological conditions. The results of many studies, e.g., dehydration, water immersion, head-down tilting (62–67), provide evidence that in addition to the renin–angiotensin-aldosterone system, ADH is the key hormone for volume control. The antidiuresis during exercise is due to an increased ADH secretion (68–71). The water conserving mechanism of ADH in the intravascular space is of particular importance to the water binding capacity of the intravascular protein mass.

C. Red blood cell changes after long-term physical exercise

In contrast to short-term physical exercise, severe long-lasting exercise is well-known to produce intravascular hemolysis (53,72–75), possibly leading to hemoglobinuria. The question is what are the reasons for this phenomenon? Based on the view of Rous and Robertson (76) that the destruction of erythrocytes is normally accomplished by mechanical fragmentation, Broun (77) proposed that vigorous exercise favors such hemolysis by both the b12

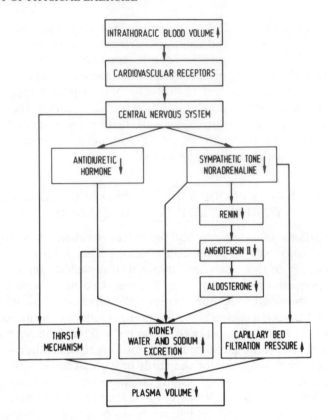

Figure 1. Mechanisms involved in the neuro-humoral control of plasma volume according to the concept of Gauer and Henry (61)

increased rate of blood flow and the violent muscular contraction. However, his studies (77–80) did not present experimental proof to support this hypothesis. A better documented explanation was provided by Davidson (81). He reported that intravascular hemolysis appeared in the soles of the feet of subjects who ran on hard roadways. From experiments with a compressible PVC tube filled with heparinized blood samples and inserted into the runners' shoes, he suggested that mechanical damage of RBC within the microcirculation of the soles of the feet is responsible for the intravascular hemolysis in runners. Such hemolytic changes could be reduced by the use of 'Sorbo'-rubber inner-soles in the shoes (82).

Whereas hemolytic changes are a common feature during or after long-distance runs, hemoglobinuria is seen in only a few subjects. Hemoglobinuria occurs when the Hb binding capacity of plasma, or, specifically, of haptoglobin, is exceeded. Under exercise conditions the so-called exertional (march) hemoglobinuria occasionally appears. According to Davidson (81) and Buckle (82), mechanical destruction is the primary factor causing exertional hemoglobinuria and similar interpretations can be given to other studies where hemoglobinuria was found after karate (83) and conga-drum play (84). In addition, if the erythrocyte membrane has structural defects (85) the mechanical alterations during exercise became of greater importance.

In some instances low haptoglobin levels and disorders of the Hb-binding sites of haptoglobin are also predisposing factors for hemoglobinura (73). However, under normal conditions, exercise induced intravascular hemolysis does not lead to significant hemoglobinuria.

III. ADAPTATION OF BLOOD VOLUME AND RED BLOOD CELL MASS TO REPEATED PHYSICAL EXERCISE

Under conditions of acute physical exercise—whether in well-trained or untrained subjects—the RCM remains constant. This generalization does not necessarily apply to those subjects involved in repeated exercise. Steinhaus (86) demonstrated a higher activity in the red bone marrow of trained dogs compared to untrained dogs. Furthermore, the increased RBC destruction in some forms of repeated exercise, e.g., running, has to be considered.

The effect of chronic physical exercise on BV will be discussed with the help of data from cross-sectional as well as from longitudinal studies. Cross-sectional studies are appropriate for the study of highly-trained athletes. On the other hand the results of longitudinal studies have the advantage that an intra-individual comparison is possible. Furthermore, changes at the beginning of physical training in formerly sedentary subjects can be followed.

A. Cross-sectional studies

The effect of physical exercise on blood volume has been known for a long time. Gibson and Evans (87) reported that physically active subjects have a larger BV than their untrained counterparts. This finding has been confirmed in numerous subsequent investigations (88–102) and, the opposite, long inactivity, e.g., bed rest, was shown to result in a decrease in BV (88,89,92,94,103–105). Most studies reported lower Hct and Hb values in athletes compared to untrained subjects despite an increased RCM and increased total amount of circulating Hb. Clement *et al* (106) investigated the Hb concentration of members of the 1976 Canadian Olympic team in comparison to the values of the general Canadian population in 1975. The Canadian male and female athletes had significantly lower ($p < 0.01$) Hct and Hb values than the general population. Comparative studies from our own laboratory (101, 102) also revealed that well-trained athletes have lower Hct and Hb concentrations than untrained subjects. However, RCM, total circulating Hb, and PV were increased in the endurance athletes. Since the PV was disproportionally larger than the RCM the diminished Hb concentration was due to hemodilution. In addition, blood viscosity and colloidal osmotic pressure were found to be lower in well-trained athletes compared to their untrained counterparts.

Dill *et al* (107) suggested that the lower Hb concentration in endurance athletes is related to a high training status without a disadvantage. From the physiological point of view these changes may imply a definite advantage for thermoregulatory function and capillary perfusion. As an example, an athlete could lose approximately 200 ml of plasma before his Hct and colloidal osmotic pressure reaches the same level as found in sedentary subjects. At this point it could be suggested that the notion of a so-called 'optimal' Hct is probably more appropriate in athletes. The statement of Dill *et al* (107): 'Clearly, championship performance in distance running is not associated with thick blood', is supported by the above mentioned data and suggests that hemodilution may be a primary adaptational event to repeated exercise despite the increased RCM. The causal mechanisms of the larger BV in athletes are poorly understood. Hypoxia during exercise may be the stimulus for an increased erythropoietin level in the blood leading to increased erythropoiesis and increased RCM and total Hb. Non-specific hormones, e.g., testosterone, which has been found to be increased after long-lasting exercise (108), might amplify this effect. The increase in BV may be considered a two-step process (109) in which the dimensions of the heart and vascular bed first increase, and the ensuing demand for a greater filling volume is satisfied as a second step. The increased volume requirement is mediated by stretch receptors in both atrias of the heart which are sensitive to changes in central venous pressure. Stimulation of these receptors results in hormonal and nervous responses which effect water and electrolyte excretion by the kidney. However, it is not known whether the same mechanism controls BV over a long period of time (67).

In recent studies it could be shown that endurance-trained athletes have a significantly larger intravascular plasma protein mass than their untrained counterparts. From this finding it was postulated that endurance training stimulates the synthesis of plasma protein in the liver resulting in a considerable expansion of PV. The relationship between PV and intravascular protein mass is shown in Figure 2. Although data from sedentary subjects and athletes lie on the same regression line, the athletes generally have larger PV and intravascular protein masses than the non-athletes (101).

Differences between athletes and untrained subjects are inter-individual comparisons and may therefore be due not only to physical training, but also the result of other influences. For that reason, longitudinal studies are needed to confirm the above described findings.

B. Longitudinal studies

From many longitudinal studies it can be shown that the exercise-induced increases of BV depend on the intensity and duration of physical exercise as well

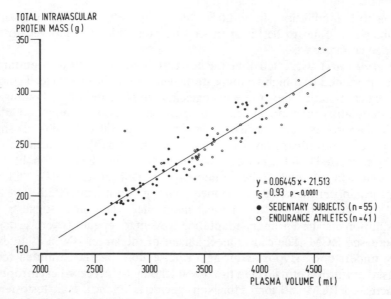

Figure 2. Relationship between plasma volume and intravascular protein mass

as on the pre-training fitness. Furthermore, the type of exercise has to be considered. It is well known that especially endurance exercise, e.g. jogging, cycling, swimming, cross-country skiing, has an impact on RCM and PV.

Physical training of low intensity was not accompanied by changes of BV (110). After a six-week sedentary period, five young men undertook an exercise regimen for three weeks consisting mostly of cross-country running. The intensity of the exercise program was not exactly reported. While the physical condition was improved, indicated by an increased $\dot{V}_{O_2}$ max, BV did not change after the training program (111). A six-week training program of sedentary female ($n = 15$) and male ($n = 12$) subjects in our own laboratory (43) showed a significant ($p < 0.01$) increase in the $\dot{V}_{O_2}$ max from 31.6 to 34.4 ml/kg/min and from 41.5 to 47.8 ml/kg/min, respectively, whereas BV remained unchanged. The daily training, consisting mainly of cycling and running, covered 10 min/day for two weeks, 15 min/day the following two weeks, and 20 min/day the last two weeks.

More intensive training programs (112) resulted in an increased PV while the RCM remained constant. Convertino et al (68), for example, investigated the time course of the increase in BV during isotonic exercise training on an ergometer with a short-duration high-intensity training program of about 60% $\dot{V}_{O_2}$ max for 2 hr/day for eight days. After training, BV increased by 457 ml (+ 8.1%) due to an increase in PV of 427 ml (+ 12.1%). RCM showed no significant change.

Less intensive training can also lead to an increase of BV provided that it is continued for a long time. This was shown by Holmgren *et al* (93) from studies in a long-term training program.

IV. INITIAL HEMATOLOGICAL CHANGES DURING THE ADAPTATION TO CHRONIC EXERCISE—'SPORTS ANEMIA'

Whereas in all longitudinal studies discussed above the hematological changes were noted after a rather long period of training (see above), the initial responses within the first few days, have been studied less extensively. With respect to these changes in subjects who have been kept under a sedentary state for a long time and are suddenly subject to strenuous exercise repeatedly, a number of Japanese investigators reported that an anemia appeared within the first week of daily exercise (113–125). This anemia always went hand in hand with a hypoproteinemia (113,114,118). The changes were not a reflection of an increased plasma volume because the total Hb content and the total serum protein content in the circulating blood decreased as the physical training advanced (118). The anemia was named 'sports anemia' (126). The cause of this phenomenon has been attributed to an increased susceptibility of RBC to hemolysis which is initiated by repeated hard muscular exercise (114,121,127). The hypoproteinemia was explained as a result of the protein requirement of some organs for hypertrophy during adaptation (114). To demonstrate the 'sports anemia' it was necessary to maintain a certain level of physical activity after a prolonged sedentary period (114,118,122,125) and, in the case of the athlete, the training for competitional events (121,128,129). It only appeared during the early adaptational phase. Consequently, it disappeared when the subject continued the exercise for a period longer than approximately two weeks (124). Thus, the so-called 'sports anemia' is not a feature of the well-trained athlete (118,122). As was mentioned in the previous section, the slight reduction of Hb concentration and RBC concentration in highly-trained endurance athletes is due to an increased PV and is not a case of 'sports anemia'.

Before we discuss the potential causes for 'sports anemia', a few additional characteristics of this phenomenon need to be mentioned;
1. 'Sports anemia' appears in the early stage of physical training involving strenuous muscular exercise. The severity of the anemia found after two weeks' training is directly related to the level of work (116,118,122) and is less severe during daily exercise bursts of only moderate intensity.
2. As already stated above, the anemia always appears concomitantly with hypoproteinemia (113,114,118).
3. 'Sports anemia' can be prevented by supplying a protein rich diet consisting of highly qualified animal protein (114,130).

As far as point (1) is concerned, Yoshimura (122) calculated the relation between the strength of muscular exercise and the reduction of Hb content in total circulating blood after two weeks adaptation to hard physical exercise. A significant correlation was found ($p < 0.01$). Depending on the intensity of work the reduction of total Hb content ranged between 0.5 g/kg bodyweight and 2.5 g/kg body weight.

Points (2) and (3) may suggest that a protein deficiency is responsible for the blood property changes. However, Yoshimura (116) and Yoshimura *et al* (118) found in ten out of twelve cases studied that the subjects maintained a positive nitrogen balance during development of 'sports anemia'. Thus, the reduction of serum proteins and the anemia cannot be explained by protein deficiency. On the other hand, it was observed that the nutritional status of individuals, especially protein intake, does greatly influence the course of 'sports anemia' (116,118,124).

Chapter 10 deals with the subject of protein and other nutritional factors in the regulation of erythropoiesis. Therefore, this point will only be discussed as far as its relevance to the erythropoietic effect of exercise.

The normal level of blood Hb is maintained when the destruction and the formation of RBC are well-balanced. By measuring the osmotic fragility of the RBC, as an index of their sensitivity to destruction, and the reticulocyte count, as a measure of the rate of RBC formation, one can separate the two main causes of 'sports anemia': an increased RBC destruction on the one hand, and a decreased rate of regeneration of erythrocytes in the bone marrow on the other hand. Furthermore, the possibility of iron deficiency as a cause of 'sports anemia' must be taken into consideration.

A. Red blood cell destruction in the early stage of physical training

Yoshimura (22) studied the osmotic fragility of RBC in previously untrained subjects who exercised on a bicycle ergometer for 2 hr daily for two weeks. The work intensity was kept on a constant level and the protein intake was maintained at about 75 g/day throughout the study. The extra energy expenditure required for exercise was covered by supplying carbohydrates. Blood samples were taken and the osmotic fragility of RBC was measured using a series of hypotonic saline solutions (131) and the results expressed by the concentration of NaCl giving 50% hemolysis. This point is termed the half hemolysis rate. Shown in Figure 3 are the changes of the half hemolysis rate in one subject who was representative of the group as a whole. A shift of the hemolysis curve to the left side indicates an increased osmotic fragility of the erythrocytes and that the membrane resistance of RBC decreased. As shown in the figure, the osmotic fragility of RBC membranes decreased on the third day of training and was gradually restored as the training continued. Similar results have been reported by Hiramatsu (121) who conducted a series of experiments with dogs. The animals were forced to run daily for 3 hr at a speed of 12 km/hr after a two-week sedentary period. The training continued for

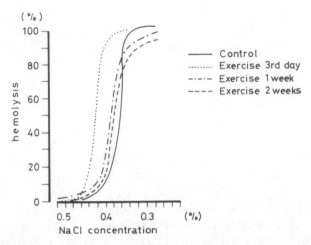

Figure 3. Changes of osmotic fragility of RBC measured successively along the course of physical training in muscular exercise. Each curve represents the measurements made on successive days after the start from the sedentary period. The day of measurement is indicated for the corresponding line of curve (122)

three weeks and then the animals were returned to a sedentary state. The fragility of erythrocytes was measured not only in hypotonic saline solution but also by mechanical shaking in an isotonic saline solution at a rate of 180 cpm for 50 min. The rate of mechanical hemolysis was accelerated during the first week of exercise. Then the mechanical resistance of the erythrocytes increased gradually and returned to the control level two weeks after the cessation of running. Measurements of the Hb binding capacity of haptoglobin (132) and measurements of free Hb in plasma (124) revealed that the increased RBC fragility during exercise results in an increased intravascular hemolysis. The mechanism of erythrocyte destruction is as yet unclear. The question now is what are the factors causing the RBC to become more fragile during the adaptation to hard physical exercise? Two main theories have been presented in the past. One is the hypothesis of a physical or mechanical factor already discussed in the previous section. The alternative is the hypothesis of a chemical hemolytic factor in the blood during hard muscular training.

1. Mechanical erythrocyte destruction

The mechanisms leading to a mechanical destruction of erythrocytes during exercise have already been discussed. However, Yamada *et al* (133) showed that a traumatic alteration of the RBC did not occur following daily training sessions with a bicycle ergometer. They investigated two groups of young male students during a two week training period. One group of subjects pedalled with bare feet, while the other pedalled with rubber shoes and the pedals were covered by rubber cushions. Yamada *et al* (133) found a similar rate of osmotic fragility and the same extent of anemia independently of the experimental design. Thus, a traumatic alteration of the RBC membrane cannot be the only mechanism underlying 'sports anemia'.

2. Chemical erythrocyte destruction

The question of erythrocyte destruction by a humoral factor in the early stages of physical training has occasioned a great deal of speculation. Shiraki (127) demonstrated that a hemolysing substance in the splenic blood is involved in the decreased osmotic fragility of the erythrocytes during the adaptation to a high level of physical activity. This information has raised many questions about an enhanced erythrocyte hemolysis due to basic physiological mechanisms. On the other hand, a number of observations (117,122,134,135) have led to the suggestion that the sympathetic nervous system, activated by stressful daily repetition of vigorous exercise, also plays a role in the chemical erythrocyte destruction.

The following sections attempt to evaluate these different theories.

a. Role of the spleen as a factor involved in the mechanism causing 'sports anemia'. Shiraki (127) investigated the relevance of the spleen to RBC fragility during hard physical exercise. Four dogs which stayed in a sedentary state prior to the experiments were trained to run for 4 hr/day at a speed of 12 km/hr. After five days a distinct increase in osmotic fragility of the RBC appeared. Total circulating Hb content was considerably reduced (6.0 ± 1.8 g/kg bodyweight) compared to the Hb in a control group of sedentary dogs (8.5 ± 2.4 g/kg bodyweight). On the other hand, with four dogs splenectomized prior to the experiments no change with respect to the fragility and no anemia was observed. By separating the plasma from the erythrocytes of intact exercising dogs 5–7 days after the onset of training and incubating this plasma with erythrocytes of an intact resting dog, Shiraki (127) found that the osmotic fragility of the erythrocytes increased significantly. Performing the experiment the other way round—erythrocytes of an intact exercising dog with plasma of an intact resting dog—the fragility of the RBC was restored to the normal range. From additional results of subsequent measurements of plasma and RBC from all of his dogs—intact exercising and resting dogs, splenectomized exercising and resting dogs— Shiraki (127) concluded that some hemolytic factors must be increased in the serum or plasma by strenuous exercise, but that it is not in sufficient concentrations in the plasma of splenectomized dogs to increase the osmotic fragility of RBC. Shiraki (127) further performed an experiment to estimate the fragility in splenic blood as compared with the blood in the peripheral circulation. He collected blood, from anaesthetized dogs, from both the

V.lienalis and the *V.femoralis* at the same time. After this blood was taken, adrenaline (0.3 mg/kg) was injected intravenously, and a contraction of the spleen was observed. When the contraction started, another sample was taken from the *V.lienalis*. The highest erythrocyte fragility was found in the *V.lienalis* after adrenaline injection, the lowest fragility in the peripheral circulation and intermediate osmotic fragility in the erythrocytes from the *V.lienalis* prior to the adrenaline injection. Shiraki (127) therefore concluded that a hemolytic factor is stored in the spleen, and it is forced out by contraction of the spleen *via* sympathetic activation.

b. Role of the sympathetic nervous system as a factor involved in the mechanism causing 'sports anemia'. As far as the sympathetic nervous system is concerned, Ootsuka (134) performed a series of experiments with rats. One group received daily injections of isotonic saline solution subcutaneously, the second one subcutaneous injections of cortisone and the third group, injections of adrenaline. Osmotic fragility of the RBC was estimated by the half hemolysis rate before and ten days after the beginning of the experiments. Ten days of continuous injections of adrenaline induced an increase of erythrocyte fragility and brought about a slight anemia, while cortisone injections decreased RBC osmotic fragility. Since it is well-established that the plasma catecholamine concentration in man can increase during exercise (136–139), and the magnitude of increase is less after training (136,137,139,140), the results of Ootsuka (134) support the concept of a role of catecholamines in the RBC hemolysis of 'sports anemia' (113–125). Winder *et al* (140), in a longitudinal study of human subjects, followed the plasma catecholamine response to exercise. Six untrained subjects exercised vigorously 30–50 min/day for seven weeks. Resting catecholamine levels were not significantly altered by training. However, plasma levels of epinephrine and norepinephrine during exercise were considerably lower after seven weeks of training. These data are compatible with the hypothesis of stress as a causal factor in 'sports anemia', although the data of Winder *et al* (140) are not entirely in accordance with catecholamines causing the increase in RBC osmotic fragility. In addition, as no hematological measurements were done in their study, the correlation between catecholamine response during exercise and the appearance of 'sports anemia' remains uncertain. In this connection it is worth mentioning the study of Usami (117). Four previously sedentary subjects were submitted to daily vigorous exercise and urinary 17-hydroxysteroids excretion as a parameter of catabolic steroid production was measured. Besides a typical 'sports anemia', Usami (117) found that the urinary excretion of 17-hydroxysteroids increased in the early period of physical training and was restored to normal as the training advanced. The pioneering studies of Selye (141) indicated that under the influence of systemic stress the organism responds with a general-adaptation-syndrome.

Among a variety of non-specific damaging agents, muscular exercise may be one by which the syndrome is occasioned. During the initial phase of the general-adaptation-syndrome an increased production of catabolic hormones by the adrenals appears. Thus, an increased urinary 17-hydroxysteroid excretion in face of a total Hb reduction may indicate that stress is a factor involved in the mechanism causing 'sports anemia'. Yoshimura *et al* (142) suggested a hypothesis that the organism is stressed by daily repetition of vigorous muscular exercise during the adaptation period to a high level of physical fitness. Thereby adrenaline secretion is promoted and the contraction of the spleen may be accelerated. Thus, the hemolysing factor flows out into the circulating blood. Consequently the RBC fragility is increased and 'sports anemia' is established. Their view is supported by the facts that no significant anemia appears in well-trained subjects who do not feel any stress in face of a heavy work load, while the anemia appears only among subjects who spent a rather sedentary life before the experiments (118,122). Furthermore, these sedentary subjects develop no anemia if performing physical activities of weaker strength (118,122).

c. Nature of the hemolytic factor stored in the spleen. In 1936 Bergenhem and Fåhraeus (143) found a hemolytic substance in blood which was incubated for several hours at body temperature. They concluded that this hemolytic substance was either identical with the so-called lysolecithin or very closely related to it. Singer (144) developed a micromethod for measurements of lysolecithin in serum. Singer *et al* (145) found that in six out of 14 splenectomized subjects studied the lysolecithin content of the unincubated serum from peripheral blood was considerably lower than in normal individuals. In eight out of 14 cases studied a lack of increase of lysolecithin in the serum upon incubation was observed. Singer *et al* (145) concluded that splenectomy frequently leads to a disturbance of the whole mechanism of lysolecithin production. Since Bergenhem and Fåhraeus (143) believed that this substance is produced in the spleen, the observations made by Singer *et al* (145) were in general confirmation of their findings.

Yoshimura *et al* (125) demonstrated in three sedentary subjects that the lysolecithin content in both serum and RBC increased and cholesterol in serum and RBC decreased in the early stage of physical training. At the same time erythrocyte fragility increased most remarkably. From the blood samples taken before the training and from those taken at the third, fifth, seventh, and tenth day of exercise they calculated the correlation between the half hemolysis rate and the concentration of lysolecithin. They found a positive correlation with both serum lysolecithin and RBC lysolecithin. The higher correlation ($r = 0.844$, $p < 0.01$, $N = 15$) was that between lysolecithin in RBC and the half hemolysis rate. A significant negative correlation ($r = 0.679$, $p < 0.01$, $N = 14$) appeared between cholesterol in serum and the half hemolysis rate. Based on the knowledge of lysolecithin as a hemolytic substance (143) and of cholesterol as a substance stabilizing RBC membranes (146) they concluded that the causal factor of increased RBC fragility in the early period of exercise may be the increased lysolecithin in serum and RBC in association with the decreased cholesterol in serum and RBC. Shiraki and Sagawa (147) found that a decreased pH increased the fragility of RBC. Furthermore, the reduction of pH of the blood increased the lysolecithin in the plasma and decreased its free cholesterol content. Similar changes appeared in the lipid profile in RBC. By restoring pH to the normal, cholesterol content of RBC readily returned to the normal value, whereas the restoration of lysolecithin in RBC and plasma was slow.

Based on available experimental data, Yoshimura and Shiraki (151) suggested a hypothetical outline of the mechanism of 'sports anemia'. Free cholesterol of the RBC membrane can rapidly exchange with free cholesterol in plasma (148,149), whereas phospholipids exchange more slowly (150). In muscular exercise lactic acid accumulates in the venous blood and the blood pH tends to decrease. This change is rapidly reversed during recovery and the changes of lipid profile of systemic blood should be restored the next morning. The splenic blood, however, stagnates after exercise, leading to an accumulation of acidic metabolites. Further changes in the lipid profile of both the RBC and the plasma of splenic blood may thereby be promoted. The splenic blood is pushed out by the contraction of the spleen caused by stressful exercise the following day. Due to the liberation of this blood in combination with the changes induced by the reduction of venous pH during exercise, the lipid profile changes of systemic blood are accelerated day by day until they cannot be restored by resting overnight. This may be an explanation for the lack of hematological changes during the very first days of training. However, it is still a matter of speculation what kind of adaptive changes appear in systemic blood which result in a subsequent return of RBC fragility to normal as the training advances.

As explained above, certain links in the chain of events which are believed to be responsible for 'sports anemia' have not been fully proven. Others may have to be replaced in the future. In this connection some brief considerations shall be made as far as the origin of the lysolecithin is concerned. According to Switzer and Eder (152) lysolecithin comprises 9.6% of the phospholipids of human plasma. They demonstrated that the major portion of the plasma lysolecithin is present in association with plasma proteins other than lipoproteins. Their findings strongly suggested that the lysolecithin is bound to albumin. Since lysolecithin is a potent hemolytic agent (143), its binding is of physiological importance. Klibansky and DeVries (153) demonstrated that the changes in erythrocytes exposed to lysolecithin could be reversed by the addition of albumin which bound the lysolecithin. The production of lysolecithin in plasma can occur by the conversion of lecithin *via* the activity of the lecithin-cholesterol acyltransferase (154,155). Lysolecithin in plasma was shown to exchange instantaneously with the RBC membrane (156). According to Jaffé and Gottfried (157) lysolecithin comprises 1.4 ± 1.4% of the total amount of membrane phospholipids in the human erythrocyte. From experimental data of several studies (154,158,159) a cycle can be constituted, with lysolecithin from plasma albumin entering the RBC membrane and forming lecithin which in turn is released into plasma to combine with lipoproteins, where lysolecithin is again formed and transferred to plasma albumin. Exercise physiology may take advantage of these findings from the field of lipid research to further elaborate the physiological reasons for 'sports anemia' in the near future.

B. Reticulocyte count in the early stage of physical training

It has been mentioned that a decreased rate of production of erythrocytes in the bone marrow may be another reason contributing to the 'sports anemia'. However, there is no evidence in the literature that the reticulocyte count drops below control level after the onset of physical trianing. Yoshimura *et al* (125) and Yamada *et al* (133) found an elevated reticulocyte count throughout a training period of daily strenuous work with a bicycle ergometer. Hiramatsu (121) investigated the reticulocyte count in students training for rugby and volleyball. The daily training averaged 4–4.7 hr. After the training period a significant increase of the reticulocyte count was observed. In all of the three studies the elevated reticulocyte count occurred in the face of an anemia and, indeed, may represent an appropriate physiological response. Therefore, it is unlikely that a decreased RBC production in the bone marrow is the primary cause of 'sports anemia'. In this connection it is worth mentioning Broun's work from 1923 (79). He investigated hematological changes in five vigorously exercising dogs over a period of five days. The dogs had been kept in a sedentary state two months prior to the experiments. A pronounced drop in total circulating Hb occurred up to the end of the five days training session. However, the reticulocyte count increased considerably throughout the time of the experiments. Similar data regarding an increased reticulocyte count in response to 'sports anemia' in exercising dogs were given by Shiraki (127). Broun (79) discussed in his paper that there is at first a period in which blood destruction is proceeding more rapidly than blood formation and an anemia therefore appears.

C. Iron deficiency as a cause of 'sports anemia'?

Yamada *et al* (123) investigated whether or not 'sports anemia' is related to iron deficiency. Twelve students were subjected to a 4 hr running program for seven days after staying in a sedentary state for one week. They were divided into two groups. The students of the experimental group were supplied with 1000 mg $FeSO_4$ daily, those of the control group did not receive the iron supplement. It was demonstrated that even with supplementation of iron, and with significantly higher serum iron levels, the 'sports anemia' appeared similarly to the anemia of the control group. Initial Hb concentration was 14.61 g/100 ml and 14.59 g/100 ml for the iron supplemented (experimental) and non-supplemented (control) group respectively. After two weeks (sedentary period seven days/training period seven days) the Hb concentration had decreased to 13.18 g/100 ml (experimental group) and 13.43 g/100 ml (control group), respectively. Thus, the Hb reduction in the early stage of adaptation to physical exercise is probably not due to iron deficiency.

In the previous section the phenomenon of 'sports anemia' has been mentioned. However, at this point it should be noted that 'sports anemia' was not noticed in a study by Deitrick et al (160). They subjected eight untrained healthy men to a training program for three weeks. The program consisted of 10 min/day of high intensity aerobic exercise four times a week. The main concern was to evaluate the relationship between the phenomenon of retrogression in physical performance and the phenomenon of 'sports anemia' during the early phase of the training. The protocol of Deitrick et al (160) did not cause the anticipated exercise-induced anemia. Despite this, retrogression did occur on the fifth training day. Unfortunately blood was not drawn during that day. Therefore, Deitrick et al (160) discussed the possibility that the brief anemic period which subsequently led to the temporary decrease in performance might have been missed. However, the most likely explanation is that the exercise training program was not of the proper proportions to elicit the proposed-exercise induced anemia. Indeed, 10 min of exercise per day, four times a week is considerably less than the training programs of 2 hr daily in the studies of Yoshimura (122) and Yoshimura et al (115,118,125), respectively. Therefore, the contradictory results may be at least partly due to methodology, and for the time being it seems to be well established that 'sports anemia' is caused by an increased susceptibility of RBC to hemolysis rather than by an insufficient erythrocyte production or by iron deficiency.

D. Protein metabolism in the early stage of physical training

It was mentioned above that 'sports anemia' can be prevented by supplying a protein rich diet consisting of highly qualified animal protein. Since the prevention of anemia is of considerable interest to the athlete this dietary problem will be briefly discussed.

Shiraki et al (124) investigated the influence of three different dietary protocols on total circulating Hb, RBC count, RBC fragility, and reticulocyte count. For three weeks 14 students underwent a daily vigorous physical training with a bicycle ergometer. Prior to this training program control

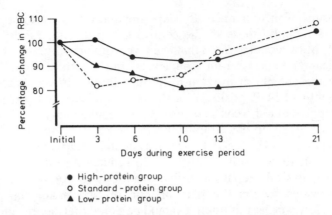

Figure 4. Percentage changes in RBC count during the exercise period. Each point indicates the mean value. Reproduced with permission from the Center for Academic Publications, Japan (124)

measurements of all the parameters studied were done during a sedentary period of one week. Thereafter the subjects were divided into three groups of high protein diet (2.0 g/kg/day), standard protein diet (1.25 g/kg/day), and low protein diet (0.5 g/kg/day). Standard protein diet was identical with that during the control period. In the high protein group a negligible reduction of the total circulating Hb occurred after one week of exercise (12.9 ± 2.3 g Hb/kg bodyweight to 12.8 ± 2.1). However, a significant reduction ($p < 0.05$) was observed in the standard protein group (13.4 ± 1.2 g Hb/kg bodyweight to 11.8 ± 1.2). In the low protein group a reduction from 12.3 g Hb/kg bodyweight to 10.9 appeared. Since only two subjects participated in this group, no statistical analyses were made.

Shown in Figure 4 are the changes in RBC count of the three groups during the exercise period. In the high protein group the RBC count was reduced slightly in the early period and then it tended to be restored around two weeks after the beginning of the exercise. Moreover, it increased above the initial value after three weeks. In the standard protein group, the reduction was 20% on the third to sixth days, and after two weeks the RBC count tended to recover to the initial level and finally at the third week it became higher than that of the initial level. In the low protein group, the RBC count decreased gradually until weeks one to two of the experiment, and did not return to the initial value.

In Figure 5 the changes in reticulocyte counts during the exercise period are given. On the third day, reticulocytes increased remarkably in the high protein group, while the increase was very slight or absent in the standard and low protein groups. From the sixth to tenth day, the responses were similar in

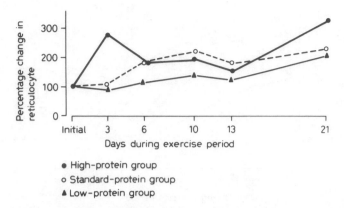

Figure 5. Percentage changes in reticulocyte count during the exercise period. Each point indicates the mean value. Reproduced with permission from the Center for Academic Publications, Japan (124)

both standard and high protein groups, and a sharp rise of reticulocytes was seen in the third week with both groups, while the response was still very low in the low protein group.

The changes in osmotic fragility of RBC are shown in Figure 6. The results are expressed as percentage changes in half hemolysis rate from the initial value. Osmotic fragility increased from the third to the tenth day in the standard and low protein groups, and after two weeks the fragility decreased below the initial level in the standard protein group, but in the low protein group it remained at the initial level. On the other hand, in the high protein group osmotic fragility decreased gradually until the tenth day and remained depressed thereafter.

In this experiment it was therefore confirmed that the reduction of erythrocytes and total circulating Hb, the response of reticulocytes in the circulating blood, and the changes in osmotic fragility of the RBC during the exercise period were closely related to the protein intake from the diet.

The dependence of RBC count and Hb changes on the quality of dietary protein was shown by Yoshimura et al (130). Non-athletic students were subjected to daily vigorous physical exercise with a bicycle ergometer. The amount of dietary protein was about the same as in the standard protein group of the study by Shiraki et al (124). However, the proportion of animal protein was 57% in the experiment of Yoshimura et al (130) whereas it was only 30% in that of Shiraki et al (124). Yoshimura et al (130) found that the Hb concentration and the RBC count tended to decrease while the total Hb in circulating blood was maintained at the normal level during and after two weeks of training. According to Yoshimura et al (130), the reduction of Hb concentration and the decreased RBC count can be explained by increases in

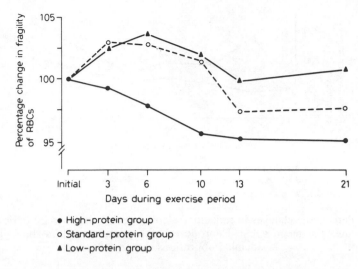

Figure 6. Percentage changes in osmotic fragility of RBC during the exercise period. Osmotic fragility of RBC is expressed as half hemolysis rate which is the concentration of NaCl causing 50% hemolysis. Points are mean values. Reproduced with permission from the Center for Academic Publications, Japan (124)

PV. Thus, 'sports anemia' can be prevented by providing a high qualified protein in a usual amount. However, the underlying mechanisms by means of which amount and quality of the dietary protein prevent this kind of anemia are not fully understood.

E. The physiological role of increased RBC destruction and serum protein metabolism in the early stage of physical training

It was pointed out in the introduction that many systems are involved in the adaptation of the human organism to physical exercise. It has been reported by Åstrand and Rodahl (42) that maximum oxygen uptake has a linear relationship with the total amount of Hb. From this point of view, a reduction of RBC during training may have a negative influence on the improvement of physical fitness in the process of training. Thus, it is clear that the transient 'sports anemia' is unfavorable in the early stage of adaptation (161). However, the developing anemia and hypoproteinemia goes hand in hand with a re-utilization of Hb and serum proteins in certain organs to meet the demand imposed by physical exercise. This was shown by Hiramatsu (162). He transfused ^{59}Fe-labeled RBC into resting and exercising rats. The exercising group ran for 2 hr/day on a treadmill with a speed of 1.3 km/hr.

Three rats were sacrificed at time intervals of two to seven days during the four weeks of the experiment. The blood was collected and skeletal muscle, heart, liver, spleen, and bone marrow were excised. Specific activity of radioactive ^{59}Fe incorporated into hemin molecules of these organs was determined. The same experiments were done on rats injected with serum labeled with radio-iron. Aside from a shortened lifespan of the erythrocytes in the exercising rats, it was demonstrated that the rate of incorporation of ^{59}Fe into tissue hemin in resting rats was higher from erythrocyte hemin than from serum protein in the spleen, bone marrow, and skeletal and heart muscles. The rate in the liver, however, was higher from serum protein than from erythrocyte hemin. Also in the exercising group the rate of incorporation of hemin ^{59}Fe from erythrocytes was accelerated in all tissues, especially in the skeletal and heart muscles, spleen, and bone marrow. Thus, Hiramatsu (162) concluded that erythrocyte hemin may be utilized more easily or more effectively in these organs than serum iron, and its utilization may be promoted by the availability of Hb from the destruction of erythrocytes during physical training. In this connection, it should be mentioned that Whipple (163) appears to have been the first to suggest that exercise might increase the concentration of myoglobin in muscle. Pattengale and Holloszy (164) performed a series of experiments to obtain information, under controlled conditions, regarding the effect of regularly performed exercise on the concentration of myoglobin in skeletal muscle. Rats were subjected to a vigorous program of treadmill running of progressively increasing intensity lasting 15 weeks. The myoglobin content of the quadriceps muscles was found to be approximately 75% higher in the exercising group than in sedentary controls. Less pronounced increases of myoglobin content in the hind limb muscles of exercising rats after a daily treadmill program of ten days were reported by Ashida (165). In 16 rats fed on a standard protein diet (casein 16% *ad libitum*) the myoglobin content was significantly higher in the exercising group (4.7 ± 0.63 mg/g wet weight) compared with the resting group (3.5 ± 0.80 mg/g wet weight). Taking the above mentioned data (162–165) together, one may conclude that the Hb in RBC is utilized to produce muscle protein and new RBC. The acceleration of muscle hypertrophy through repeated exercise (166) may, therefore, benefit from a temporary increase in the destruction of RBC, and this may be regarded as an adaptive process. However, 'sports anemia' is only transient and the exercising subject finally reaches a level of total circulating Hb and total circulating serum proteins that is significantly higher than in sedentary subjects (102). Thus, it can be assumed that the time required for the adaptation of the organs to physical exercise differs and that the increase of Hb as well as the increase of serum protein are rather gradually brought into play.

V. CONCLUSIONS

It was the aim of this article to describe the hematological changes in response to acute and repeated physical exercise.

The hematological changes during and after acute exercise are mainly due to a redistribution of plasma fluid resulting in hemoconcentration or hemodilution, respectively.

A marked decrease of PV is seen particularly in response to short-term strenuous exercise, whereas smaller decreases or even increases are seen after prolonged physical exercise. However, after long-lasting severe exercise, hemolysis due to mechanical RBC destruction is regularly found.

Another goal of this chapter was to describe the adaptation of BV and RCM to endurance (aerobic) exercise in subjects who changed from a sedentary life to a high level of physical activity. The adaptation to endurance exercise finally leads to an increased RCM and a disproportional larger increase of PV resulting in subnormal values of Hb concentration and Hct.

After the first weeks of training the increase of BV was found to be totally due to an increased PV.

However, if the exercise schedule is too strenuous, a so-called 'sports anemia' may develop in the early stage of training. The extensive literature dealing with the phenomenon of 'sports anemia' is discussed. However, this kind of anemia is only a temporary effect. In the course of longer periods of endurance training an increased RCM in addition to an increased PV can be found.

VI. ACKNOWLEDGMENT

The help of Mrs L. Schepeler in the preparation of this chapter is gratefully acknowledged.

VI. REFERENCES

1. Barcroft, J., Harris, H. A., Orahovats, D., and Weiss, R. (1925). 'A contribution to the physiology of the spleen', *J. Physiol. (Lond)*, **6**, 443–456.
2. Nylin, G. (1947). 'The effect of heavy muscular work on the volume of circulating red corpuscles in man', *Am. J. Physiol.*, **149**, 180–184.
3. Nylin, G. (1955). 'Zirkulationsstudien mit radioaktiven Isotopen', *Münch. med. Wschr.*, **97**, 4–10.
4. Hoffman, G., Kleiderling, W., Schmidt, H. A. E., and Schoeppe, W. (1958). 'Zur Frage der aktiven Blutmenge', *Klin. Wschr.*, **36**, 864–865.
5. Ühlinger, A., and Bühlmann, A. (1961). 'Das Verhalten des Blutvolumens während kurzfristiger körperlicher Arbeit. Bestimmung mit Cr^{51}- und I^{131}-Albumin', *Cardiologia*, **38**, 357–370.
6. Åstrand, P.-O., and Saltin, B. (1964). 'Plasma and red cell volume after prolonged severe exercise', *J. Appl. Physiol.*, **19**, 829–832.

7. Fricke, G. (1965). 'Über das Verhalten des Zellfaktors bei körperlicher Arbeit. Bestimmungen mit T-1824 (Evansblau) und radioaktivem Chromat', *Cardiologia*, **47**, 25–44.
8. Costill, D. L., and Saltin, B. (1974). 'Changes in the ratio of venous to body hematocrit following dehydration', *J. Appl. Physiol.*, **36**, 608–610.
9. Starling, E. H. (1896). 'On the absorption of fluids from the connective tissue spaces', *J. Physiol. (Lond.)*, **19**, 312–326.
10. Landis, E. M., and Pappenheimer, J. R. (1963). 'Exchange of substances through the capillary walls', in *Handbook of Physiology Section 2: Circulation* (Eds. W. F. Hamilton and P. Dow), American Physiology Society, Washington, D. C., vol. 2, pp. 961–1034.
11. Keys, A., and Taylor, H. (1935). 'The behavior of the plasma colloids in recovery from brief severe work and the question as to the permeability of the capillaries to proteins', *J. Biol. Chem.*, **109**, 55–67.
12. Cassels, D. E., and Morse, M. (1942). 'Blood volume and exercise', *J. Pediat.*, **20**, 352–364.
13. Cullumbine, H., and Koch, A. C. E. (1949). 'The changes in plasma and tissue fluid volume following exercise', *Quart. J. Exp. Physiol.*, **35**, 39–46.
14. König, E., and Zöllner, N. (1961). 'Veränderungen des Plasmavolumens während und nach körperlicher Arbeit bei Rechtsinsuffizienz', *Verh. Dtsch. Ges. Kreisl.-forsch.*, **27**, 334–337.
15. Ekelund, L. G., and Holmgren, A. (1964). 'Circulatory and respiratory adaptation, during long-term, non-steady state exercise, in the sitting position', *Acta Physiol. Scand.*, **62**, 240–255.
16. Bartley, S. H. (1965). 'Fatique. Mechanism and Management', in *American Lectures in Living Chemistry* (Ed. I. Newton Kugelmass), Charles C. Thomas, Springfield, IL., pp. 45–58.
17. König, E., and Lemp, A. (1966). 'Plasmavolumenänderungen durch alltägliche Belastungen bei Herzgesunden und Herzinsuffizienten', *Klin. Wschr.*, **44**, 862–870.
18. König, E., and Zöllner, N. (1966). 'Veränderungen des Plasmavolumens durch Tretarbeit im Liegen bei Herzgesunden und Rechtsinsuffizienten', *Z. ges. exp. Med.*, **140**, 268–286.
19. Ekelund, L.-G. (1967). 'Circulatory and respiratory adaptation during prolonged exercise of moderate intensity in the sitting position', *Acta Physiol. Scand.*, **69**, 327–340.
20. Morehouse, L. E., and Miller, A. T., Jr. (1971). 'Body fluid changes in exercise', in *Physiology of Exercise*, The C.V. Mosby Company, St.Louis, pp. 128–136.
21. van Beaumont, W., Greenleaf, J. E., and Juhos, L. (1972). 'Disproportional changes in hematocrit, plasma volume, and proteins during exercise and bed rest', *J. Appl. Physiol.*, **33**, 55–61.
22. Lundvall, J., Mellander, S., Westling, H., and White, T. (1972). 'Fluid transfer between blood and tissues during exercise', *Acta Physiol. Scand.*, **85**, 258–269.
23. van Beaumont, W. (1973). 'Red cell volume with changes in plasma osmolarity during maximal exercise', *J. Appl. Physiol.*, **35**, 47–50.
24. van Beaumont, W. Strand, J. C., Petrofsky, J. S., Hipkind, S. G., and Greenleaf, J. E. (1973). 'Changes in total plasma content of electrolytes and proteins with maximal exercise', *J. Appl. Physiol.*, **34**, 102–106.
25. Novosadová, J. (1977). 'The changes in hematocrit, hemoglobin, plasma volume and proteins during and after different types of exercise', *Europ. J. Appl. Physiol.*, **36**, 223–230.

26. Thompson, W. O., Thompson, P. K., and Dailey, M. E. (1928). 'The effect of posture upon the composition and volume of the blood in man', *J. Clin. Invest.*, 5, 573–604.
27. Waterfield, R. L. (1931). 'The effects of posture on the circulating blood volume', *J. Physiol. (Lond.)*, 72, 110–120.
28. Fawcett, J. K., and Wynn, V. (1960). 'Effects of posture on plasma volume and some blood constituents', *J. Clin. Path.*, 13, 304–310.
29. Dill, D. B., Talbott, J. H., and Edwards, H. T. (1930). 'Studies in muscular activity. VI. Response of several individuals to a fixed task', *J. Physiol. (Lond.)*, 69, 267–305.
30. Ebert, R. V., and Stead, E. A., Jr. (1941). 'Demonstration that in normal man no reserves of blood are mobilized by exercise, epinephrine, and hemorrhage', *Am. J. Med. Sci.*, 201, 655–664.
31. Holmgren, A. (1956). 'Circulatory changes during muscular work in man. With special reference to ˙arterial and central venous pressures in the systemic circulation', *Scand. J. Clin. Lab. Invest.*, 8, Suppl. 24, 1–97.
32. Cobbold, A., Folkow, B., Kjellmer, I., and Mellander, S. (1963). 'Nervous and local chemical control of pre-capillary sphincters in skeletal muscle as measured by changes in filtration coefficient', *Acta Physiol. Scand.*, 57, 180–192.
33. Kjellmer, I. (1964). 'The effect of exercise on the vascular bed of skeletal muscle. *Acta Physiol. Scand.*, 62, 18–30.
34. Arturson, G., and Kjellmer, I. (1964). 'Capillary permeability in skeletal muscle during rest and activity', *Acta Physiol. Scand.*, 62, 41–45.
35. Folkow, B., Heymans, C., and Neil, E. (1965). 'Integrated aspects of cardiovascular regulation', in *Handbook of Physiology, Section 2: Circulation*, (Eds. W. F. Hamilton and P. Dow), American Physiology Society, Washington, D.C., vol. 2, pp. 1787–1823.
36. Fahey, T. D., and Rolph, R. (1975). 'Venous and capillary blood hematocrit at rest and following submaximal exercise', *Europ. J. Appl. Physiol.*, 34, 109–112.
37. Margaria, R. (1930). 'The vapour pressure of normal human blood', *J. Physiol. (Lond.)*, 70, 417–433.
38. Mellander, S., Johansson, B., Gray, S., Jonsson, O., Lundvall, J., and Ljung, B. (1967). 'The effects of hyperosmolarity on intact and isolated vascular smooth muscle: Possible role in exercise hyperemia', *Angiologica*, 4, 310–322.
39. Lundvall, J. (1972). 'Tissue hyperosmolality as a mediator of vasodilatation and transcapillary fluid flux in exercising muscle', *Acta Physiol. Scand.*, Suppl. 379.
40. Kjellmer, I. (1965). 'Studies on exercise hyperemia', *Acta Physiol. Scand.*, 64, Suppl. 244, 1–27.
41. Folkow, B., Haglund, U., Jodal, M., and Lundgren, O. (1971). 'Blood flow in the calf muscle of man during heavy rhythmic exercise', *Acta Physiol. Scand.*, 81, 157–163.
42. Åstrand, P. O., and Rodahl, K. (1970). *Textbook of Exercise Physiology*, McGraw-Hill, New York.
43. Röcker, L. (1979). *Das Verhalten von Plasmavolumen und Plasmaproteinen nach körperlichen Leistungen, körperlichem Training und Hitzeeinwirkung*, Habilitationsschrift, Berlin.
44. Hawk, P. B. (1904). 'On the morphological changes in the blood after muscular exercise', *Am. J. Physiol.*, 10, 384–400.
45. Ekeland, L.-G. (1967). 'Circulatory and respiratory adaptation during prolonged exercise', *Acta Physiol. Scand.*, 292, Suppl. 70, 9–38.
46. Pugh, L. G. C. E. (1969). 'Blood volume changes in outdoor exercise of 8–10 hour duration', *J. Physiol.*, 200, 345–351.

47. Keller, H. M., Imhof, P., Howald, H., Imhof, U., and Turri, M. (1971). 'Veränderungen von Plasmavolumen, Hämatokrit und Körpergewicht bei Skilangläufern', *Schweiz. Z. Sportmed.*, **19**, 61–74.
48. Dill, D. B., Yousef, M. D., and Nelson, J. D. (1973). 'Responses of men and women to two-hour walks in desert heat', *J. Appl. Physiol.*, **35**, 231–235.
49. Costill, D. L., and Fink, W. J. (1974). 'Plasma volume changes following exercise and thermal dehydration', *J. Appl. Physiol.*, **37**, 521–525.
50. Dill, D. B., and Costill, D. L. (1974). 'Calculation of percentage changes in volumes of blood, plasma, and red cells in dehydration', *J. Appl. Physiol.*, **37**,. 247–248.
51. Harrison, M. H. (1975). 'Plasma volume change during work in a hot environment', *J. Physiol.*, **245**, 102P–103P.
52. Harrison, M. H., Edwards, R. J., and Leitch, D. R. (1975). 'Effect of exercise and thermal stress on plasma volume', *J. Appl. Physiol.*, **39**, 925–931.
53. Refsum, H. E., Jordfald, G., and Stromme, S. B. (1976). 'Hematological changes following prolonged heavy exercise', in *Advance in Exercise Physiology, Medicine and Sport*, (Eds. E. Jokl, R. L. Anand, and H. Stoboy) Karger, Basel, New York, vol. 9, pp. 91–99.
54. Saltin, B., and Stenberg, J. (1964). 'Circulatory response to prolonged severe exercise', *J. Appl. Physiol.*, **19**, 833–838.
55. Costill, D. L., Coté, R., Miller, E., Miller, T., and Wynder, S. (1975). 'Water and electrolyte replacement during repeated work in the heat', *Aviat. Space Environ. Med.*, **46**, 795–800.
56. Saltin, B. (1964). 'Aerobic work capacity and circulation at exercise in man', *Acta Physiol. Scand.*, **62, Suppl. 230.**
57. Jacobsson, S., and Kjellmer, I. (1964). 'Accumulation of fluid in exercising skeletal muscle', *Acta Physiol. Scand.*, **60**, 286–292.
58. Senay, L. C., Jr. (1972). 'Changes in plasma volume and protein content during exposures of working men to various temperatures before and after acclimatization to heat: Separation of the roles of cutaneous and skeletal muscle circulation', *J. Physiol.*, **224**, 61–81.
59. Senay, L. C., and Kok, R. (1977). 'Effects of training and heat acclimatization on blood plasma contents of exercising men', *J. Appl. Physiol.*, **43**, 591–599.
60. Scatchard, G., Batchelder, A. C., and Brown, A. (1944). 'Chemical, clinical, and immunological studies on the products of human plasma fractionation. VI. The osmotic pressure of plasma and of serum albumin', *J. Clin. Invest.*, **23**, 458–464.
61. Gauer, O. H., and Henry, J. P. (1976). 'Neurohormonal control of plasma volume', *Intern. Rev. Physiol. Cardiov. Physiol.*, **II, 9**, 145–190.
62. Collins, K. J., and Weiner, J. S. (1968). 'Endocrinological aspects of exposure to high environmental temperatures', *Physiol. Rev.*, **48**, 785–839.
63. Segar, W. E., and Moore, W. W. (1968). 'The regulation of antidiuretic hormone release in man. I. Effects of change in position and ambient temperature and blood ADH levels', *J. Clin. Invest.*, **47**, 2143–2151.
64. Epstein, M. (1978). Renal effects of head-out water immersion in man: implications for an understanding of volume homeostasis', *Physiol. Rev.*, **58**, 529–581.
65. Blomqvist, C. G., Nixon, J. V., Johnson, R. L., Jr., and Mitchell, J. H. (1981). 'Adaptation to zero gravity as simulated by head-down tilt', *Human Cardiovascular Adaptation to Zero Gravity*, Symposium, 20 April 1979, University of Copenhagen, August Krogh Institute, European Space Agency, Paris, pp. 6–7.

66. Röcker, L. (1981). 'Volume regulating hormones and their role in the cardiovascular adaptation to zero gravity', *Human Cardiovascular Adaptation to Zero Gravity*, Symposium, 20 April 1979, University of Copenhagen, August Krogh Institute, European Space Agency, Paris, pp. 18–20.
67. Röcker, L., Kirsch, K., and Agrawal, B. (1982). 'Long-term observations on plasma antidiuretic hormone levels during and after heat stress', *Europ. J. Appl. Physiol.*, (in press).
68. Convertino, V. A., Brock, P. J., Keil, L. C., Bernauer, E. M., and Greenleaf, J. E. (1980). 'Exercise training-induced hypervolemia: role of plasma albumin, renin, and vasopressin', *J. Appl. Physiol.*, **48**, 665–669.
69. Melin, B., Eclache, J. P., Geelen, G., Annat, G., Allevard, A. M., Jarsaillon, E., Zebidi, A., Legros, J. J., and Gharib, Cl. (1980). 'Plasma AVP, neurophysin, renin activity, and aldosterone during submaximal exercise performed until exhaustion in trained and untrained men', *Europ. J. Appl. Physiol.*, **44**, 151–171.
70. Wade, C. E., and Claybaugh, J. R. (1980). 'Plasma renin activity, vasopressin concentration, and urinary excretory responses to exercise in men', *J. Appl. Physiol.*, **49**, 930–936.
71. Wade, C. E., Dressendorfer, R. H., O'Brien, J. C., and Claybaugh, J. R. (1981). 'Renal function, aldosterone, and vasopressin excretion following repeated long-distance running', *J. Appl. Physiol.*, **50**, 709–712.
72. Gilligan, D. R., Altschule, M. D., and Katersky, E. M. (1943). 'Physiological intravascular hemolysis of exercise. Hemoglobinemia and hemoglobinuria following cross-country runs', *J. Clin. Invest.*, **22**, 859–869.
73. Bichler, K. H., Lachmann, E., and Porzsolt, F. (1972). 'Untersuchungen zur mechanischen Hämolyse bei Langstreckenläufern', *Sportarzt und Sportmed.*, **23**, 9–14.
74. Heilmann, E., Blumenberg, G. R., Behr, J., Lunke, G., and Schmidt, J. (1976). 'Die mechanische Hämolyse bei Langstreckenläufern', *Sportarzt und Sportmed.*, **27**, 27–31.
75. Poortmans, J. R., and Haralambie, G. (1979). 'Biochemical changes in a 100 km run: proteins in serum and urine', *Europ. J. Appl. Physiol.*, **40**, 245–254.
76. Rous, P., and Robertson, O. H. (1917). 'The normal fate of erythrocytes. I. The findings in healthy animals', *J. exp. Med.*, **25**, 651–664.
77. Broun, G. O. (1922). 'Blood destruction during exercise. I. Blood changes occurring in the course of a single day of exercise', *J. exp. Med.*, **36**, 481–500.
78. Broun, G. O. (1923). 'Blood destruction during exercise. II. Demonstration of blood destruction in animals exercised after prolonged confinement', *J. exp. Med.*, **37**, 113–130.
79. Broun, G. O. (1923). 'Blood destruction during exercise. III. Exercise as a bone marrow stimulus', *J. exp. Med.*, **37**, 187–206.
80. Broun, G. O. (1923). 'Blood destruction during exercise. IV. The development of equilibrium between blood destruction and regeneration after a period of training', *J. exp. Med.*, **37**, 207–220.
81. Davidson, R. J. L. (1964). 'Exertional haemoglobinuria: a report on three cases with studies on the haemolytic mechanism', *J. Clin. Path.*, **17**, 536–540.
82. Buckle, R. M. (1965). 'Exertional (march) haemoglobinuria. Reduction of haemolytic episodes by use of sorbo-rubber insoles in shoes', *Lancet*, **i**, 1136–1138.
83. Streeton, J. A. (1967). 'Traumatic haemoglobinuria caused by karate exercise', *Lancet*, **ii**, 191–192.
84. Kaden, W. S. (1970). 'Traumatic hemoglobinuria in congo-drum players', *Lancet*, **i**, 1341–1342.

85. Hornbostel, H., Huenges, R., Montz, R., and Osburg, K. (1970). 'Neuere Erkenntnisse bei der Marschhämoglobinurie', *Dtsch. med. Wschr.*, **95**, 458–462.
86. Steinhaus, A. H. (1933). 'Chronic effects of exercise', *Physiol. Rev.*, **13**, 103–147.
87. Gibson, J. G., 2nd., and Evans, W. A., Jr. (1937). 'Clinical studies of the blood volume. II. The relation of plasma and total blood volume to venous pressure, blood velocity rate, physical measurements, age and sex in ninety normal humans', *J. Clin. Invest.*, **16**, 317–328.
88. Kjellberg, S. R., Rudhe, U., and Sjöstrand, T. (1950). 'Increase of the amount of hemoglobin and blood volume in connection with physical training', *Acta Physiol. Scand.*, **19**, 146–151.
89. Sjöstrand, T. (1953). 'Volume and distribution of blood and their significance in regulating the circulation', *Physiol. Rev.*, **33**, 202–228.
90. Sjöstrand, T. (1955). 'Das Sportherz', *Dtsch. med. Wschr.*, **80**, 963–966.
91. Sjöstrand, T. (1956). 'Blutverteilung und Regulation des Blutvolumens', *Klin. Wschr.*, **34**, 561–569.
92. Gregersen, M. I., and Rawson, R. A. (1959). 'Blood volume', *Physiol. Rev.*, **39**, 307–342.
93. Holmgren, A., Mossfeldt, F., Sjöstrand, T., and Ström, G. (1960). 'Effect of training on work capacity, total hemoglobin, blood volume, heart volume and pulse rate in recumbent and upright positions', *Acta Physiol. Scand.*, **50**, 72–83.
94. Schmidt, H. A. E., Musshoff, K., Reindell, H., König, K., Burchard, D., Held, E., and Keul, J. (1962). 'Die Beziehungen zwischen Blutvolumen, Herzvolumen und körperlicher Leistung', *Z. Kreisl.-Forsch.*, **51**, 165–176.
95. Albert, S. N. (1963). *Blood Volume* (Ed. J. Adriani), Charles C. Thomas, Springfield, IL., p. 24.
96. Bevegård, S., Holmgren, A., and Jonsson, B. (1963). 'Circulatory studies in well trained athletes at rest and during heavy exercise, with special reference to stroke volume and the influence of body position', *Acta Physiol. Scand.*, **57**, 26–50.
97. Scholer, H. (1964). 'Das Blutvolumen, eine Klinisch relevante Betriebs-größe, ein extracardialer Parameter der Zirkulation', *Cardiologia*, **45**, 231–250.
98. Gebhardt, W., Wierig, U., Keul, J., and Reindell, H. (1966). 'Kreislaufzeiten und Blutvolumen von Sportlern in Beziehung zu anderen Meßgrößen des Kreislaufs', *Arch. Kreisl.-Forsch.*, **49**, 188–214.
99. Saltin, B., Blomqvist, G., Mitchell, J. H., Johnson, R. L., Jr., Wildenthal, K., and Chapman, C. B. (1968). 'Response to exercise after bed rest and after training. A longitudinal study of adaptive changes in oxygen transport and body composition', *Circulation*, **38, Suppl. 7**, 1–78.
100. Brotherhood, J., Brozović, B., and Pugh, L. G. C. (1975). 'Haematological status of middle- and long-distance runners', *Clin. Sci. Molecular Med.*, **48**, 139–145.
101. Röcker, L., Kirsch, K. A., and Stoboy, H. (1976). 'Plasma volume, albumin and globulin concentrations and their intravascular masses. A comparative study in endurance athletes and sedentary subjects', *Europ. J. Appl. Physiol.*, **36**, 57–64.
102. Röcker, L. (1977). 'Der Einfluß körperlicher Aktivität auf das Blut', in *Zentrale Themen der Sportmedizin* (Ed. W. Hollmann), Springer-Verlag, Berlin, Heidelberg, New York, vol. 2, pp. 91–111.
103. Miller, P. B., Johnson, R. L., and Lamb, L. E. (1964). 'Effects of four weeks of absolute bed rest on circulatory functions in man', *Aerospace Med.*, **35**, 1194–1200.
104. Taylor, H. L., Erickson, L., Henschel, A., and Keys, A. (1945). 'The effect of bed rest on the blood volume of normal young men', *Am. J. Physiol.*, **144**, 227–232.

105. Vogt, F. B., Mack, P. B., Johnson, P. C., and Wade, L., Jr. (1967). 'Tilt table response and blood volume changes associated with fourteen days of recumbency', *Aerospace Med.*, **38**, 43–48.
106. Clement, D. B., Asmundson, R. C., and Medhurst, C. W. (1977). 'Hemoglobin values: comparative survey of the 1976 Canadian Olympic team', *CMAJ.*, **117**, 614–616.
107. Dill, D. B., Braithwaite, K., Adams, W. C., and Bernauer, E. M. (1974). 'Blood volume of middle-distance runners: effect of 2.300-m altitude and comparison with non-athletes', *Med. Sci. Sports*, **6**, 1–7.
108. Komadel, L., Mikulaj, L. and Repceková, D. (1980). 'Einfluß der Belastung auf den Testosteronspiegel des Blutes' in *Sportmedizin, 26. Deutscher Sportärztekongreß Bad Nauheim 1978* (Eds. P. E. Nowacki and D. Böhmer), Thieme Verlag, Stuttgart, New York, p. 114–117.
109. Guyton, A. C., Coleman, T. G., and Granger, H. J. (1972). 'Circulation: overall regulation', *Ann. Rev. Physiol.*, **34**, 13–46.
110. Glass, H. I., Edwards, R. H. T., Garetta de, A. C. and Clark, J. C. (1969). '[11]Co red cell labelling for blood volume and total hemoglobin in athletes: effect of training', *J. Appl. Physiol.*, **26**, 131–134.
111. Bass, D. E., Buskirk, E. R., Iampietro, P. F., and Mager, M. (1958). 'Comparison of blood volume during physical conditioning, heat acclimatization and sedentary living', *J. Appl. Physiol.*, **12**, 186–188.
112. Oscai, L. B., Williams, B. T., and Hertig, B. A. (1968). 'Effect of exercise on blood volume', *J. Appl. Physiol.*, **24**, 622–624.
113. Yamaji, R. (1951). 'Studies on protein metabolism in muscular exercise. I. Nitrogen metabolism in training of hard muscular exercise', *J. Physiol. Soc. Jap.*, **13**, 476–482, (in Japanese).
114. Yamaji, R. (1951). 'Studies on protein metabolism in muscular exercise. II. Changes of blood properties in training of hard muscular exercise', *J. physiol. Soc. Jap.*, **13**, 483–489, (in Japanese).
115. Yoshimura, H., Yamaji, R., Yamamoto, Y., Hayashi, M., Fukuda, M., Niiyama, Y., Koishi, H., Inoue, T., and Kirimura, K. (1951). 'Effects of muscular work on protein metabolism', *J. Jap. Soc. Food Nutr.*, **3**, 2–7, (in Japanese).
116. Yoshimura, H. (1955). 'The protein metabolism and protein requirement in muscular training', *J. Jap. Soc. Food Nutr.*, **7**, 199–207, (in Japanese).
117. Usami, S. (1957). 'Protein metabolism in strenuous muscular exercise and stress theory. IV. Studies on protein metabolism in muscular exercise', *J. Physiol. Soc. Jap.*, **19**, 468–481, (in Japanese).
118. Yoshimura, H., Usami, S., Koshitani, J., and Yoshioka, T. (1957). 'Studies on protein requirement of heavy workers. V. Studies on protein metabolism in muscular exercise', *Seikagaku*, **29**, 143–153, (in Japanese).
119. Yamada, T. (1958). "Resistance of erythrocyte in hard muscular exercise', *Jap. J. Phys. Fitness*, **7**, 242–251, (in Japanese).
120. Yamada, T. (1958). 'Studies on properties of erythrocyte during physical training. I', *Jap. J. Phys. Fitness*, **7**, 231–241, (in Japanese).
121. Hiramatsu, S. (1960). 'Studies on the cause of erythrocyte destruction in muscular exercise. (Changes in erythrocyte properties in sports training and their physiological significance. Report I)', *Acta Haem. Jap.*, **23**, 843–851, (in Japanese).
122. Yoshimura, H. (1965). 'Studies on protein metabolism in hard muscular work in relation to its nutritional requirement', in *Proceedings of a Symposium on Arctic Biology and Medicine*, Aeromedical Laboratory, Fort Wainwright, Alaska, pp. 439–476.

123. Yamada, T., Shiraki, K., and Yoshimura, H. (1975). 'Sports anemia and nutrition', in *Annual Report of Japanese Malnutrition Panel in US-Japan Cooperative Medical Program*, National Institute of Nutrition, Tokyo, pp. 55–59, (in Japanese).
124. Shiraki, K., Yamada, T., and Yoshimura, H. (1977). 'Relation of protein nutrition to the reduction of red blood cells induced by physical training', *Jap. J. Physiol.*, **27**, 413–421.
125. Yoshimura, H., Inoue, T., and Yamada, T. (1977). 'Changes of osmotic fragility of erythrocyte related to change of lipid profile in serum during hard physical training to muscular exercise', in *Annual Report of Japanese Malnutrition Panel in US-Japan Cooperative Medical Program*, National Institute of Nutrition, Tokyo, pp. 69–80, (in Japanese).
126. Yoshimura, H. (1959). 'Studies on anemia during physical training', *Jap. J. Phys. Fitness*, **8**, 167–168, (in Japanese).
127. Shiraki, K. (1968). 'The effect of splenectomy on sports anemia', *J. Physiol. Soc. Jap.*, **30**, 1–13, (in Japanese).
128. Yoshimura, H., Yamaoka, S., Usami, S., Yamada, T., Morishima, M., Hachisuka, H., Yoshioka, T., Tateishi, M., Ikeda, K., Tanaka, N., Saito, S., and Hattori, K. (1961). 'Studies of the "sports anemia" on the athletes and its countermeasures. I', *J. Jap. Soc. Food Nutr., (Eiyoto Shokuryo)*, **14**, 224–229, (in Japanese).
129. Horiguchi, S., Miyashita, K., Ideta, S., and Asaka, K. (1975). 'Peripheral blood findings of young female through the result of blood tests of students of a women's college. 2. Calory intake during camp training and athlete's anemia', *Osaka City Med. J.*, **21**, 79–83.
130. Yoshimura, H., Usami, S., and Hiramatsu, S. (1959). 'Studies on protein requirement of the heavy workers', *Med. Biol.*, **51**, 26–30, (in Japanese).
131. Hisaoka, F., and Shiraki, K. (1974). 'The effect of splenectomy and dietary protein on erythrocyte survival and fragility in rats', *J. Nutr. Sci. Vitaminol.*, **20**, 375–382.
132. Ashida, T., Yamada, T., and Yoshimura, H. (1972). 'Effect of protein nutrition on the Hb-binding capacity of haptoglobin in the muscular training', *J. Jap. Soc. Food Nutr., (Eiyoto Shokuryo)*, **25**, 633–639, (in Japanese).
133. Yamada, T., Shiraki, K., and Yoshimura, H. (1976). 'Studies on the mechanism causing the sports anemia', in *Annual Report of Japanese Malnutrition Panel in US-Japan Cooperative Medical Program*, National Institute of Nutrition, Tokyo, pp. 73–79, (in Japanese).
134. Ootsuka, A. (1967). 'Effect of adrenal hormones, especially adrenaline as a cause of sports anemia', *Bull. Doshisha Womens' Coll.*, **18**, 157–166, (in Japanese).
135. Tsutumi, T., Goto, Y., and Aoki, K. (1968). 'Catecholamine metabolism of man in ordinary life and the effect of physical exercise on it', *Bulletin of the Physical Fitness Research Institute—The Meiji Life Foundation of Health and Welfare*, **14**, 1–12, (in Japanese).
136. Hartley, L. H., Mason, J. W., Hogan, R. P., Jones, L. G., Kotchen, T. A., Mougey, E. H. Wherry, F. E., Pennington, L. L., and Ricketts, P. T. (1972). 'Multiple hormonal responses to graded exercise in relation to physical training', *J. Appl. Physiol.*, **33**, 602–606.
137. Hartley, L. H., Mason, J. W., Hogan, R. P., Jones, L. G., Kotchen, T. A., Mougey, E. H., Wherry, F. E., Pennington L. L., and Ricketts, P. T. (1972). 'Multiple hormonal responses to prolonged exercise in relation to physical training', *J. Appl. Physiol.*, **33**, 607–610.
138. Galbo, H., Holst, J. J., and Christensen, N. J. (1975). 'Glucagon and

catecholamine responses to graded and prolonged exercise in man', *J. Appl. Physiol.*, **38**, 70–76.

139. Cousineau, D., Ferguson, R. J., de Champlain, J., Gauthier, P., Côté, P., and Bourassa, M. (1977). 'Catecholamines in coronary sinus during exercise in man before and after training', *J. Appl. Physiol.*, **43**, 801–806.

140. Winder, W. W., Hagberg, J. M., Hickson, R. C., Ehsani, A. A., and McLane, J. A. (1978). 'Time course of sympathoadrenal adaption to endurance exercise training in man', *J. Appl. Physiol.*, **45**, 370–374.

141. Selye, H. (1946). 'The general adaptation syndrome and the diseases of adaptation', *J. Clin. Endocr.*, **6**, 117–230.

142. Yoshimura, H., Inoue, T., Yamada, T., and Shiraki, K. (1980). 'Anemia during hard physical training (sports anemia) and its causal mechanism with special reference to protein nutrition', *Wld. Rev. Nutr. Diet.*, **35**, 1–86.

143. Bergenhem, B., and Fåhraeus, R. (1936). 'Über spontane Hemolysinbildung im Blut unter besonderer Berücksichtigung der Physiologie der Milz', *Z. exp. Med.*, **97**, 555–587.

144. Singer, K. (1941). 'Lysolecithin and hemolytic anemia. The significance of lysolecithin production in the differentiation of circulating and stagnant blood', *J. Clin. Invest.*, **20**, 153–160.

145. Singer, K., Miller, E. B., and Dameshek, W. (1941). 'Hematologic changes following splenectomy in man, with particular reference to target cells, hemolytic index and lysolecithin', *Am. J. Med. Sci.*, **202**, 171–187.

146. Cooper, R. A., and Jandl, J. H. (1968). 'Bile salts and cholesterol in the pathogenesis of target cells in obstructive jaundice', *J. Clin. Invest.*, **47**, 809–822.

147. Shiraki, K., and Sagawa, K. (1979). 'Changes of membrane properties of RBC due to the reduction of plasma pH', Data presented at *56th Annual Meeting of Physiol. Soc. of Japan*.

148. Hagerman, J. S., and Gould, R. G. (1951). 'The in vitro interchange of cholesterol between plasma and red cells', *Proc. Soc. Exp. Biol. Med.*, **78**, 329–332.

149. Quarfordt, S. H., and Hilderman, H. J. (1970). 'Quantitation of the in vitro free cholesterol exchange of human red cells and lipoproteins', *J. Lipid. Res.*, **11**, 528–535.

150. Reed, C. F. (1968). 'Phospholipid exchange between plasma and erythrocyte in man and the dog', *J. Clin. Invest.*, **47**, 749–760.

151. Yoshimura, H., and Shiraki, K. (1980). 'Role of red blood cells in adaptation to hard muscular exercise with special reference to protein nutrition-physiological meaning of sports anemia', in *Environmental Physiology: Aging, Heat and Altitude* (Eds. S. M. Horvath and M. K. Yousef), Elsevier North-Holland, New York, Amsterdam, Oxford, pp. 147–177.

152. Switzer, S., and Eder, H. A. (1965). 'Transport of lysolecithin by albumin in human and rat plasma', *J. Lipid. Res.*, **6**, 506–511.

153. Klibansky, C., and DeVries, A. (1963). 'Quantitative study of erythrocyte-lysolecithin interaction', *Biochim. Biophys. Acta*, **70**, 176–187.

154. Glomset, J. A. (1963). 'Further studies of the mechanism of the plasma cholesterol esterification reaction', *Biochim. Biophys. Acta*, **70**, 389–395.

155. Glomst, J. A. (1968). 'The plasma lecithin: cholesterol acyltransferase reaction', *J. Lipid. Res.*, **9**, 155–167.

156. Tarlov, A. R. (1966). 'Lecithin and lysolecithin metabolism in rat erythrocyte membranes', *Blood*, **28**, 990–991.

157. Jaffé, E. R., and Gottfried, E. L. (1968). 'Hereditary nonspherocytic hemolytic disease associated with an altered phospholipid composition of the erythrocytes', *J. Clin. Invest.*, **47**, 1375–1388.

158. Oliveira, M. M., and Vaughan, M. (1964). 'Incorporation of fatty acids into phospholipids of erythrocyte membranes', *J. Lipid. Res.*, **5**, 156–162.
159. Robertson, A. F., and Lands, W. E. M. (1964). 'Metabolism of phospholipids in normal and spherocytic human erythrocytes', *J. Lipid. Res.*, **5**, 88–93.
160. Deitrick, R. W., Ruhling, R. O., and Deitrick, D. W. (1980). 'Retrogression and the red blood cell', *J. Sports Med.*, **20**, 67–74.
161. Shiraki, K., Yamada, T., Ashida, T., and Yoshimura, H. (1975). 'Protein nutrition and physical fitness in relation to sports anemia', *Proc. 10th Intern. Congress of Nutrition Science, Kyoto*, 181–182.
162. Hiramatsu, S. (1960). 'Changes in erythrocyte properties in muscular exercise and their physiological significance', *Acta Haem. Jap.*, **23**, 852–861, (in Japanese).
163. Whipple, G. H. (1926). 'The hemoglobin of striated muscle. I. Variations due to age and exercise', *Am. J. Physiol.*, **76**, 693–707.
164. Pattengale, P. K., and Holloszy, J. O. (1967). 'Augmentation of skeletal muscle myoglobin by a program of treadmill running', *Amer. J. Physiol.*, **213**, 783–785.
165. Ashida, T. (1972). Sports anemia and protein nutrition', *J. Jap. Soc. Food Nutr., (Eiyoto Shokuryo)*, **25**, 380–392, (in Japanese).
166. Goldberg, A. L. (1967). 'Work-induced growth of skeletal muscle in normal and hypophysectomized rats', *Am. J. Physiol.*, **213**, 1193–1198.

Current Concepts in Erythropoiesis
Edited by C. D. R. Dunn
© 1983 John Wiley & Sons Ltd.

CHAPTER 12

The erythropoietic effects of weightlessness

P. C. JOHNSON

Medical Research Branch
Lyndon B. Johnson Space Center
National Aeronautics and Space Administration, Houston

Contents

I. HISTORICAL ASPECTS

Prior to the initial space flight, lists were made of the possible physiological abnormalities expected when man entered a near zero gravity environment. As

279

an example, there was concern that the near zero gravity state might affect the fluid dynamics of the eye and adversely affect vision. In fact, flight experience from the earliest U.S.S.R. orbital flights and the U.S.A. Mercury flights indicated that the lack of an atmosphere decreased light dispersion with the result that vision was actually improved and that many of the other concerns were also unfounded.

Some of the predicted changes did occur. There was a redistribution of fluid and a loss of vascular and extravascular fluid no longer sequestrated in the dependent portions of the body by gravitational force. On return to Earth, the Mercury crew members showed the predicted weight loss and cardiovascular response to an extracellular fluid volume adequate for space flight no longer adequate for standing on the Earth's surface. One crew member had near syncope even though he had been in the weightless state for less than two days.

Because of the concern that the fluid volume decrease might be an operational problem to the crewmen and the medical recovery team, NASA allowed Dr Craig Fischer and myself the opportunity to perform a plasma volume (PV) determination (^{125}I-human serum albumin) on the crewmen before and after the Gemini 4 mission. These determinations showed that space flight caused a decrease in circulating PV, and that this decrease was at least partially responsible for the cardiovascular manifestations in the upright position upon return to Earth's gravity. These include increased pulse rate, decreased pulse pressure, and changed blood pressure. When the determined PV was subtracted from the calculated blood volume, we noted that the derived red blood cell mass (RCM) had decreased during the mission. This was totally unexpected and could not be explained on the basis of anything other than some factor relating to the mission had caused the RCM to decrease. The calculated changes were considerably greater than the relatively small amount of blood withdrawn from the crewmembers for the pre- and post-flight blood chemistry and hematology studies. As might be expected, there was doubt that a change in RCM had occurred. We, the generators of the data, worried that something about space flight might have caused a change in the ratio of the peripheral to total body hematocrit and that this was the explanation for the decrease in the calculated RCM. Because of the initial findings and because NASA flight surgeons were still interested in documenting the change in PV, we were allowed to perform both a PV and a RCM determination pre- and post-flight for the crew members of Gemini 5 and 7. Gemini 7, a dedicated 14-day medical mission, included an elaborate balance study to measure calcium changes and nearly all of the medical measurements made during that mission were elevated to the status of 'medical experiments'. However, the PV, RCM, and red blood cell (RBC) survival determinations (^{51}Cr) continued to be justified as operational procedures necessary only to protect and monitor the health of the crewmen. As a consequence, we were limited to a series of operationally-practical study points rather than scientifically more desirable duplicate measurements pre-flight and multiple post-flight determinations.

showed a modestly shortened ^{51}Cr RBC survival (1).

With the start of the Apollo moon landing program, a decision was made to forego all medical experimentation so that the crews could give their full attention to the problems of landing and returning safely from the moon. Medical operations under Dr Charles E. Berry agreed to allow only the operational pre- and post-flight medical procedures, done for Gemini crews, to continue during Apollo. Since the RCM determinations had never reached the status of a medical experiment additional measurements were allowed during Apollo. The result was a series of determinations which verified that a RCM decrease occurs when man is exposed to a near zero-G state (2).

The next project after the Apollo moon landings was the Skylab program consisting of three missions, each longer in duration than the previous one. A major purpose of these three missions was to prove that man could exist and work in orbit for periods of up to three months in duration. During Skylab a variety of medical studies were performed, including measurements of the RCM. Because the hematology studies were elevated to experiment status, [^{14}C]glycine RBC lifespan, and ^{59}Fe-iron kinetic studies were performed along with the usual RCM and PV measurements (3).

With the Skylab program, came a major change in atmosphere breathed by the crew members. The launch to the Skylab in an Apollo command module spacecraft was under conditions identical with those of previous Apollo space ships. The atmospheres in the Gemini and Apollo craft were 100% oxygen at 5 pounds per square inch (psi) pressure, resulting in an oxygen partial pressure 60% greater than sea level. In contrast, the Skylab maintained atmospheric pressure at 5 psi but the atmosphere contained 30% nitrogen producing a near sea level oxygen partial pressure. Since the high oxygen pressure of the Apollo cabin atmospheres had been used to explain the post-flight decreases in RCM, it was predicted that an RCM decrease would not be recorded after the Skylab missions. As the data were calculated and each individual showed a decrease, it was realized that the hyperbaric oxygen exposure could not be the only explanation for the space flight induced decreases in circulating RCM.

Two to three post-flight RCM measurements were made for the Skylab crew members, and we learned that the RCM deficit is made up within four to six weeks post mission. The Skylab data were peculiar in that the immediate post-flight RCM deficit was greatest after the shortest mission and least after the longest mission. This led to theories that recovery of the deficit would begin after 60 days whether the crewman returned to Earth or stayed in flight (3).

Since Skylab, the U.S.S.R. has flown a reusable space laboratory, Salyut 4, which has been the home of crewmen who have remained in orbit up to 175 days. Using carbon monoxide to measure RCM, the U.S.S.R. investigators found decreases post-flight of a magnitude similar to those found in the U.S. program. More importantly, their data indicate no inflight recovery during these long duration flights. From this we can assume that the relationship between flight duration and 'recovery' of the RCM loss in the Skylab missions was fortuitous and not a physiological fact or mechanism. If indeed 'recovery' of the RCM does not occur in flight, it is important from a crew health viewpoint, to understand the mechanisms which apparently prevent the RCM from dropping below approximately 75% of the preflight RCM. The U.S.S.R. data indicated that the post-flight recovery of the RCM after long duration flights takes over 30 days and that a decrease in reticulocyte numbers can be expected postflight. The U.S.S.R. has not used a low pressure hyperoxic atmosphere as has the U.S.A. so that hypobaria and hyperoxia cannot be implicated in the RCM decrease found by their investigators and by inference is probably not the only cause of the changes noted after the U.S.A. flights.

The accumulated data indicate that a decrease in RCM occurs whenever man attempts weightless flight. The decrease in mass is a result of decreased numbers of RBC in the circulation rather than a decrease in mean cell volume (MCV), which is generally increased post-flight. For example, the mean MCV actually increased slightly from 88.3 to 90.5 during the Apollo missions. A decrease in circulating RBC can occur only if production is inhibited or if destruction or loss are enhanced or through a combination of these mechanisms.

Enhanced destruction is, of course, synonymous with a shortened RBC lifespan. Early in the program, hemolysis was thought to occur since the calculated ^{51}Cr RBC half-times were shortened after the Gemini missions (1). Additionally, hyperoxia is known to cause RBC hemolysis, and, as has been noted, the cabin atmospheres during the early missions were hyperoxic although not to the level used experimentally to produce hemolysis in laboratory animals. Additionally, later missions did not include a hyperoxic atmosphere. The possibility cannot be completely excluded that the level of hyperoxia, while insufficient to cause hemolysis, may have been sufficient to suppress erythro-poiesis by an 'excess oxygen' mechanism. Evidence of RBC loss through bleeding was not found either externally, e.g., GI tract, or internally, e.g., dermis or ocular fundi.

When hemolysis was no longer adequate to explain the results, bone marrow inhibition became the more popular explanation of the decrease in the RCM found after a space flight. Lowered post-flight reticulocyte counts were the major evidence in support of this theory. Plausible causes of bone marrow inhibition include: Inadequate caloric or protein intake; relative increase in the total body hematocrit as a result of the early inflight decrease in PV, and, as a result of an increased plasma phosphorus, a shift in the hemoglobin P_{50} causing the RBC to more readily give up bound oxygen.

II. HYPEROXIA AS A CAUSE OF THE RCM DECREASE

The percentage decreases in the ^{51}Cr RCM in the various missions of the Gemini and Apollo series is shown in Table 1. The mean decrease during Apollo was

Table 1. ^{51}Cr Red Cell Mass change

		Mission duration (days)	% Decrease for each crewman		
Gemini	4	4	12.0	13.0	
	5	8	20.0	22.0	
	7	14	19.0	7.0	
Apollo	7	11	0.5	9.4	0.3
	8	6	+2.3	2.2	4.0
	9	10	4.3	7.2	10.2
	14	9	1.7	9.1	4.0
	15	12	13.7	7.0	9.6
	16	11	13.6	11.9	17.0
	17	13	8.4	14.9	10.4

Mean Apollo Results

	% Decrease*	
21 crewmen (all above Apollo missions)	7.5 ± 1.1	
		$p < 0.05$
18 control subjects	0.01 ± 0.7	
12 crewmen of Apollo moon landing missions (Apollo 14–17)	10.1 ± 1.3	$p < 0.05$
6 crewmen with nitrogen in atmosphere (Apollo 7 and 8)	2.4 ± 1.7	

*Mean ± S.E.

7.5%. To rule out procedural problems and effects from drawing the blood specimens, concurrent control subjects were used. Generally, the determinations for the control subjects were done a day before the crew members at the launch site, recovery carriers, or the Johnson Space Center. These control subject values indicate that the decreases found in the crew members were due to flight-related factors and not due to the volume of blood drawn or to drawing blood at remote operational sites.

Table 2 shows that the peripheral hematocrits of returning crew members were essentially identical to the pre-flight peripheral hematocrits. This indicates there was a correspondence between the RCM decrease and the PV decrease so that the peripheral hematocrit at recovery was very similar to the pre-flight hematocrit. After the missions the RBC counts, hemoglobins, and hematocrits were very close to the pre-flight values with no consistent change. However, the calculated MCV tended to be increased slightly post mission. This indicates that the RCM drop was not a result of a decrease in MCV. When hematocrits were obtained 1–2 days later, there was a general decrease with

Table 2. Peripheral hematocrit data for crew members of Apollo missions 14–17

Mean individual pre-flight hematocrit	Change at recovery	Change 1 or 2(*) days later
46	0	−2
42	−1	−2
46	+1	0
47	0	−4*
46	0	−3*
43	+1	0*
42	−1	−2
44	+1	−2
43	+1	−3
46	−4	−4
44	0	−3
41	+1	−1
Mean difference	−0.1 ± 0.4†	−2.2 ± 0.4†

†$p < 0.05$

reference to the immediate post-flight values. The decrease in the hematocrit was a result of an expanding PV which rapidly returns the blood volume to a level equal to pre-flight values.

Table 3 shows the RCM of the crewmen who flew in the Apollo missions in whom the RCM was measured 14 days before launch and in the first 2 hr after the ocean landing. In this table, the RCM is corrected for bodyweight and indicates that the RCM decrease was greater for most of the missions than could be accounted for by the invariable weight decrease of the returning crewmen. For at least 3 hr prior to launch, the crewmen breathed 100% oxygen at sea level pressure. On the launch pad the command module atmosphere was at sea level pressure, but it contained 40% nitrogen. Apollo 7 to 9 were test missions which were performed to make sure that the equipment was adequate to perform a moon landing. Traces of the nitrogen added prior to launch remained in the command module atmosphere throughout the Apollo 7 and 8 missions (at a concentration of less than 5%). Shortly after each launch, the atmosphere was automatically bled from sea level to 5 psi, which was the operational pressure thereafter. Subsequently, all cabin atmosphere leaks were made up with 100% oxygen. From Apollo 9 on, the extravehicular activities allowed the residual nitrogen to escape into space. From that time on, the Apollo crewmen, as did the Gemini crewmen, breathed 100% oxygen at 5 psi. For those moon landing missions, Apollo 14–17, in which RCM determinations were made for the crews, the lunar module was attached to the command module early in the mission. The interior volume of the lunar module (6.7 m³) diluted any residual nitrogen in the command module

Table 3. Red Cell Mass of Apollo crew members

Crew member	1	2	3	
Apollo mission				Mission duration days
Pre-flight RCM (in ml/kg B.W.)*				
7	30.5	27.8	23.7	11
8	28.9	27.0	26.2	6
9	33.7	31.0	28.4	10
14	30.6	28.0	26.2	9
15	33.5	29.9	27.7	12
16	33.0	26.7	27.0	11
17	29.5	25.9	25.5	13
Post-mission RCM (% Change in ml/kg B.W.)				
7	−3.2	+3.9	+3.7	
8	+3.1	+1.8	+7.6	
9	−4.2	−6.8	−0.1	
14	−1.0	−0.4	+0.3	
15	−11.3	−8.0	−2.9	
16	−12.4	−7.9	−8.9	
17	−12.5	−6.2	−2.7	
Mean % change				
Moon Landings	Apollo 14–17	−6.2 ± 1.3† $p = 0.05$		
Non-moon Landings	Apollo 7–8	+2.8 ± 1.4†		

*Mean ± s.d. = 28.6 ± 0.6
†Mean ± s.e.

(5.95 m³) by a factor of two. Extravehicular activity on the moon's surface, as occurred during these missions, released the entire atmosphere of the lunar module which, when reoccupied, was replenished with 100% oxygen at 5 psi. Analysis of the RCM data from the lunar landing missions showed no difference between the mean change of the crew members who remained in the command module circling the moon from the mean change of the crew members who descended to the moon.

Table 4 shows the results of an altitude chamber study performed under NASA auspices by the USAF (4). In it, eight subjects were exposed to 100% oxygen at 5 psi. Only minute traces of nitrogen remained in the atmosphere. Table 4 shows the percentage decrease in the total body hemoglobin calculated by the carbon monoxide method. Half of the subjects were at bedrest while the other half were allowed to be up and about. Both groups remained in the chamber for 30 days. Also shown is the percentage change in RCM as

Table 4. Results of USAF study 100% O_2–5 psi atmosphere

Days of exposure	Mean % decrease in total body hemoglobin (CO method)	
	Bedrest	Controls
10	1	2
15	7	6
21	10	10
30	14	12
+14*	5	2
Mean % decrease in ^{51}Cr RCM		
28†	16	—

*14 days post exposure
†Bedrest day

measured by the ^{51}Cr-labeled RBC technique. The ^{51}Cr measurement was made pre-exposure and on exposure day 28.

The data from the ground-based study combined with the RCM decreases of the Apollo missions using 10% oxygen; the Gemini missions; and the lesser effect in the Apollo missions in which some nitrogen remained, Apollo 7 and 8, led to a hypothesized toxic effect of 100% oxygen at 5 psi on the circulating RBC (2). Two other NASA sponsored studies, in which a 5 psi atmosphere was used but with oxygen percentages consistently less than 95%, showed mean RCM decreases of 3.0% (5). Taken together then, these studies seem to prove that 100% oxygen in a 5 psi atmosphere, when breathed over a period of several days, will cause a decrease in the circulating RCM. However, results from the U.S.S.R. missions and the U.S. Skylab missions are evidence that something about a weightless flight other than a hyperoxic atmosphere causes a decrease in the RCM. Several theories have been proposed to explain this space flight induced phenomenon. These are discussed below.

III. BONE MARROW INHIBITION AS A CAUSE OF THE RCM DECREASE

Following the Apollo program, NASA flew three long duration missions using a large laboratory vehicle made from a Saturn IVB shell. For Skylab, the atmosphere was changed to an oxygen partial pressure equivalent to sea level but with a reduced nitrogen partial pressure. The total atmospheric pressure continued to be 5 psi, as in previous programs. The crews experienced a hyperoxic environment only in the prebreathing, prelaunch phase (minimum of 3 hr at 1 atmosphere) and when in their Apollo command module, until they

Table 5. Skylab results

Mission duration (days)	Recovery day	Percentage change (in ml of red cell mass)			
		Weeks after recovery			
		2	4	6	9
28	−15	−18		−8	−3
	−16	−16		—	+2
	−12	−13		−2	+2
59	− 6	− 3		+3	
	−20	−14		+2	
	−11	− 6		+3	
84	− 5	−4	+5		
	− 8	−4	+2		
	− 7	−6	+4		

Mean cell volume (MCV) change +4.2 ± 1.6*.
^{51}Cr RBC half-life (days); pre-mission 26.1 ± 0.9; post-mission 24.2 ± 0.7; difference −1.9 ± 1.0†.
[^{14}C]glycine mean RBC lifespan throughout the mission (days); crew members 123 ± 2; control subjects 121 ± 4†.
*Mean ± s.e..
†$p > 0.05$.

had opened the hatch connecting to Skylab. The lack of hyperoxic exposure led the investigators to predict that a smaller decrease or no change in RCM would be found. NASA performed a 56-day simulation in preparation for Skylab. It was performed in an altitude chamber designed to faithfully duplicate the Skylab equipment, experiments, food, and living arrangements. The atmosphere was the same as was planned for Skylab. It was hypobaric (5 psi), but not hyperoxic. The three subjects who participated showed percentage decreases in RCM of 2.9, 1.9, and 3.4 for a mean decrease of 2.7%. Although these changes were less than those seen after the Skylab missions, they indicate that there may be an effect of hypobaria in addition to that due to weightless flight (3,5). The Skylab data are shown in Table 5. The mean percentage decrease in the RCM of the 28-day mission was greater than the decrease after the 84-day mission. Repeat studies were performed post-flight. The timing of the recovery in the RCM seemed earlier after the 84-day missions than after the 28-day mission. However, RCM determinations were not performed at four weeks post-recovery after the first two missions. The mean ^{51}Cr RBC half-time and mean RBC lifespan were unaffected by the missions. This is evidence against hemolysis during the periods monitored.

Shown in Table 6 are the reticulocyte counts for the nine Skylab crew members. At recovery, the reticulocyte percentage and number were less than the pre-flight mean. On the following day (R + 1), two of the three crew members of the 84-day mission had reticulocyte counts above the pre-flight

Table 6. Reticulocyte counts of Skylab crew members
(Reticulocytes × 10^{-3}/mm^3 blood)

Mission duration	28 days			59 days			84 days		
	Commander	Scientist pilot	Pilot	Commander	Scientist pilot	Pilot	Commander	Scientist pilot	Pilot
Pre-mission Mean	37	37	27	32	33	43	48	43	44
± s.D.	2	1	3	6	3	2	5	7	3
Recovery day (R)	17	19	8	25	21	29	41	38	40
R + 1 day	18	24	12	—	—	—	46	45*	67*
R + 3 days	24	30	14	29	24	41	38	48	31
R + 1 week	29	30	22	42*	55*	102*	66*	55	72
R + 2 weeks	28	38*	21	38	81	126	77	88	83
R + 3 weeks	33	35	26	88	74	91	77	78	88

*First value greater than pre-mission mean.

IRON TURNOVER AT RECOVERY.

Mission duration days	(µg/kg body weight per day) Crew members	Controls
28	0.22	0.38
	0.35	0.33
	0.38	0.35
59	0.39	0.29
	0.24	0.30
	0.21	0.29
84	0.30	0.21
	0.38	0.23
	0.42	0.32
Mean ± s.e.	0.32 ± 0.03†	0.30 ± 0.01

†$p > 0.05$

Table 7. Long duration U.S.S.R. missions

Mission duration Days	Crew member	%Decrease in Red Cell Mass	
		Early post-flight	Late post-flight
96	1	24 (day 1)*	4 (day 32)*
	2	26	3
140	1	16 (day 3)*	—
	2	16	17 (day 7)*
175	1	19 (day 3)*	6 (day 36)*
	2	18	4

*The post mission day on which determination was made.

mean. This was quite different from the post mission reticulocyte counts of the six crew members from the two shorter Skylab missions. These values were used as evidence that the bone marrow is inhibited during weightless flight and that this inhibition is the cause of the RCM decrease. Unfortunately, we will have to wait for Spacelab and additional Shuttle missions before we can determine if the space flight induced decrease in reticulocytes is associated with a decrease in erythropoietin activity.

The U.S.S.R. spacecraft use an atmosphere equivalent to sea level. Three of their missions have lasted longer than the longest Skylab mission. The U.S.S.R. investigators determine RCM by the carbon monoxide method. Their results are shown in Table 7. Significant decreases in RCM were found. The weight loss of these crew members was slight with a small weight gain found in one of the two crewmen of the 175-day mission. As in the Skylab data, it appears that there is a considerable delay between the return to Earth and recovery of the RCM loss.

Taken together, the Skylab and U.S.S.R. data indicate that during space flight the RCM decreases, and this cannot be related to hyperoxia since the hyperoxic exposure of the Skylab crew members was of short duration prior to lift off and the U.S.S.R. cosmonauts are not exposed to a hyperoxic environment. After the long duration missions, there was a delay between the time the crewmen return to Earth and the return of their RCM to pre-flight levels. This delay, combined with the noted decrease in the reticulocyte numbers, suggests that the basic mechanism for the change is bone marrow inhibition. The only data against this are;

1. No prolongation of the post-flight plasma iron turnover (see Table 6).
2. The RCM decrease found after the short Gemini 4 and 5 missions was too great to be due only to bone marrow inhibition.

Both may not be entirely correct. First, the iron turnover was obtained during

Table 8. Initial Shuttle results obtained from routine hematology determinations

Mean	Pre-flight	Landing + 0	+ 3 days
RBC Count	4.8 ± 0.2*	5.2	4.6
Hemoglobin concentration	14.4 ± 0.4*	15.8	14.3
Hematocrit	0.42 ± 0.01*	0.46	0.42
Reticulocyte Number	32 ± 3*	34	32
MCV	87.5	88.5	91.3

*Mean ± s.e.
Four crew members.
The first two Shuttle missions lasted less than three days each.

the early post-flight phase. At that time, the PV was rapidly increasing during readaptation of the cardiovascular system to gravity. This would shorten the ^{59}Fe disappearance time. Second, the Gemini atmosphere was hyperoxic. Therefore, in the short Gemini missions we could postulate a hemolytic component due to hyperoxia.

The recently completed Shuttle missions lasted less than three days each. RCM determinations were not made; however, routine hematology (CBC) was performed. At landing, the RBC count, hemoglobin concentration, and hematocrit were increased (Table 8). This suggests a disproportionate loss of plasma. Also, these crewmen were relatively dehydrated on landing. Three days after landing, the RBC count and hemoglobin were below mean pre-flight levels while the MCV was increased. The mean changes were slight but in the right direction to indicate both PV and RCM changes. The reticulocyte numbers were not decreased, so there was no evidence of bone marrow inhibition.

If the Gemini, Apollo, Skylab, and Russian missions are considered, no relationship is observed between mission duration and the extent of the RCM decrease. If there was a change early after insertion into a weightless orbit, then marrow inhibition could not be the only cause, since marrow inhibition could not result in a rate of RCM decrease greater than 1% per day. A rate of loss less than 0.5% per day, representing partial inhibition, seems more reasonable. The changes found in the shorter Gemini and Apollo missions indicate a rate somewhat greater than 0.5%, with some missions exceeding 1% per day. It is still possible that the combination of a space flight effect combined with hyperoxia could have caused the greater than 1% per day loss of RCM during the Gemini flights.

Table 9. Effect of environmental temperature on plasma volume

Mean temperature (°C)	Red Cell mass	Plasma volume	Hematocrit
21	2008	3180	43
29	2003	3620	37
% Change*	-0.1 ± 1.0	$+13.3 \pm 1.8$	-12.3 ± 2.3

Studies done two weeks apart.
*Mean ± s.e. of mean.
Six subjects.

IV. POSSIBLE MECHANISMS OF BONE MARROW INHIBITION

As a result of the Skylab and U.S.S.R. data, the hyperoxia theory could be ruled out as the only cause of the RCM decrease. Several reasons for bone marrow inhibition have been proposed. These include the following possibilities;
1. Inflight response to a hematocrit rise as a result of the decreased PV which is known to occur within the first two days of flight.
2. Response to an increased plasma phosphorus shifting the hemoglobin P_{50}.
3. Decreased caloric and protein intake inhibiting bone marrow function.

A. Hematocrit increase

There is strong circumstantial evidence to suggest that a PV decrease follows the redistribution of fluids during weightless flight. Thus, the hemoglobin concentration during the early phases of the Skylab missions was increased approximately 10%. Assuming no change in the RCM, this could produce an hyperoxic tissue state and, consequently, suppressed erythropoiesis might occur if there were no shift in the oxyhemoglobin dissociation curve or change in the arterial blood flow. If a change in hemoglobin concentration of the order of 10% is capable of stimulating or inhibiting erythropoiesis, this should be provable and would need only inflight substantiation. Against it, however, is the fact that a 10% change in hemoglobin occurs regularly in normal subjects alternately exposed to hot and cold environments. As an example, our studies showed a 12% decrease in hematocrit from 43 to 37 between a cold winter day in Philadelphia and the warm environment of the Virgin Islands, yet, no acute change in RCM (6). These data are shown in Table 9. In a further attempt to test the hemoconcentration hypothesis, Dunn (7) has reduced the PV in mice by water deprivation and shown inhibition of erythropoiesis commencing prior to declining erythropoietin titers.

B. Response to increased plasma phosphorus

Any displacement of the oxyhemoglobin dissociation curve (ODC) profoundly affects the amount of oxygen available to the tissues. Qualitatively, a decrease in the affinity of hemoglobin for oxygen can be considered comparable to an increase in blood flow, hemoglobin concentration, or arterial pO_2. Shifts of the ODC are produced by changes in pH, CO_2 concentration, and temperature. Additional factors are the concentrations of intracellular phosphate compounds, particularly 2,3-diphosphoglyceric acid (2,3-DPG). Skylab measurements did not suggest that there was an increase in 2,3-DPG (8), but plasma phosphorus was increased during flight (9). In addition, the possibility exists that blood pCO_2 levels may have increased because ambient levels of carbon dioxide were above usual Earth concentrations. Each of these factors decrease hemoglobin's affinity for oxygen and would cause unloading of additional oxygen at the tissue level. Such a change might inhibit erythropoiesis, thus, leading to the RCM decrease of space flight.

C. Insufficient caloric or protein intake

During the Gemini missions, the crew members' mean daily caloric intake was kept below the usual 2800 kcal pre-flight intake on the assumption that the relatively inactive crew would require less calories. The rationale being that to prevent a weight gain required the reduction of caloric intake by approximately 300 kcal/day. As the crew members continued to return from flight several kilograms below pre-flight weight, attempts were made to increase caloric intake during the flights. Menus were calculated and designed on an individual basis for each Apollo crew member. Due to inflight workloads and space sickness, some crew members voluntarily ate less than had been planned. The data in Table 10 show that there was no relationship between mean daily caloric intake and the percentage change in RCM on a ml or a ml/kg body weight basis. In Table 10, the caloric intakes are arranged in increasing order. The Skylab data showed similar results, and even though daily caloric intake was as much as double that of some Apollo crew members, a significant weight loss was seen post flight undoubtedly partly due to a fluid loss. These data, shown in Table 11, indicate that the decrease in reticulocytes seen post mission was not entirely the result of an inadequate caloric intake. The same is true of the crew members in the U.S.S.R. long-duration flights.

In a study to determine if some unknown factor in the diet could be the cause of the RCM decrease found in the Apollo crew members, six paid volunteers (young males of college age) were maintained on a diet of Apollo flight food for one week (10). The caloric intake was planned to be isocaloric so that the subjects would not lose weight. However, subjects found the diet relatively unpalatable and consumed less than planned amounts (mean intake 2360

Table 10. Caloric intake and Red Cell Mass decrease in crew members of Apollo
missions 14 to 17

Weight (kg)	Mean (kcal/day)	% Decrease in RCM	% Change in RCM (ml/kg B.W.)
63	1565	11.9	−8.9
75	1720	9.1	−0.4
81	1805	8.4	−2.7
76	2007	10.4	−6.2
77	2284	14.9	−12.5
78	2310	1.7	+0.3
83	2330	4.0	−1.0
73	2366	17.0	−12.4
80	2403	13.6	−7.9
74	2492	7.0	−2.9
74	2572	9.6	−8.0
81	2903	13.7	−11.3

Table 11. Caloric intake and Red Cell Mass decrease in crew members of Skylab
missions

Mission duration (days)	Mean (kcal/day)	Body weight Decrease (kg)	% Decrease in red cell mass	
			(ml)	(ml/kg B.W.)
59	2784	4.5	6.1	0.7
28	2811	3.6	12.1	5.5
28	2831	1.5	15.2	11.9
59	2844	3.1	19.8	15.9
28	2972	2.8	15.6	10.9
84	3081	1.2	8.3	6.4
84	3201	0.1	4.8	5.3
84	3287	0.7	7.4	5.6
59	3879	4.2	10.6	9.3

kcal/day). During the one-week duration of the study, 100 ml of blood was
withdrawn from each subject. The results are shown in Table 12. The mean
body weight loss was 1.7 kg. PV decreased 113 ml (3.7%), and the RCM
decreased 104 ml (5.1%). While only 100 ml of blood had been withdrawn for
hematology and serum chemistry determinations, the total blood volume
decrease was 218 ml. Thus, the study showed a weight loss and a blood
volume loss. Both the mean weight loss and RCM decrease were approximately equal to those found after the Apollo space flights. This indicates that

Table 12. Results of the Apollo food evaluation study

	Pre	Post	% Decrease
Weight (kg)	72.1	70.4	2.4
Red cell mass (ml/kg)	28.3	27.5	2.8
Plasma volume (ml/kg)	42.3	41.7	1.4
Red cell mass (ml)	2043	1939	5.1
Plasma volume (ml)	3051	2938	3.7
Hematocrit	44	44	0.0

Mean of six subjects

reduced caloric intake can cause a decrease in RCM, but it could not be the total explanation for the decreases found after space flights, since even when adequate caloric intake was maintained, decreases in RCM were found, e.g., Skylab.

The effect of short-term protein deprivation on hematopoietic functions of healthy volunteers has been studied by Catchatourian et al (11). Protein intake was decreased to 8–10 g/day from 60–95/g day in three subjects. After eating the protein deficient diet for eight days, a hematocrit decrease of 3.0% was found. At the end of the diet period, a 500 ml phlebotomy was performed, and a delay in the post phlebotomy reticulocyte response was noted. PV and RCM were not measured so that it cannot be determined from these data whether the hematocrit drop included an increase in PV or a change in the peripheral/total body hematocrit ratio. Protein intake approaching the low values used in the Catchatourian study occurred during Gemini V. This might help account for the 21% decrease in RCM found after that mission, which was the greatest mean loss yet recorded in the U.S. program.

In the Apollo missions, protein intake varied from a low of 51 g/day to a high of 112 g/day with the mean being 76 g/day. Protein intake was even greater during Skylab. Therefore, it seems likely that protein deprivation is not a cause of the RCM and reticulocyte decreases.

Dunn et al have used the Skylab data to obtain a multi-variate regression analysis which includes three factors possibly related to the RCM decrease (12). These include changes in dietary intake during the flight (compared with absolute protein or caloric intake inflight—discussed above), changes in lean body mass (LBM) inflight, and the exercise performed by the crewmen on the bicycle ergometer. A highly significant correlation was found (r = 0.81). The equation is;

$$\Delta RCM = 11.0 \ (\Delta diet) + 0.0004 \ (\Delta LBM) - 169.1 \ (exercise) - 325.9$$

Of the three terms, the change in LBM contributed most to the over-all correlation which was much less sensitive to the change in diet. This is perhaps further evidence that a decrease in dietary intake *per se* is not of prime importance to the RCM decrease. It seems to suggest that the invariable space flight induced loss of LBM may be an etiological factor in the RCM decrease. The decrease in LBM has been shown to include atrophy of the antigravity muscles and may or may not include a component related to changes in dietary intake.

V. OTHER IDEAS ABOUT THE CAUSE OF THE RCM DECREASE

A. Prolonged excretion of hypertonic urine causing hemolysis due to the hypertonic renal medulla

Leon and Fleming noted that there was a statistically significant increase in urine osmolality in the inflight urine specimens of the Skylab crew members (13). They note that: 'Alexander *et al* proposed that prolonged excretion of a hypertonic urine leads to increased RBC destruction'. To test this hypothesis, Leon and Fleming decreased the water intake of laboratory rats by 66% for a 20-day period. The rats responded by decreasing food consumption 40%. The percentage reticulocytes decreased during the first five days to levels below 1% from the control level of about 3%. When water was again available, the reticulocyte percentages increased to twice control within three days. Measuring ^{14}CO derived from $[^{14}C]$glycine incorporated into the hemoglobin of the RBC, these authors found no difference in mean RBC lifespan or in the random hemolysis rate. (The glycine was injected 22 days before the 20-day dehydration period.) The osmolality of the animals' urine increased 70%. Thus, as in the experiments of Dunn (7), erythropoiesis was inhibited during dehydration but there was no evidence of enhanced RBC destruction. However, in both studies, one in mice and the other in rats, water deprivation caused the animals to decrease their food intake. The combination caused an inhibition of erythropoiesis. Although crewmen are never actively deprived of water, calculation indicates that all crew members go into negative water balance on the first day of weightless flight and this continues for a variable period thereafter (14). This is probably an iso-osmolar fluid loss as there was no increase in plasma sodium post-mission in the Apollo and Skylab crew members, and no increase in serum osmolality during or after Skylab (9). Thus it is possible that a negative water balance, with or without concomitant reduction in food intake, may contribute to the decrease in RCM.

B. RBC shape changes and the question of hemolysis

Kimzey *et al* used the scanning electron microscope to study the RBC shape to determine how this is affected by space flight (15). It is believed that RBC shape abnormalities might have an effect on the rate of removal of the RBC by the reticuloendothelial system. No significant change in shape was found after the moon landing Apollo 17 mission with the percentage of discocytes (normal configuration) showing a statistically insignificant change from 90% to 84%. Similar findings occurred after Skylab with the mean percentage of discocytes (nine crewmen) showing no change, being 83% both inflight and post-flight. During and after Skylab, the percentage of echinocytes increased from a pre-flight mean of 1% to about 15% in two crew members, 2% to 5% in three crew members and showed no essential change in the other four. These data suggest that space flight may cause an increase in echinocytes but with little change in the percentage of discocytes. Attempts have failed to correlate the increase in percentage of echinocytes with the changes in plasma electrolytes (e.g., Na, K, Ca), cellular ATP or 2,3-DPG (15).

The increase in echinocytes might cause premature removal of RBC from the circulation which would be seen as a shortened mean cell survival. However, decreased RBC lifespan was not found in the [14C]glycine determinations done on the nine crew members of Skylab including the three crewmen who showed the largest increase in the percentage of echinocytes. Therefore, the RCM decrease occurring after space flight in which hyperoxia is not a factor does not seem to be a hemolytic event. Nevertheless, it should be noted that a small change in RBC survival (whether ^{51}Cr or [14C]glycine is used) would be difficult to observe in the data collected. Daily blood samples were not obtained so any estimate of the half-time has a variance great enough to obscure 5% to 10% changes.

VI. HEMOLYSIS IN LABORATORY RATS FLOWN IN THE U.S.S.R. PROGRAM

Leon and Landlaw studied laboratory rats flown in the Cosmos 782 and 936 missions. The animals were injected with [14C]glycine pre-flight. The expired [14]CO was measured from the flight animals, some of which had been caged on an inflight centrifuge to produce a simulated gravity by using $1 \times g$ rotational force. The data indicate a three-fold increase in the rate of random hemolysis in the flight animals. This was largely attenuated in the animals flown on the $1 \times g$ centrifuge. The centrifuged inflight animals showed a random hemolysis rate similar to that of the ground-based vivarium control animals (16,17). These data are shown in Table 13.

VII. CONCLUSION

The results obtained to date from U.S. and U.S.S.R. crew members seem to have proven that space flight will cause the individual to decrease his circulating RCM. This decrease is a direct result of space flight and appears independent of factors such as the volume of blood drawn and the cabin

Table 13. Red blood cell survival parameters of laboratory rats flown on U.S.S.R. —
Cosmos 936 (17)

	K* (%/day)	% S*	T* (days)
Vivarium control	0.3 ± 0.1	85 ± 6	53 ± 2
Simulated flight	0.3 ± 0.2	83 ± 7	53 ± 2
Ground centrifuged	0.3 ± 0.3	86 ± 12	55 ± 4
Flight	1.0 ± 0.4	61 ± 12	43 ± 4
Flight centrifuged	0.2 ± 0.1	90 ± 5	53 ± 2

*For the ^{14}C-labeled RBC: K = rate of random hemolysis: % S = percentage which live to
senescence; T = mean lifespan

atmosphere. The cause of this decrease is still unknown and is probably
multifactorial with several factors differing qualitatively and quantitatively
from flight-to-flight.

A. Factors known to have been involved

These include:
1. Relative hyperoxia.
2. Hypobaria.
3. Insufficient protein and/or caloric intake.
4. Space flight induced decrease in LBM.

B. Factors possibly additive

These include:
1. Increased plasma phosphorus with a shift in the RBC hemoglobin P_{50}.
2. Relative lack of exercise performed during the mission.
3. Inflight increase in RBC echinocytes.
4. Renal blood flow changes associated with weightlessness.
5. Increased inflight total body and/or peripheral hematocrit.

C. Factors probably not involved

These include:
1. Dehydration in flight.
2. Toxic substances.
3. Radiation exposure.
4. Decreased bone marrow stimulation from testosterone.

Some of the above factors have not been discussed in this chapter because there
is insufficient data available or because the hypothesis has not yet been tested.

For example: in the correlation found by Dunn *et al*, daily exercise levels on the bicycle ergometer contributed to the correlation. Unfortunately, the effect of exercise on the RCM, even in a $1 \times g$ environment, depends on the type and duration of exercise (see Chapter 11) so the influence of work on the RCM in microgravity remains speculative. Renal blood flow changes are believed to occur, but to the present, have not been measured directly. Calculated creatinine clearance can be estimated from the Skylab data and show a slight increase suggestive of increased renal blood flow. Urinary ADH was decreased during the Skylab flights but, somewhat paradoxically, plasma osmolality, sodium and uric acid were also decreased perhaps confirming an increase in renal blood flow (9). The changes in renal function may be great enough to affect erythropoietin production.

The radiation exposure to date has been so small, it can be ruled out as a factor. The mission mean skin dose radiation exposure during Apollo varied between 0.16 and 1.14 rads. During Skylab, exposure of the blood-forming organs was greatest during the 84-day mission. The doses for the three crew members were 7.9, 7.3, and 6.7 rem. Toxic substances were looked for and all but eliminated by pre-flight out-gasing studies. Minute amounts of toxins have been found in the recycled cabin atmosphere; however, none approach levels known to have an effect on the RBC. Conceivably, the combination of several toxins could be a cause, but there is little reason to believe that the U.S.S.R. craft contain the same mix of hydrocarbons as do the U.S. space vehicles. Additionally, several different types of spacecraft have been flown. It would seem unlikely that we could find a toxin at elevated levels common to all situations unless the toxin is excreted by the crew member himself. Changes in testosterone levels have been looked for and not found. The data, however, are sparse and it could be that additional results could change the seeming unimportance of this factor.

The mechanism by which the change in RCM occurs is not yet known. Intravascular hemolysis seems to have been ruled out since there is no reported change in haptoglobin levels after the Apollo or Skylab missions (2,15). Enhanced trapping of the RBC by the reticuloendothelial system is an attractive hypothesis for the decrease. It has not been investigated. Bone marrow function has not been studied except by indirect measures such as iron turnover and incorporation and by reticulocyte counts (3). The iron studies may not be valid because of the PV changes occurring early post mission. The reticulocyte numbers may have been influenced by decreases in Vitamin E levels. Decreases in this vitamin may have been sufficient to increase reticulocyte lifespan and/or increase RBC sensitivity to damage by hyperoxia. Either directly or as a response to hemolysis, these mechanisms may explain why no post-flight decreases in reticulocytes were seen after the Gemini and Apollo missions (hyperoxic cabin atmospheres), but were observed in the crews of the Skylab and U.S.S.R. missions where the cabin atmospheres were essentially normoxic. Erythropoietin levels have yet to be measured in flight.

In summary, much has been learned of the inflight RCM decrease, but the cause in the human has yet to be proven to be absence of gravitational force. The mechanism by which it occurs is also unproven. From what is known, we can predict that every crew member will lose part of his measurable RCM during space flight. This loss of circulating RBC will be made up post-mission by a post-flight stimulation of the bone marrow. This stimulation will last long enough to return the RCM to normal. No residual ill effect is known to remain. Whether this decrease in RCM and later increase in bone marrow function will be correlatable with eventual pathology is now unknown.

VIII. REFERENCES

1. Fischer, C. L., Johnson, P. C., and Berry, C. A. (1967). 'Red blood cell mass and plasma volume changes in manned space flight'. *J. Am. Med. Assoc.*, **200**, 579–583.
2. Kimzey, S. L., Fischer, C. L., Johnson, P. C., Ritzman, S. E., and Mengel, C. E. (1975). 'Hematology and immunology studies', in *Biomedical Results of Apollo* (Eds. R. S. Johnston, L. F. Dietlein and C. A. Berry), National Aeronautics and Space Administration, Publication SP-368, Washington, D.C., pp. 197–226.
3. Johnson, P. C., Driscoll, T. B., and LeBlanc, A. D. (1977). 'Blood volume changes', in *Biomedical Results from Skylab* (Eds. R. S. Johnston and L. F. Dietlein), National Aeronautics and Space Administration, Publication SP-377, Washington, D.C., pp. 235–241.
4. Larkin, E. C., Adams, J. D., Williams, W. T., and Duncan, D. M. (1974). 'The hematologic responses to hypobaric hyperoxia; Hematologic responses to a continuous 30-day exposure to hypobaric hyperoxia', in *Report to the National Aeronautics and Space Administration from Defense Contract MIP-744016*, Washington, D.C.
5. Johnson, P. C. (1973). 'Blood volume and RBC lifespan', in *Final Report of the Skylab Medical Experiments Altitude Test (SMEAT)*, National Aeronautics and Space Administration, Publication TMX-58115, Houston, TX.
6. Johnson, P. C., Driscoll, T. B., and Fischer, C. L. (1971). 'Blood volume changes in divers of Tektide I', *Aerospace Med.*, **42**, 423–426.
7. Dunn, C. D. R. (1980). 'The effect of food and water restriction on erythropoiesis in mice: Relevance to the anemia of space flight', *Am. J. Physiol.*, **238**, R301–R305.
8. Mengel, C. (1977). 'Red cell metabolism studies on Skylab', in *Biomedical Results from Skylab* (Eds. R. S. Johnston and L. F. Dietlein), National Aeronautics and Space Administration, Publication SP-377, Washington, D.C., pp. 242–248.
9. Leach, C. S., and Rambaut, P. C. (1977). 'Biochemical responses of the Skylab crewmen: An overview', in *Biomedical Results from Skylab* (Eds. R. S. Johnston and L. F. Dietlein), National Aeronautics and Space Administration, Publication SP-377, Washington, D.C., pp. 204–216.
10. Handler, E. W., Leach, C. S., Johnson, P. C., Fischer, C. L., Rummel, J., and Rambaut, P. C. (1971). 'Biochemical and physiological consequences of the Apollo flight diet', *Aerospace Med.*, **42**, 1192–1195.

CURRENT CONCEPTS IN ERYTHROPOIESIS

11. Catchatourian, R., Eckerling, G., and Fried, W. (1980). 'Effect of short-term protein deprivation on hemopoietic functions of healthy volunteers', *Blood*, **55**, 625–628.
12. Dunn, C. D. R., Johnson, P. C., and Leonard, J. I. (1981). 'Erythropoietic effects of spaceflight re-evaluated', in *Proceedings of the 3rd Annual Meeting of the International Union of Physiological Sciences Commission on Gravitational Physiology*, Innsbruck, Austria, September–October 1981. *The Physiologist*, **24**, (**Suppl**), S5–S6.
13. Leon, H. A., and Fleming, J. E. (1980). 'Extremes of urine osmolality: Lack of effect on red blood cell survival', *Am. J. Physiol.*, **239**, C27–C31.
14. Leach, C. S., Leonard, J. I., Rambaut, P. C., and Johnson, P. C. (1978). 'Evaporative water loss in man in a gravity-free environment', *J. Appl. Physiol.*, **45**, 430–436.
15. Kimzey, S. L. (1977). 'Hematology and immunology studies', in *Biomedical Results from Skylab* (Eds. R. S. Johnston and L. F. Dietlein), National Aeronautics and Space Administration, Publication SP-377, Washington, D.C., pp. 249–281.
16. Leon, H. A., Serova, L. V., Cummins, J., and Landlaw, S. A. (1978). 'Alterations in erythrocyte survival parameters in rats after 19.5 days aboard Cosmos 782', *Aviat. Space Environ. Med.*, **49**, 66–69.
17. Leon, H. A., and Landlaw, S. A. (1978). 'Effect of weightlessness and centrifugation on erythrocyte survival in rats subjected to prolonged space flight', in *Final Reports of U.S. Experiments flown on the Soviet Satellite Cosmos 936* (Eds. S. N. Rosenzweig and K. A. Souza), National Aeronautics and Space Administration, Technical Memorandum 78526, Ames Research Center, Moffett Field, C.A., pp. 60–77.

Current Concepts in Erythropoiesis
Edited by C. D. R. Dunn
© 1983 John Wiley & Sons Ltd.

CHAPTER 13

Nuclear events during differentiation of erythroleukemia cells

WILLIAM SCHER*, BARBARA M. SCHER†, and SAMUEL WAXMAN*

Departments of Medicine and Microbiology†,
Cancer Chemotherapy Foundation Laboratory,
Mount Sinai School of Medicine of the City University of New York.*

Contents

I. INTRODUCTION

Since the finding, in 1971, that mouse erythroleukemia (MEL) cells in tissue culture could be induced to differentiate along the erythrocytic pathway by the addition of dimethyl sulfoxide (DMSO) to the medium (1) this system has been used extensively for the study of erythrodifferentiation (see references 2–7 for reviews). Due to limitations of space as well as the availability of several other fairly recent reviews, a complete review of all events that have been studied in MEL cells during differentiation that might involve nuclear acitivities is not being attempted, nor is a complete listing of all pertinent references included. However, it is hoped that this chapter touches on most of the events that have been studied in MEL cells that directly pertain to nuclear structure or function and therefore will be useful in the planning of future research.

DMSO, and many other agents, induce increased levels of several erythrocytic-specific and erythrocytic-compatible characteristics in these cells. The specific erythrocytic markers include three types of globin mRNA and their translated globin chains, fully assembled hemoglobin, and spectrin. When treated with some inducers the cells mature morphologically from approximately a pronormoblast stage to an orthochromatophilic normoblast stage. Under certain conditions an enucleated, reticulocyte-like stage has been reported (8,9) although this finding has not been further substantiated. The time course of the induction of hemoglobin synthesis in MEL cells has similarities to the time course of erythrocytic cell production *in vivo*. Slight increases in hemoglobin levels are seen after one day of inducer treatment. By three days there is a modest increase; by five days there is nearly a maximum response and by seven days a maximum level is noted. With certain inducers, such as hexamethylene bisacetamide (HMBA), 98% of the cells may produce enough hemoglobin to be detected by benzidine–hydrogen peroxide staining.

Friend leukemia virus (FLV)–transformed cells that can be cloned and maintained, apparently indefinitely, in suspension culture, have been used for the majority of these studies and the following discussion will review investigations primarily carried out with this system. However, rat carcino-gen-transformed erythroleukemia (EL) cell lines (10–12), mouse Rauscher leukemia virus (RLV)-infected EL lines (13–17) and human cell lines capable of erythrodifferentiation (18,19) also have been developed. To our knowledge evidence for viral-association with EL cell lines has only been reported for mouse lines although it was suggested that the rat line also contained viral particles (10). The physiologic erythrocytic hormone, erythropoietin (EPO) has not been shown to have a major effect on FLV-infected MEL cells. EPO was shown to induce a slight stimulation of heme synthesis after three days of culture in one FLV-infected MEL cell line (20) and to augment the effect of DMSO on heme synthesis (also after three days of culture) (21,22). However, RLV-infected MEL cells, which have only been grown in semi-solid medium, do respond to EPO with erythrodifferentiation, including increases in hemoglobin levels (13,14), in much the same fashion that FLV-infected cell lines respond to DMSO. None of the long-term EL cell lines has yet been shown to respond to 'burst-promoting activity' the other major physiologic erythrocytic hormone (23).

II. DNA AND SOME DNA-ASSOCIATED COMPONENTS

The molecular mechanisms that control cellular differentiation are poorly understood. MEL cell differentiation is one of the model systems that is being utilized to gain insight into this process. Most of the hypotheses suggested to explain this process have centered upon either membrane or nuclear effects. Although the initial regulatory sites may reside in the membrane there is evidence that at least some of the critical steps occur in the nucleus. All of the inducing agents known increase the level of globin mRNA (2–7). The levels of all three adult-type globin mRNAs are increased. Increases in both nuclear and cytoplasmic globin mRNAs have been documented. Therefore at least one control step in the process of formation of each type of globin is pretranslational. Studies with 5-bromo-2'-deoxyuridine (BRdU), a compound that is incorporated into DNA in place of thymidine, have shown that control over globin mRNA and hemoglobin synthesis probably can occur at the level of transcription (24–27). This is thought to be the case since, BRdU markedly inhibits the DMSO-induced increase in heme synthesis and in globin mRNA and hemoglobin levels (24–27). This inhibition occurs only during the time that BRdU is being incorporated into DNA and the simultaneous addition of thymidine partially reverses the inhibition due to BRdU. However, because BRdU can inhibit thymidine transport as well as the incorporation of thymidine into DNA this theory has been controversial (28,29).

Furthermore, induction of differentiation in MEL cells seems to be associated with a transmitted change. MEL cells can undergo five or six cell divisions following commitment (3–6,30,31). Commitment was defined for this purpose as being the ability to produce hemoglobin and have a limitation in cell multiplication in the absence of an inducing agent following a suitable period of time in contact with an inducing agent (31). (This type of 'terminal' commitment should not be confused with the fact that MEL cells are erythrocytic and therefore are 'committed' to erythrocytic, rather than lymphocytic, for example, maturation if they are stimulated to do so.)

Commitment can be detected after approximately 20 hr of treatment with many inducers. Events that are initiated prior to this time are generally considered 'early events' in the erythrodifferentiation program of MEL cells, while those initiated after this time are considered to be 'late events' (9).

MEL cells appear to undergo at least one, or at most a few, cycles of DNA replication after being treated with an inducer prior to their becoming terminally committed. However, since 90% or more of the cells can and always do become induced to produce hemoglobin under certain conditions, the induction cannot be due to a rare, random, point mutation in a single cell. Since induction in a majority of the cells can occur after an inducer has been removed from the cells, there must be a change in the cells that occurs which is transmissible for five or six cell divisions. The transmissible change can be due to any of three processes;

1. A regulated change in sequence, modification or configuration of the DNA.
2. A marked reduction in the level of a critical regulatory molecule, the level of which cannot be regenerated in up to five cell divisions in the absence of an inducer.
3. A marked increase in the level of a regulatory molecule, the level of which can be maintained through up to five cell divisions in the absence of an inducer.

In normal mammalian erythrocytic maturation the nucleus becomes smaller and is finally ejected from the cell (see reference 32 for a discussion). It was noted in the first report on the induction of differentiation of MEL cells that the nucleus and the nuclear-cytoplasmic ratio become smaller during this process (1). Subsequently this has been studied in more detail by several investigators (33,34). The nucleus becomes hetero-pyknotic and resembles the nucleus of an orthochromatophilic normoblast. This occurs even if the cell does not become smaller during the induction process, which occurs with certain selected inducers (35).

A. DNA and Chromatin Structure

As mentioned above, during MEL cell maturation there is an increase in the level of total as well as translatable globin mRNA sequences (3–6). Therefore, at least in so far as globin synthesis is concerned, a regulatory site exists that is pretranslational, i.e., either at or prior to transcription of globin mRNA or during post-transcriptional globin mRNA processing. Studies of MEL cell globin gene region characteristics have therefore been undertaken. It was reported that either isolated nuclei or chromatin from DMSO-treated cells have a greater capacity to code for globin mRNA in an *in vitro* cell-free transcription system than have similar preparations from untreated cells (3,36–38). Concentrations of DMSO or other inducing agents, that are higher than those required for the stimulation of MEL cell erythrodifferentiation, have been shown to stimulate general transcription of chromatin when added to an MEL cell-free system (39). DMSO, at an even higher concentration, 2.5 M, was shown to stimulate both total RNA and *gal* RNA synthesis in cell-free systems that utilized bacterial and bacteriophage components (40–42). It is not known if all of these findings have the same or different biochemical *raison d'être*.

Several alterations in MEL cell DNA and/or chromatin that may occur during differentiation have been studied. Genes that code for differentiation-related proteins are in a different configuration in the differentiated cell than in the undifferentiated parent cell. For example, in the nucleated red blood cell of the chick the globin gene is more sensitive to treatment with DNAase I than it is in the chick oviduct (43). This appears to be a specific change related to differentiation since the ovalbumin gene is preferentially sensitive to DNAase I in the oviduct, but not in the erythrocyte. When the globin genes in MEL cells were examined for their DNAase I sensitivity, it was found that they were equally sensitive prior to and following DMSO treatment of the cells (38,44). This was the case in both inducible and DMSO-resistant, non-inducible variant cell lines. However, the globin genes of all of the MEL cell cultures examined were more sensitive to DNAase I than were the globin genes of adult mouse liver (44). Therefore, it was surmised that MEL cells, which are erythrocytic precursors, have their globin genes already in a configuration that is primed for further erythrocytic differentiation and awaiting biochemical signals to progress along this pathway. Following the same general train of thought other investigators have examined the globin genes in differentiating MEL cells using DNAase II as the test agent, but the results are controversial (discussed in 44).

It is possible, although it has not been definitely demonstrated, that the 'erythrocytic-type' of DNAase I-sensitive configuration of DNA can be introduced into the DNA from cells of non-erythrocytic lineage which then allows the transcription of globin genes. That is, cells that are hybrids, produced by the fusion of MEL cells with mouse teratocarcinoma, human fibroblast or human B-lymphoblast cells can be induced to express not only the globin genes of the MEL cell parent, but of the other parent cell as well (see 45,46). Presumably the globin genes in the parent lines for these cell fusions were not in a DNAase I-sensitive configuration prior to cell fusion except for those in the MEL cells. Mouse lymphoblasts are one of the various types of cells shown not to have their globin genes in a DNAase I-sensitive configuration (44). Therefore, if this 'configuration' is necessary for this phenomenon then the non-MEL cell globin genes that were introduced into hybrid cells and then became expressed, presumably were altered to this type of configuration after cell fusion.

Other experiments have focused on the effect of the X-chromosome on hemoglobin formation. The mouse X-chromosome contains a regulatory locus (loci) that inhibits DMSO-induced heme synthesis and therefore hemoglobin formation. Hybrid cell lines formed from MEL cells (line FTG3CI which does not contain an X-chromosome) and either mouse primary bone marrow cells or lymphoma cells (which both contained mouse X-chromosomes) neither synthesize heme or hemoglobin in response to DMSO unless hemin is added to the medium or the X-chromosome is eliminated by segregation techniques (46). However, globin mRNA levels are increased by DMSO treatment in these hybrids. Therefore, a locus on the mouse X-chromosome appears to control the DMSO induction of heme synthesis that is required for hemoglobin synthesis (e.g. 47). However it was also reported that several hybrid lines formed from the same line of MEL cells and human lymphoblasts in which 48–64% of the metaphases examined contained a human X-chromosome were capable of increasing hemoglobin production in 39–54% of the cells in response to DMSO (46,48). Therefore, it is not clear whether or not the human X-chromosome contains a similar regulatory locus. It may actually have been present and operative in only approximately half of the cells in the hybrid lines tested. Hybrids formed from tetraploid MEL cells and non-erythrocytic cells (human fibroblasts or non-erythrocytic peripheral blood mononuclear cells) respond to DMSO by activation of some of the globin genes from the non-erythrocytic parent (45,49,50). Similar hybrids formed utilizing diploid MEL cells did not respond to DMSO. These findings could be related to the gene dosage of the X-chromosome of the non-erythrocytic parent line in relation to the dose of critical factors supplied by the tetraploid MEL cells.

There appears to be no globin gene amplification during the MEL cell differentiation process (51). However, since this study was performed with a radiolabeled DNA probe complimentary to globin mRNA it would only detect opposite sense, (non-coding strand of) DNA globin sequences. Therefore, it is possible, although unlikely, that an amplification of globin-coding single-stranded DNA sequences occurred and was not detected by these methods.

Morphologic changes in the nucleus are prominent features of DMSO-induced differentiation of MEL cells as they are of normal mammalian erythrocyte maturation *in vivo* (mentioned above). In general, as MEL cells mature not only do the cells themselves and the nuclei become smaller, but the chromatin assumes a more clumped, condensed appearance (1). MEL cell nuclear condensation does not appear to be related to the nucleosome repeat length in chromatin since it does not change during DMSO treatment when the cultures are in the late logarithmic and stationary phases of multiplication (52). In untreated cultures a change has been noted in this aspect shortly after DNA synthesis begins. The internucleosome spacer of newly replicated (10 min) MEL cell chromatin is approximately 20 bases longer than that of total chromatin (53).

The binding of intercalating compounds to the chromatin has been used as a probe for differences in chromatin structure which occur after treatment with DMSO. It has been reported that the binding of fluorescent compounds that intercalate between the bases of DNA in MEL cell chromatin is decreased in cells undergoing induced differentiation when compared to uninduced cells. This was found when either propidium iodide (54) or acridine orange was utilized as the intercalating agent (55). An increase in the sensitivity of the chromatin of DMSO-treated MEL cells to acid denaturation has also been noted using acridine orange as a probe. These changes in denaturability, thought to be related to chromatin condensation in other systems, have been seen as early as 24 hr after culture with DMSO and are well established by 48 hr (55).

In addition to these changes other alterations have also been noted during DMSO-induction of MEL cells. The DNA synthesized in cells after their treatment with DMSO or other inducing agents has a lower single-strand molecular weight (as judged by alkaline sucrose gradient centrifugation) than the DNA synthesized during the same time period in untreated cells (56). Pre-radiolabeled DNA, formed before addition of DMSO to the cells, also decreases in single-strand molecular weight (also determined in alkaline sucrose gradients) after the addition of DMSO to the cells (57).

Rotationally-constrained DNA (nucleoids or 'folded genomes') isolated from DMSO-treated cells has a slower sedimentation velocity (57) and a lower superhelical density (58) when compared to untreated cells. These chromatin changes are consistent with an accumulation of nicks or gaps in the DNA from induced cells. In keeping with this idea, treatment of the cells with known DNA-damaging agents, such as ultraviolet light and X-rays, modestly induces MEL cell erythrodifferentiation (56,57). In contrast, in another study it was reported that DNA strand breaks could not be detected in differentiating MEL, K-562, or HL-60 cells by the alkaline elution technique (59). It is not known, however, if the size of the products of DNA breakage are in a range measurable by the alkaline elution technique (molecular weight approximately $0.29–4.1 \times 10^9 D$) (60).

Explanations not involving pre-existing DNA discontinuities, are possible for at least some of the findings noted. For example, depurination or depyrimidation can also lead to strand breakage in alkali. Changes in the sedimentation properties of the nucleoids could also be due to changes in the protein content of chromatin. The changes seen in DNA and/or chromatin structure could be due to increased instability of the chromatin which then undergoes degradation during isolation. Increased susceptibility of the chromatin to the action of both exogenous and endogenous nucleases has been noted in DMSO-treated MEL cells (61). Differences in nuclease-sensitivity have also been noted in the chromatin of FLV-infected cells of different malignant stages (62). However, mixtures of either differentially-radiolabeled DNA or nucleoids from DMSO-treated and untreated cells were not modified in their respective sedimentation properties as a consequence of the mixing (57). This would seem to rule out the presence of a diffusable cellular substance from the cells of one culture, untreated or DMSO-treated, whose presence during the isolation procedure could change the sedimentation behavior of DNA or nucleoids from the cells of the other culture.

There may be a possible link between the apparent appearance of an increase in single-stranded regions in DNA during DMSO treatment and an alteration in transcription. Single-stranded DNA isolated from MEL cells as well as from other cell types is enriched in sequences that are being actively transcribed (63). The occurrence of such sequences was slightly enriched in DMSO-induced cells compared to untreated ones. Cross-hybridization experiments indicated that 10% of the single-stranded, transcriptionally-active DNA sequences of the DMSO-treated cells were specific to these cells and were not present in untreated MEL cells (63).

B. Methylation of DNA

Gene expression in higher organisms has been related at least in part, to the extent of methylation and DNAase I-sensitivity of actively transcribed regions. The incorporation of 5-azacytidine, a cytosine analog, which cannot be methylated at the 5-position, into a retrovirus gene has been shown to be associated with the acquisition of DNAase I-hypersensitive sites, undermethylation of DNA, and gene expression (64).

Hemoglobin gene expression in the developing chick embryo has also been correlated with regions of preferential DNAase I-digestion, DNAase I-hypersensitive sites and undermethylation of DNA (65). How the chemically-induced differentiation of MEL cells and other erythroleukemia cells relates to this postulated program is not clear. The sensitivity of the globin genes of MEL cells to DNAase I digestion was elevated both in uninduced and induced MEL cells when compared to non-erythrocytic cells (44). Recently experiments by Sheffery et al. (44a) have indicated that there was an increase in site-specific cleavages by DNAase I (DNAase I-hypersensitive sites) in chromatin regions near both α- and β-major globin genes after HMBA-mediated erythrocytic differentiation. There was, however, no discernible change in the pattern of DNA methylation around either gene during this induction. Similarly, induction of K-562 cells with hemin to yield hemoglobin-producing cells did not cause the methylation pattern in and around the (flanking) β-globin gene to change from the pattern of the uninduced state (66).

The DNA produced by DMSO-induced MEL cells is, however, undermethylated and agents known to interfere with methylation (such as ethionine) can weakly induce differentiation in these cells (67,68). The undermethylation of DNA is apparently due to a lack of exposure sites for, or activity of DNA methyltransferase(s) since no DNA demethylating enzyme activity has been described. The DNA methyltransferase of MEL cell chromatin is primarily associated with the internucleosomal, transcriptionally less active, regions of chromatin (69). Undermethylation of DNA has been noted as early as 24 hr after addition of inducer. It may be that the undermethylation causes the activation of additional signals required for the initiation of the transcription of the β-globin genes and of other proteins. It is also possible that this more extensive undermethylation is the harbinger of a more general alteration of chromatin structure which leads ultimately to chromatin condensation and the terminally differentiated state.

Many of the changes affecting chromatin structure in DMSO-treated MEL cells become evident in the period from 20 hr to 27 hr after the addition of DMSO. This is also the approximate time when the prolongation of the G1 phase is noted in inducer-treated cells and is close to the time when 'commitment' is first observed in DMSO-treated cells (31,70).

There are several reasons why chromatin structure could be altered in erythrocytic differentiation. Any of the above changes could be related to the initiation of the expression of certain genes or, conversely, gene expression could result in changes in chromatin-related functions which would lead ultimately to a shift in the conformation of the chromatin to a more condensed state. The result of this chromatin condensation could then lead to a gradual shutdown in the expression of certain genes which could further modify chromatin structure and/or function, and could lead ultimately to the loss of proliferative capacity seen in the differentiating cells. The structural changes seen could be related to any of the above events.

It is of interest to note that a low degree of superhelical structure has been observed in nucleoids prepared from hen erythrocytes (71), cells in which the chromatin is highly condensed and non-functional (72). In contrast, the nucleoids prepared from embryonic erythrocytes in which the chromatin is active and not highly condensed, had more pronounced superhelicity (71).

C. DNA synthesis

Cytokinesis is not required for the induction of MEL cell differentiation (73–75). However, it appears that some DNA replication or DNA synthesis is essential or enhances the magnitude of induction of erythrodifferentiation in MEL cells (4–6,76–78).

DNA synthesis is affected by most inducers in usually two ways. Firstly, there is generally an early lag in the rate of DNA synthesis after treatment of a culture with an inducer (79). In cells that are in late logarithmic or early stationary phase and have just been placed in fresh medium with and without an inducer, there is a rapid increase in DNA synthesis (4,6,76,77). In untreated cultures the increase in rate continues for about 10 hr and then reaches a plateau for about 30 hr. In treated cultures the increased rate stops by 4 hr to 6 hr and a decrease in DNA synthesis sets in that lasts for 20 hr to 30 hr. The rate of DNA synthesis again increases as treated cultures enter logarithmic phase and reach a maximum during the second or third day. Later in the third day it decreases as the treated cultures also reach stationary phase. The induced lag in DNA synthesis (or the transient prolongation of the G1 state of the cell cycle) may be important for the differentiation process. Most inducers that have been tested cause this lag. However, since two potent inducers, actinomycin D and hypoxanthine, did not prolong G1 (6,80), it does not seem to be essential. Furthermore, if a culture in early logarithmic growth is subcultured into fresh medium with and without added DMSO there is little or no initial lag in cell multiplication rate in either condition.

The early portion of the S-phase may be particularly important in the initiation of MEL cell erythrodifferentiation. The replication of both α- and β-globin chromosomal DNA sequences appears to occur preferentially in line DS-19 cells during the first quarter to third of the S-phase when compared to the replication of non-globin sequence regions of the genome (81,82). However, this does not seem a universal phenomenon since in line T3-Cl-2 globin genes were found to be replicated during the latter portion of the middle third of the S-phase (83).

Although DMSO treatment may result in a lag in DNA synthesis and cell multiplication, it frequently causes a small increase (approximately 10%) in final cell concentration after five days of growth. This is apparently due to the fact that the treated cells have a smaller modal volume and a lower total protein content (6,84,85; see below). Therefore, treated cultures can yield more cells with the nutritional components available in non-replenished media than can untreated cultures.

Secondly, and perhaps more importantly, during the later stages of MEL cell differentiation the rate of DNA synthesis decreases (78,87). At first appraisal this might appear to be due to the catabolization of nutritional components in the medium and the entrance of the culture into the stationary phase of growth due to the depletion of medium nutrients. This accounts however, for only part of the phenomenon. Cultures entering or in the stationary phase of growth that are treated with 2% DMSO and reseeded into fresh medium do not subsequently enter another normal logarithmic growth phase. In contrast, cells that are reseeded into medium free of an inducer (after a slight lag interval) enter the S-stage of the cell cycle and the culture again grows logarithmically. For example, it was reported that a concentration of DMSO less than optimal for inducing differentiation (1.0%, vol/vol, 140 mM) severely reduced MEL cell multiplication rate when the cells were serially reseeded daily into fresh medium containing the inducer compared to cells reseeded into medium without DMSO (86). In this experiment the cells were not allowed to enter the stationary phase of multiplication due to lack of nutritional components since the medium was constantly replenished. This induced limitation of cell multiplication and of replicative DNA synthesis has been termed 'commitment' as defined above (31). Using a commitment assay performed in liquid medium it was demonstrated that the cells once induced to commit to hemoglobin synthesis by four days of DMSO treatment undergo no further cell division when replated into fresh medium without DMSO. The 'uncommitted' cells in the very same culture flask do re-enter a logarithmic growth phase. (e.g., see Figure 3 in reference 30).

D. DNA polymerases

The alterations in DNA synthesis due to DMSO treatment could be related to altered activities of DNA polymerases. Three laboratories have examined DNA-dependent DNA polymerases during the differentiation of MEL cells. The specific activity of DNA polymerase I (α) was found to rise during the first two days of treatment of the cells with 1.5% DMSO relative to that in untreated cells at that time and then to decrease for the next three days. The activity of this polymerase in DMSO-treated cells did not fall below that in untreated cells until the fifth day. At that time the activity was approximately 60% of that in untreated cells (88). Subsequently studies in MEL cells of the three eukaryotic cell DNA polymerases (α, β and γ, generally regarded as responsible for replicative DNA synthesis, repair DNA synthesis and mitochondrial DNA synthesis, respectively) have been carried out. Lacatena *et al.* demonstrated that the activity per cell of DNA polymerase α in MEL cells followed that of the general cellular DNA synthesis rate, being highest during logarithmic growth in both untreated and inducer-treated cells (89). These investigators found that the activity per cell of DNA polymerase γ remained unchanged during DMSO treatment, but that the activity of DNA polymerase β in induced cultures was approximately 50% of that in untreated ones for the first 24 hr of growth. However, at 48 hr and 72 hr of growth the levels in the treated cultures increased and were nearly as high as in the untreated ones. The DMSO-induced alteration in the activity of DNA polymerase β did not occur in a variant cell line that was resistant to DMSO-induced differentiation. This suggests that there may be a relative lack of ability to repair DNA strand breaks during DMSO treatment. Giri *et al.* (90) found the same pattern of DNA polymerase α activity in untreated and induced MEL cells synchronized by thymidine treatment or by elutriation; that is, it was highest in the S-phase of the cell cycle (89, and discussion in 6). However, in this study no changes were noted in the β polymerase activity Giri *et al.* also reported that if after four days of growth in replenished medium in the presence or absence of HMBA the cells were reseeded again into fresh medium the α polymerase activity recovered in the untreated cells, but not in the HMBA-treated ones. This suggests that at least a portion of the limitation in DNA synthesis that occurs in terminally differentiating, committed MEL cells may be due to a decrease in the activity of DNA polymerase α.

E. DNA ligase

Another enzymatic change which may be related to the limitation of cell multiplication seen in the DMSO-treated MEL cells is the marked decrease in the level of DNA ligase activity observed in cells grown for three or more days in DMSO-containing medium (91). When MEL cells were induced to differentiate by culturing in the presence of 1.8% DMSO the apparent specific activity of the DNA ligase decreased to approximately 12% of the value of that in untreated MEL cells. When strain DR-10, a variant cell line resistant to DMSO, was treated with DMSO in similar fashion the DNA ligase activity remained the same as that in untreated cells. When DNA ligase-containing extracts of untreated and DMSO-treated cells were mixed, the activities in the two types of extract were additive. Therefore, there was no evidence for the presence of an inhibitor of DNA ligase activity in the extracts from DMSO-treated cells.

The DMSO effect seems to be relatively specific for DNA ligase. The specific activity of a DNAase I-like enzyme in the MEL cells increased slightly with DMSO-treatment, while the specific activity of acid phosphatase remained unchanged. These data would indicate that a change of some sort is occurring in the nucleus of the DMSO-treated MEL cells such that the extractable DNA ligase activity is reduced in amount. It seems unlikely that the DNA ligase activity is simply bound more tightly in the nuclear fraction. Several chromatin proteins have been found to be more easily extracted from the nuclei of DMSO-treated MEL cells than those from nuclei of untreated MEL cells (92). The lack of DNA ligase activity could be due to a change in the rate of synthesis or breakdown of the enzyme(s) in the cell or could be due to the sequestering of the DNA ligase activity in some inactive form in the extracts.

MEL cells were grown in the presence or absence of DMSO and samples of the cells tested for DNA ligase activity at various intervals (Table 1). The cells grown in the absence of DMSO contained a specific activity of DNA ligase which varied from 0.6 to 1.3 units/mg protein in cells cultured for 0–113 hr. The cells grown in the presence of 1.8% DMSO contained a high specific activity of DNA ligase (0.6–1.3 units/mg) for the first 43 hr of culture. After 67 hr in culture, however, the specific activity of the extracts had decreased to 0.13 units/mg and remained at 0.1 units/mg or less for the remainder of the experiment (113 hr in culture).

This loss of extractable DNA ligase activity occurred after about five doublings of the cells in the presence of DMSO. It is known that after commitment due to DMSO treatment as well as other inducers the cells generally undergo no more than five or six cell divisions (6,31,93). These data suggest that the lack of DNA ligase activity could be directly or indirectly related to the loss of proliferative capacity seen in 'committed' MEL cells.

Table 1. DNA ligase and DNAase activity in extracts of MEL cells grown in the presence or in the absence of DMSO

Addition to medium	Time in culture*	DNA ligase activity†		DNAase activity‡	
	(hr)	units per mg protein	units per 10^8 cells	units per mg protein	units per 10^8 cells
None	0	0.58	1.8	21	62
	19	0.65	2.8	23	98
	43	1.33	4.5	21	71
	67	0.58	1.8	21	62
	95	0.74	2.2	15	51
	113	1.10	3.0	24	65
DMSO, 1.8% (vol/vol)	0	0.58	1.8	21	62
	19	1.08	3.6	26	86
	43	1.27	3.6	29	82
	67	0.13	0.29	29	66
	95	0.09	0.18	27	68
	113	<0.04	<0.11	20	56

*Cells were grown for the number of hours indicated in medium plus 15% fetal bovine serum with or without DMSO and then cell-free extracts were prepared as described (91).
†Enzyme assays were performed as described (91). DNA ligase activity was determined by following the ligation of the cohesive termini of bacteriophage ϕ105 DNA. Each incubation mixture (40 µl) contained 10 mM Tris-HCl (pH 7.6), 0.12 M KCl, 10 mM MgCl$_2$, 0.15 mM ATP, 15–30 µg G-actin, 2.4 µg ϕ105 DNA, and 3–50 µg protein from cell-free extracts. Incubation was carried out for 30 min at 37 °C. Assay products were deproteinized, subjected to ethidium bromide-agarose gel electrophoresis and quantitated by scanning the gels with a fluorescence reflectance scanner. One unit of enzyme is defined as the quantity required to ligate 1 pmol of cohesive termini of ϕ105 DNA per 30 min at 37 °C.
‡Endodeoxyribonuclease activity was determined by following the cleavage of PM2 DNA from Form I (supercoiled DNA) to Form II (nicked, circular DNA) (91). Each incubation mixture (50 µl) contained 0.02 M Tris-HCl (pH 8.0), 0.01 M MgCl$_2$, 1.23 µg PM2 DNA, and 1-3 µg protein from cell-free extracts. Incubations were carried out for 20 min at 37 °C. Assay products were analyzed as described for the DNA ligase assay. One unit of enzyme is defined as the quantity required to cleave 1 pmol of Form I DNA to yield Form II per 30 min at 37 °C.

DNA synthesis in several types of eukaryotic cells including MEL cells (94) has been shown to proceed by a stepwise process which involves the synthesis of individual DNA segments which are then thought to be joined by DNA ligase (95,96). Studies performed with isolated MEL (and other) cell nuclei indicated that several cytoplasmic factors are required for optimal DNA synthesis (94). DNA ligase appears to be one of these factors (97). DNA ligase has been shown to be present in cytoplasm (at least partially) due to its leakage from nuclei during cell fractionation procedures (95).

Whether, in fact, the DNA ligase level in cell-free extracts reflects the state of the cell in culture, whether these observations are related to the loss of multiplication capacity and what the exact mechanism is for the apparent decrease in DNA ligase activity are questions that await further experimentation.

F. Deoxyribonucleases (DNAases)

In a preliminary report (61) an endogenous chromatin-bound Ca^{2+}-activated nuclease activity that may be similar to one previously described by Hewish and Burgoyne (98) has been observed in DMSO-treated MEL cells. This activity was not detected in untreated MEL cells. This result could be explained by one or more mechanisms. For example, there could be a change in the enzyme level itself, in the availability of susceptible sites for cleavage in the chromatin DNA and/or in the level of poly(ADP)-ribosylation of chromatin proteins. A rat liver chromatin-bound, Ca^{2+}, Mg^{2+}-dependent endonuclease has been shown to be inactivated by poly(ADP-R) polymerase activity (99).

In contrast to these results, the actin-inhibitable DNAase activity per cell was relatively unchanged by DMSO treatment (Table 1). The slight elevations in specific activity (40–80%) which were seen were probably due to the lowered content of extractable protein seen in DMSO-treated cells (100). These slight variations in actin-inhibitable DNAase activity could not be ascribed to changes in the G-actin levels of the extracts since these levels were not markedly altered by DMSO treatment of the cells (101).

III. NUCLEAR PROTEINS

A. Synthesis

The first thorough screening for possible alterations in MEL cell nuclear proteins during differentiation was reported in 1976 (102). Four days of DMSO treatment of clone 745 resulted in changes of 50% or more in the rate of synthesis of eight [^{35}S]methionine-containing nuclear proteins compared to those in untreated cells as detected by two-dimensional polyacrylamide gel electrophoresis (PAGE). Two chromatin proteins with molecular weights of approximately 25,000 and 27,000D and two nucleoplasmic proteins with molecular weights of about 18,000D, but with different isoelectric points, were found to increase after DMSO treatment. Four chromatin proteins with molecular weights of approximately 20,000, 40,000, 47,000, and 54,000D were demonstrated to decrease after this treatment. The decrease in some of these nuclear proteins may account for part of the lower levels of non-histone nuclear proteins noted in differentiating MEL cells (see below). In a subclone of this line (745-PC-4) the incorporation of radioactive leucine into nuclear proteins remained constant during the first 48 hr of DMSO treatment, but markedly declined in the next 72 hr as the cells became committed to limitation of cell multiplication (103). During the first 48 hr period DMSO induced increases in the synthesis of 46,000 and 280,000D molecular weight proteins and a slight increase in the synthesis of a protein with a molecular weight of 65,000D (103).

In a different cell line (T3-C1-2) which was derived from a DDD mouse (line 745 was derived from a DBA/2J mouse) Lau and Ruddon found the synthesis of only two nuclear proteins, of approximately 23,000 and 50,000D, markedly increased after five days of DMSO treatment (104). It is possible that the 23,000 and 50,000D proteins identified in this study represent the same or similar proteins of 25,000D and either 47,000 or 54,000D proteins detected by Peterson and McConkey (102). Of these nuclear proteins demonstrated to increase following DMSO treatment only the one of about 25,000D (termed IP25) has been studied further (see below).

Using the same type of PAGE procedures and also a related cell line (745A) as Peterson and McConkey, Reeves and Cserjesi demonstrated that one day of butyrate treatment led to the detectable synthesis of at least 30 additional nuclear proteins (calculated from Figure 8 in reference 105) and the reduction in the synthesis of several other proteins (105,106). The differences in the appearances of newly synthesized proteins in the nuclei of DMSO-treated and butyrate-treated cells may reflect possible differences in the mechanisms of induction due to these two agents as mentioned above (107–111). In this regard one report suggests that DMSO and butyrate-induction follow the same or similar paths (112).

B. Histones

The levels of all of the histones (except H1°, see below) and their rates of synthesis appear to remain constant relative to one another during MEL cell differentiation (103–105,113). However, the binding to chromatin of the core histones, both forms of H1 histone along with IP25 and many other nuclear non-histone proteins decreases during DMSO-treatment of the cells (92).

One known nuclear biochemical effect that butyrate produces in many systems (106,114) including MEL cells, that is not shared by DMSO, is the stimulation of hyperacetylation of histones (106,114). The hyperacetylation in all systems appears to be due to inhibition of histone deacetylase activity (106,114–117). Butyrate treatment of MEL cells for 24 hr increased the levels of the mono-, di-, tri- and tetra-acetylated forms of histone H4 and evidence for an increase in hyperacetylated forms of H3 was also presented (106,114). No hyperacetylated form of either of the two major forms of H1 (106) or of H2A or H2B were noted. Longer treatment (96 hr) with DMSO did not increase the levels of any hyperacetylated histones (106,114). Studies of shorter time periods of DMSO treatment have not been reported, but they were presumed to have the same effects as following the 96 hr treatment since DMSO was continually present. A theory that links histone hyperacetylation and MEL cell differentiation has been presented (118). It has also been shown that the non-histone chromatin high mobility group proteins HMG 14 and HMG 17, which are present in MEL cells are, like butyrate, capable of partially inhibiting histone deacetylase (119). An increase in the chromatin content of these proteins might be expected during MEL cell differentiation, but to date it has not been demonstrated. The levels of most, if not all, HMG proteins decrease during MEL cell differentiation (see Section III C).

A histone change in FLV-infected cells that has some similarities to the DNAase I-sensitivity of MEL cell chromatin—in that it is present prior to the induction of terminal differentiation by DMSO (44)—has been reported (120,121). A difference was found in the ratio of histone $H2A2_1$ to $H2A2_2$ in mouse splenic cells *in vivo* shortly after FLV infection and in those that had progressed in their FLV-induced transformation sufficiently to have the ability to be cultured as MEL cells *in vitro*. In spleen cells in uninfected mice or in mice shortly after FLV infection the $H2A2_1$: $H2A2_2$ ratio was 3:1. In cells taken at later times after infection and cultured *in vitro* the ratio was 2:1. Induction by DMSO did not alter this ratio in this study, but Neumann *et al.* reported a shift in this ratio, in the same direction but to a lesser degree, following DMSO treatment (103). An increase in translatable H2B mRNA, but not in its translation product, during DMSO-stimulated differentiation has been noted (122).

C. Non-histone Proteins

DMSO-treatment of MEL cells resulted in a general decrease in non-histone nuclear proteins (e.g., 92,103,106,123,124, also see below). Certain fractions of non-histone proteins specifically stimulated the initiation of β-globin gene transcription in a cell-free system (125). However, the level of these fractions decreased after DMSO-treatment of the cells.

Two of the major mammalian non-histone chromosomal proteins, HMG 1 and HMG 2, have been studied specifically in MEL cells (figure 4 in reference 126). Ten days of MEL cell growth in medium containing 2.0% DMSO (without medium changes) reduced the levels of HMG 1 and HMG 2 proteins by about 67% when compared to untreated cells grown with medium replenishment every other day. The decrease in other non-histone proteins is also evident in this figure. It was suggested that the decreases in HMG 1 and HMG 2 were more related to commitment to limitation of cell multiplication due to cellular differentiation than to cessation of cell multiplication due to the depletion of medium nutrients. It is stated that this finding will be studied further.

The non-histone nuclear proteins that remained following DMSO-treatment were not as tightly bound to chromatin as they were prior to this treatment and could be eluted off at lower salt concentrations (92,103). This may be related to a general process in erythrodifferentiation since the nuclear non-histone proteins are more easily extractable from chick erythrocytes than they are from other chick tissues (127). In one study it was not determined if the loose-binding of these proteins was due to cellular differentiation or if it was related to the growth phase of the culture and nutritional depletion of the medium. Nuclear protein patterns from untreated cultures, grown for only two days and therefore ostensibly in or near the logarithmic phase of growth, were compared with those obtained from cultures treated for seven days with DMSO, and therefore in stationary growth phase (92).

Several non-histone nuclear proteins appear to be in close proximity to histones since they can be chemically linked to them prior to isolation and characterization. A lower level of such chemically linked non-histone proteins was reported in MEL cells treated with DMSO for seven days than in untreated cells grown for two days (128,129).

D. Specific Proteins

1. Induced Protein, 25000D (IP25)

The level of a nuclear protein of molecular weight approximately 25,000D was found to be increased following DMSO treatment (102,104). This protein was found to be induced by either DMSO or HMBA in cell line F4N (derived from a DBA/2J mouse) prior to the appearance of hemoglobin and was termed IP25 (130). IP25 migrates in SDS-PAGE just ahead of the most rapidly moving H1 moiety. H1 has a MW of approximately 22,100D (131,132), but as with other histones and basic proteins, has according to its MW, an abnormal mobility in SDS-PAGE (131). Neither DMSO or HMBA induced IP25 in a differentiation-resistant MEL variant cell line. Therefore, a specific role in erythrodifferentiation was thought to be possible. Alternatively, since a high level of IP25 was present a structural role in chromatin seemed more likely and a similarity between IP25 and avian erythrocytic histone H5 was suggested. Chick H5 has a molecular weight of approximately 20,600D (133–135).

In their next report Keppel et al. compared IP25 to H1 (136). Both were extracted from chromatin by NaCl concentrations above 0.45 M and by 5% perchloric acid. Neither were released from nuclei by DNAase I and they were found to be distributed differently in nucleosome monomers and dimers after micrococcal nuclease digestion. H1 also differs from IP25 in that IP25 contains methionine and neither H1-1 or H1-2 (H1-A or H1-B) do. Both the tryptic and V8 protease digest profiles in SDS-PAGE of IP25 and H1 appeared to differ (130,136,137). The complete answer to the possible structural relationships between IP25 and H1-1 and/or H1-2 will not be forthcoming until the amino acid sequences of these proteins are known. The nuclease digestion experiments suggested that 'IP25, like H1, is not located in the nucleosome core, but is rather associated with the internucleosomal linker regions' (138).

Butyrate, 6-thioguanine, and hydroxyurea treatment were also shown to markedly induce IP25 in MEL cells (106,138–141). Several other agents also induce IP25 in MEL cells (E.P.M. Candido, R. Reeves, and J. R. Davies in preparation; 106). Of all the inducers tested hemin has been reported to be least effective in inducing IP25. An increase of only about 16–27% in the level of IP25 was noted after 96 hr of hemin treatment compared to a 314% increase due to DMSO treatment for the same time period (141) and in another study no hemin induction of IP25 was found (9).

It has frequently been suggested that induction of MEL cell differentiation by hemin follows a somewhat different pathway than that due to DMSO or any other inducer (e.g., 4,6,109–112,141–146). The differences in the effects of these inducers on IP25 metabolism may be related to their different effects on the differentiation process. Several findings strongly suggest that both IP25 and hemin may be required for the limitation in cell multiplication that characterizes commitment and/or for the condensation of chromatin that is characteristic of the mature erythrocytic cell nucleus (136,138). The comparison of three sets of experimental data are sufficient to tentatively reach this conclusion.

1. Hemin, although it induces hemoglobin synthesis (see 2–7), does not induce a limitation of cell multiplication (4,6,141,142,145) or a marked increase in IP25 (9,115) in 'wild-type' MEL cells.

2. In a variant cell line (F4N + 2), DMSO (or HMBA) by itself is not able to induce hemoglobin synthesis or terminal limitation of cell multiplication, but is able to induce an increase in the level of IP25 (9). DMSO has other effects on F4N + 2 cells. It can induce spectrin and three of the enzyme activities in the heme biosynthetic pathway, but it cannot induce heme synthesis.

3. When exogenous hemin is added alone to F4N + 2 cells there is no effect on these parameters, but when hemin is added with DMSO, hemoglobin synthesis was induced as well as limitation of cell multiplication and increased levels of IP25. Therefore, it appears that in 'wild-type' MEL cells DMSO is responsible for the increase in IP25 and hemin levels and that hemin working in concert with IP25 is important in the final limitation of cell multiplication. This idea is consistent with work of several laboratories (47,146,147). It was reported that hemin plus DMSO was required to induce terminal limitation of cell multiplication in other variant cell lines that would not respond in this fashion to either hemin or DMSO alone. It also

was demonstated that it is likely that for the limitation of cell multiplication to occur heme must be present in an amount greater than that required to saturate all of the available globin molecules (47). A recent report indicates that in addition to heme and IP25 at least one other factor may be required for the terminal limitation of cell multiplication (148).

On the other hand, a recent report suggests that hemin is not required for the limitation of terminal cell multiplication (149). Imidazole treatment was shown to inhibit the DMSO-induction of increased levels of globin mRNA, heme and hemoglobin. Imidazole did not, however, inhibit the DMSO-induced increase in IP25 levels or the limitation of cell multiplication. The use of inhibitors in this type of experiment brings up the frequent problem that an inhibitor or a combination of inducer plus inhibitor may have additional effects on cell multiplication that are unrelated to differentiation. In order to control for this possibility it would be convenient to have a definitive marker of erythrodiffe-rentiation other than globin mRNA, heme or hemoglobin that could be shown to be present in the cells presumed to be committed to erythrodifferentiation.

In addition to the induction of IP25 in erythrocytic cells, a similar protein has been induced in several other non-erythrocytic cell lines by butyrate (i.e., 138,150,151).

In all cases IP25 appeared to be present in cells that were undergoing terminal differentiation or had completed differentiation and were not replicating. Many of the characteristics of IP25 are found in another protein described over a decade ago in non-replicating cells, H1° (152). IP25, like H1°, (153) has been shown to be composed of two subfractions, IP25a and IP25b, which differ slightly in charge (137). Because the similarities between IP25 and H1° are so great many investigators now refer to IP25 as H1° (e.g., 92,126,154). H1° has several characteristics, in addition to its molecular weight, that relate it to the chick erythrocytic-specific histone, H5, including sequence and serological homologies (153,155–159,160,161). However, in one study no serologic homology was detected between IP25 (H1°) and H5 (154).

2. 32,000D molecular weight Protein

An alteration in another specific chromatin protein that occurs during DMSO induction of differentiation has been reported in cell line 745A (162). The level of a chromatin protein of molecular weight approximately 32,000D begins to decrease after 12 hr of cell growth in DMSO-containing medium. After 24 hr of DMSO-treatment the material in the 32,000D peak noted on SDS-PAGE was greatly diminished and after 48 hr it was not detectable. In a cell line resistant to DMSO induction (Fw) this protein was present both before and after DMSO treatment. No information is available on the possible function or other characteristics of this protein. A similar protein was not detected in mouse yolk sac erythrocytic cell nuclei which were primarily derived from mature cells (162).

E. Protein modification

1. Phosphoproteins

Phosphorylation is another modification of nuclear proteins that occurs during MEL cell induction that has been investigated. The general rate of $^{32}PO_4$ incorporation into non-histone proteins and most histones which are nucleosome-associated decreases during MEL cell differentiation. This may, at least in part, reflect the reduced accumulation of phosphate by DMSO-treated cells compared to untreated cells (163,164). However, during the first 48 hr of treatment of the cells with DMSO there are increases in the rate of ^{32}P-incorporation into H1 and H2A (103,165,166). At the same time there is a decrease in the phosphorylation of a specific 95,000–100,000D nuclear protein.

Two chromatin-associated protein (casein) kinase activities and at least one histone kinase activity have been examined in MEL cell lysates. All of these kinases are insensitive to adenosine 3′,5′-cyclic monophosphate, but the casein kinase activities are both inhibited by hemin, while the histone kinase is not (167). They appear to all be present before and during DMSO-induced differentiation. It was suggested that these kinases may play a role in the regulation of MEL cell differentiation (118,166).

2. Poly-adenosine diphosphoribosylation

In addition to the methylation of DNA the addition of another small molecule, adenosine diphosphoribose (ADP-R), that can become covalently linked to nuclear macromolecules (proteins) has been studied in MEL cells. A chromatin-bound enzyme, poly (ADP-R) polymerase (also termed synthetase) catalyzes the transfer of single ADP-R units from ADP-ribosyl nicotinamide (NAD) to form ADP-ribosyl polymers on several different nuclear proteins in the presence of DNA (168). The number of ADP-R units polymerized at a single site may reach 100 in a linear or perhaps a branched chain configuration (169,170). Added DNA markedly stimulates the reaction (171). Histone H2B and H1 and several nuclear non-histone proteins including Mg^{2+}, Ca^{2+}-endonuclease, RNA polymerase, protein A24, HMG proteins, and protamines can be poly(ADP)-ribosylated at one or more sites (171,172).

Initial studies with MEL cell line F4N (173,174) demonstrated that as in other tissue-cultured cells (175–177) the rate of poly(ADP-R) synthesis is highest in the stationary phase of growth (due to depletion of nutrients in the medium or other causes). Diluting stationary phase cultures into fresh medium is followed by a decrease in poly(ADP-R) polymerase activity which then increases until the cultures reach stationary phase at which time the activity is high. It remains high as long as the cultures are in growth-arrest (175).

In MEL cell line 745, grown without changes of medium for five days in the presence of DMSO or HMBA the rate of ADP-ribosylation in isolated nuclei remained relatively constant and did not increase during culture. Therefore, the rate of ADP-ribosylation in inducer-treated cells became about 30–50% of that in untreated cells in late logarithmic and stationary phase cultures (178,179). This effect of DMSO and HMBA was not as marked in variant cell lines that were not stimulated to increase hemoglobin production by these agents (111,178).

The enzymatic activity increased for the first 18 hr of growth in butyrate-treated cultures when compared to untreated ones, but then activity declined to the same low level seen after DMSO or HMBA treatment (174,178). Butyrate has frequently been considered to induce differentiation in MEL cells by a somewhat different mechanism than DMSO or other inducers (106–111,114). This difference could be related to the differences between the effects of DMSO and butyrate on poly(ADP)-ribosylation in this system.

Nicotinamide, which is a specific inhibitor of poly(ADP-R) polymerase, was shown to be capable of inducing a moderate level of MEL cell erythrodifferentiation. Therefore, it was suggested that a decrease in poly(ADP-R) synthesis was correlated with MEL cell differentiation. Several pyrimidine analogs of nicotinamide were tested as inducers of MEL cell differentiation (180). In this study six new inducers were discovered. N'-methylnicotinamide was the most potent of these. In addition, three other analogs were tested that were ineffective as inducers. Of the nine nicotinamide analogs that were tested only five were shown to inhibit poly(ADP-R) polymerase activity levels in vitro. All five of the inhibitory analogs were inducers of differentiation. However, N'-methylnicotinamide (the sixth, and most potent, inducer tested) did not inhibit poly(ADP-R) polymerase activity in vitro, so this effect did not strictly correlate with the ability to induce erythrodifferentiation.

Studies of the structure of nuclear poly(ADP-R) in MEL cells have shown that DMSO or HMBA treatment for two or four days did not markedly alter nuclear poly(ADP-R) chain length (124). DMSO-treated cell nuclei may contain slightly shorter chain lengths than those in HMBA-treated cells. In the isolated nuclei, there was a substantial reduction of the average chain length of the poly(ADP-R) synthesized in induced cells compared to untreated cells (124). Approximately 95% of newly synthesized poly(ADP-R) in MEL nuclei was linked to non-histone proteins. The total non-histone content of MEL cell nuclei was reduced approximately 50.0% by 72 hr of treatment with either HMBA or DMSO. The levels of non-histone nuclear proteins are lower in most, if not all, non-proliferative cells compared to proliferating cells (181). Therefore, it was suggested that there is a decrease in poly(ADP-R) chain initiation rate due to a partial loss of available non-histone protein-acceptor sites following treatment with inducers (124).

An increase in the specific activity of histone-linked poly(ADP-R), but not in non-histone nuclear protein-linked poly(ADP-R), was found in nuclei isolated from cells grown with butyrate for 24 hr (139). It is too early for a definitive statement, but this suggests that polyADP-ribosylation of histones and of non-histone nuclear proteins could be related to MEL cell differentiation. It was also demonstrated (139) that incubation of MEL cell nuclei for 30 min with 1 mM NAD stimulated the appearance on SDS-PAGE of three proteins all migrating more rapidly than IP25 (130), but substantially slower than histone H3. The level of at least one of these three proteins appeared to be higher in NAD-treated nuclei isolated from butyrate-treated cells than in those prepared from non-butyrate-treated cells.

IV. POLYAMINES

Polyamines (putrescine, spermidine, spermine, cadaverine, and 1,3-diaminopropane), although synthesized in the cytoplasm, are thought to act, at least partially, in the nucleus. They are believed to play roles in many aspects of cell function including roles in DNA and cell replication and in cell differentiation (for reviews see 182–187). They are organic cations that bind to nucleic acids and other anions and they also become covalently attached to many cellular small molecules and macromolecules (182,183,185,187). By these or other mechanisms polyamines influence many cell functions. For example, polyamines bind to and stabilize double and single-stranded DNA as well as nucleoids yielding protection from denaturation, shearing, radiation damage, intercalation of small molecules, and possibly nucleases (183,187). In addition, polyamines stimulate protein kinase-mediated phosphorylation of chromatin non-histone proteins, but not of lysine-rich histones (188). They also stimulate poly(ADP)-ribosylation of H1 histones and acidic chromatin non-histone proteins (189).

L-ornithine decarboxylase (ODC) catalyzes the first step in the pathway of the biosynthesis of the larger polyamines. It has a short half-life (10–20 min) within the cell and appears to play a role in regulating the cellular levels of polyamines (183). Therefore, initial studies concerning polyamines in MEL cells have focused on ODC activity (190–195). Several inducers of MEL cell erythrodifferentiation (DMSO, N,N'-dimethylformamide, hypoxanthine and bis-acetyldiaminopentane) stimulated increases in ODC activity within 3–9 hr after initiating treatment (191–193). Dexamethasone and phorbol-12-myristate-13-acetate (PMA), which are potent inhibitors of induced MEL cell differentiation, were found to also inhibit the stimulation of ODC activity by these inducers (except the latter inducer which was not tested) (192,193). The effects of these inhibitors were abrogated by the further addition of a polyamine to the medium. The ornithine analogs, α-methylornithine and α-hydrazinoornithine, which inhibit ODC activity, were found to be partially effective in inhibiting DMSO- or HMBA-induced differentiation. Methyl glyoxal *bis*(guanylhydrazone), an inhibitor of S-adenosyl-L-methionine decarboxylase, another enzyme in the polyamine biosynthetic pathway, was found to also inhibit the induction of differentiation due to these inducers. Polyamines were also found to abrogate this inhibition. Therefore, there appears to be an association between differentiation due to this class of inducers and the stimulation of polyamine biosynthesis.

The effects of PMA are complex since this agent is known to stimulate ODC activity by itself. The effects of another agent, L-ethionine, are also complicated. Ethionine, as noted above, (Section II B) is a weak inducer of MEL cell differentiation (67,68). It was suggested that this effect on differentiation is related to the ability of ethionine to inhibit the production of S-adenosyl-L-methionine which is required for the methylation of bases in DNA. Therefore, ethionine treatment leads to hypomethylation of DNA, but since S-adenosyl methionine is also an intermediate in the polyamine biosynthetic pathway, ethionine treatment also leads, at least initially, to a decrease in polyamine levels (182). This dual effect of ethionine may, at least partially, explain its relative lack of potency as an inducer.

A second class of inducers of MEL cell differentiation—butyrate, actinomycin-D, and S-adenosyl-amino-9(3'-amino-3'deoxyribosyl) purine—which are thought to stimulate differentiation by a different mechanism, were not able to strongly stimulate ODC activity (192,193). Therefore, altered polyamine metabolism is not always associated with MEL cell induction of differentiation.

V. APPROACHES TO THE STUDY OF DIFFERENTIATION

In studies with MEL cells (as well as with other systems) it is frequently of interest to determine if a particular event under study is closely associated with the process of differentiation. Several events that occur after induction of MEL cell differentiation have been tentatively related to the differentiation process. However, these correlations may not be perfect for several reasons. For example, various inducers may enter the differentiation pathway(s) by different routes so that not all differentiation-related events may be modified by all inducers. Various inhibitors may also enter the differentiation pathway by different routes and therefore only block portions of the pathway. In addition, the use of chemical and physical agents alone or in combination may have toxic effects that are unrelated to differentiation. Toxic effects must be distinguished from differentiation-related effects. Some of these problems would be minimized by the availability of a variety of markers that are reliably associated with differentiation besides hemoglobin and its precursors. For example, spectrin and IP25 have been used as such additional markers (e.g., 9,149).

There is no iron-clad method of determining whether or not two different events in a biological system are related to each other short of being able to reconstitute the entire system as a cell-free one. However, if all of the following four approaches are used, a fairly strong argument can be made that an event under study is related to erythrodifferentiation.

1. The time of appearance of an event(s) under study should correlate with the time of development of erythrodifferentiation.
2. The event should occur in the same dose-related manner in response to several agents that induce differentiation at different optimal concentrations.
3. The event should occur in a cell line sensitive for induction of differentiation by a particular inducer, but not in a related cell line that is resistant to induction of differentiation by the same inducer. The use of a variant cell line such as DR-10 has two advantages (196). First, DR-10 cells are resistant to some inducers (e.g., DMSO), but not to others (e.g., HMBA) so that the association of an event with both effective and ineffective inducers can be tested within the same cell line. Second, DR-10 is apparently the only differentiation-resistant line in which the accumulation of an inducer has been studied and found not to differ in this regard from its parent differentiation-sensitive line (196). Although it is not known if an inducer must enter the cell in order to induce differentiation it is likely since it has been shown that a small amount of an inducer is effective in inducing differentiation if it is microinjected into a single cell (197).
4. The event should be inhibited by the same concentrations and time of contact with agents that can inhibit differentiation. For example, the interaction of an inhibitor such as dexamethasone with several inducers on a differentiation-related event could be studied. To have the strongest possible relationship to differentiation, the event under study should become altered after treatment of the cells with either DMSO or butyrate alone or with butyrate and dexamethasone together, but not after treatment with DMSO and dexamethasone together. This would be the case since dexamethasone is a potent inhibitor of DMSO induction, but either has no effect on, or slightly stimulates, butyrate induction (192,193,198).

VI. SUMMARY

Most MEL cell cultures contain none or only a few hemoglobin-producing cells unless they are treated with an inducing agent. Such treatment leads to increases in many erythrocytic characteristics in the cells. These changes have been divided into two categories;

1. 'Early events, (those occurring prior to commitment) and

2. 'Late events', (those following commitment, such as hemoglobin production). Two of the most striking nuclear changes seen as late events after treatment with most inducers are the decrease in the size of the nucleus and the condensation of the chromatin.

These changes plus the finding that globin mRNA levels are increased after induction indicate that alterations in nuclear components must occur to regulate differentiation-associated gene expression as well as chromatin inactivation. The relationship of the nuclear events discussed in this chapter to MEL cell differentiation, other than chromatin condensation, globin gene expression, and limitation of cell multiplication, has not yet been definitively demonstrated.

The following nuclear events have been observed during MEL cell differentiation;

1. MEL cells, which are prepared to further differentiate, have their globin genes in a DNAase I-sensitive configuration(s) and have a lower histone $H2A2_1:H2A2_2$ ratio.
2. The processes of both globin gene expression and limitation of cell multiplication are initiated within 24 hr.
3. Some chemical and/or physical changes in chromatin structure are also evident. Changes in DNA structure, such as single-stranded DNA discontinuities or lack of methylation, and/or changes in nuclear proteins have been detected at this time.
4. There is usually an early transient decrease in the rate of DNA synthesis, and possibly a decrease in DNA polymerase β activity.
5. The level of IP25 increases and those of a 32,000D protein and other non-histone nuclear proteins decrease.
6. There is a decrease in the rate of poly(ADP)-ribosylation of nuclear proteins.
7. There is an increase in the level of ODC. This may affect polyamine levels in the nucleus.
8. With some inducers (i.e., butyrate) a lack of histone deacetylation is detectable.
9. Changes in the phosphorylation of nuclear proteins occur by at least the second day of inducer treatment.

Chromatin and nuclear condensation are late events in the differentiation pathway which occur with the increases in completed heme synthesis and fully assembled hemoglobin. These late changes may be related (either by cause or effect) to the decrease in DNA α-polymerase and/or DNA ligase activities which occur after 48 hr of DMSO treatment.

VII. ABBREVIATIONS

ADP-R: adenosine diphosphoribose

BRdU:	5-bromo-2'-deoxyuridine,
DMSO:	dimethyl sulfoxide
DNAase:	deoxyribonuclease
EL:	erythroleukemia
EPO:	erythropoietin
FLV:	Friend leukemia virus
HMBA:	hexamethylene bisacetamide
HMG:	high mobility group
IP25:	induced protein 25,000D
MEL:	mouse erythroleukemia
MW:	molecular weight
NAD:	ADP-ribosyl nicotinamide
ODC:	L-ornithine decarboxylase
PAGE:	polyacrylamide gel electrophoresis
PMA:	phorbol-12-myristate-13-acetate
RLV:	Rauscher leukemia virus
SDS:	sodium dodecyl sulfate

VIII. ACKNOWLEDGMENTS

We thank Ms Joan Remy and Ms Jaclyn Silverman for assistance in the preparation of this manuscript. This work was supported by United States Public Health Service Grants CA 24402-03 from the National Cancer Institute and AM 16690–06 from the National Institute of Arthritis, Metabolism and Digestive Diseases, the Charles E. Merril Trust and the Chemotherapy Foundation, Inc. Dr William Scher is the recipient of the Irving Alpert Cancer Research Scientist Award.

IX. REFERENCES

1. Friend, C., Scher, W., Holland, J. F., and Sato, T. (1971). 'Hemoglobin synthesis in murine virus-induced leukemic cells *in vitro*: stimulation of erythroid differentiation by dimethyl sulfoxide', *Proc. Natl. Acad. Sci. U.S.A.*, **68**, 378–382.
2. Harrison, P. R. (1976). 'Analysis of erythropoiesis at the molecular level', *Nature*, **262**, 353–356.
3. Harrison, P. R. (1977). 'The biology of the Friend cell', in *Biochemistry of Cell Differentiation II* (Ed. J. Paul), University Park Press, Baltimore, Md., vol. 15, pp. 227–267.
4. Marks, P. A., and Rifkind, R. A. (1978). 'Erythroleukemic differentiation', *Ann. Rev. Biochem.*, **47**, 419–448.
5. Marks, P. A., Rifkind, R. A., Bank, A., Terada, M., Gambari, R., Fibach, E., Maniatis, G., and Reuben, R. (1979). 'Expression of globin genes during induced erythroleukemia cell differentiation', in *Cellular and Molecular Regulation of Hemoglobin Switching* (Eds. G. Stamatoyannopoulos and A. W. Nienhuis), Grune and Stratton, Inc., N.Y., pp. 437–455.

6. Reuben, R. C., Rifkind, R. A., and Marks, P. A. (1980). 'Chemically induced murine erythroleukemic differentiation', *Biochim. Biophys. Acta,* **605**, 325–346.
7. Friend, C. (1980). 'The regulation of differentiation in murine virus-induced erythroleukemic cells', in *Results and Problems in Cell Differentiation: Differentiation and Neoplasia* (Eds. R. G. McKinnel, M. A. Diberardino, M. Blumenfeld, and R. Bergad), Springer-Verlag, Berlin, vol. 11, pp. 202–212.
8. Tsiftsoglou, A. S., Barrnett, R. J., and Sartorelli, A. C. (1979). 'Enucleation of differentiated murine erythroleukemia cells in culture', *Proc. Natl. Acad. Sci. U.S.A.,* **76**, 6381–6385.
9. Eisen, H., Keppel-Ballivet, F., Georgopoulos, C. P., Sassa, S., Granick, J., Pragnell, I., and Ostertag, W. (1978). 'Biochemical and genetic analysis of erythroid differentiation in Friend Virus-transformed murine erythroleukemia cells', in *Differentiation of Normal and Neoplastic Hematopoietic Cells* (Eds. B. Clarkson, P. A. Marks, and J. E. Till), Cold Spring Harbor Laboratories Press, Cold Spring Harbor, book A, vol. 5, pp. 277–294.
10. Kluge, N., Ostertag, W., Sugiyama, T., Arndt-Jovin, D., Steinheider G., and Furusawa, M. (1976). 'Dimethysulfoxide-induced differentiation and hemoglobin synthesis in tissue cultures of rat erythroleukmia cells transformed by 7, 12-dimethylbenz (a) anthracene', *Proc. Natl. Acad. Sci. U.S.A.,* **73**, 1237–1240.
11. Yamaguchi, Y., Kluge, N., Ostertag, W., and Furusawa, M. (1981). 'Erythrodifferentiation and commitment in rat erythroleukemia cells with hypertonic culture conditions', *Proc. Natl. Acad. Sci. U.S.A.,* **78**, 2325–2329.
12. Greiser-Wilks, I., Ostertag, W., Goldfarb, P., Lang, A., Furusawa, M., and Conscience, J. F. (1981). 'Inducibility of spleen focus-forming virus by BrdUrd is controlled by the differentiated state of the cell', *Proc. Natl. Acad. Sci. U.S.A.,* **78**, 2995–2999.
13. de Both, N. J., Vermey, M., Van 'T Hull, E., Klootwijk-Van-Dijke, E., Van Griensven, L. J. L. D., Mol, J. N. M., and Stoff, T. J. (1978). 'A new erythroid cell line induced by Rauscher murine leukaemia virus', *Nature,* **272**, 626–628.
14. Sytkowski, A. J., Salvado, A. J., Smith, G. M., McIntrye, C. J., and de Both, N. J. (1980). 'Erythroid differentiation of clonal Rauscher erythroleukemia cells in response to erythropoietin or dimethyl sulfoxide', *Science,* **210**, 74–76.
15. de Both, N. J., Hagemeijer, A., Rhijnsburger, E. H., Vermey, M., Van 'T. Hull, E., and Smit, E. M. E. (1981). 'DMSO-induced terminal differentiation and trisomy 15 in a myeloid cell line transformed by the Rauscher murine leukemia virus', *Cell Diff.,* **10**, 13–21.
16. Sytkowski, A. J., and Salvado, A. J. (1981). 'Histone acetylation during erythropoietin and dimethylsulfoxide induced differentiation of Rauscher erythroleukemia cells', *Clin. Res.,* **29**, 350A.
17. Perrine, S. P., Bicknell, K. A., and Sytkowski, A. J. (1981). 'The induction of selective globin chain synthesis and heme production in Rauscher erythroleukemia cells', *Blood,* **58, Suppl, 1**, 50a, No. 12.
18. Geurrasio, A., Vainchenker, W., Breton-Gorius, J., Testa, U., Rosa, R., Thomopoulos, P., Titeux, M., Guichard, J., and Beuzard, Y. (1981). 'Embryonic and fetal hemoglobin synthesis in K562 cell line', *Blood Cells,* **7**, 165–176.
19. Martin, P., and Papayannopoulou, T. (1981). 'HEL (human erythroleukemia) cells: A new inducible cell line producing fetal and embryonic hemoglobins', *Blood,* **58**, Suppl, 1, 68a, No. 181.
20. Friend, C., Scher, W., and Rossi, G. B. (1970). 'The biosynthesis of haem in Friend virus-induced leukemic cell lines cloned *in vitro*', in *The Biology of Large RNA Viruses* (Eds. R. D. Barry and B. W. J. Mahy), Academic Press, New York, pp. 267–275.

21. Preisler, H. D., and Giladi, M. (1974). 'Erythropoietin responsiveness of differentiating Friend leukemia cells', *Nature,* **251**, 645–646.
22. Preisler, H. D., and Zanjani, E. D. (1974). 'Erythropoietin-induced stimulation of heme synthesis by dimethyl sulfoxide-treated Friend leukemic cells *in vitro*', *J. Lab. Clin. Med.,* **84**, 667–672.
23. Iscove, N. N. (1978). 'Erythropoietin-independent stimulation of early erythropoiesis in adult marrow cultures by conditioned media from lectin-stimulated mouse spleen cells', in *Hematopoietic Cell Differentiation* (Eds. D. W. Golde, M. J. Cline, D. Metcalf, and F. C. Fox), Academic Press, New York, pp. 37–52.
24. Scher, W., Preisler, H. D., and Friend C. (1973). 'Hemoglobin synthesis in murine virus-induced leukemic cells *in vitro*. III. Effects of 5-bromo 2'-deoxyuridine, dimethyl formamide and dimethyl sulfoxide', *J. Cell. Physiol.,* **81**, 63–70.
25. Preisler, H. D., Housman, D., Scher, W., and Friend, C. (1973). 'Effects of 5-bromo 2'-deoxyuridine on production of globin messenger RNA in dimethyl sulfoxide-stimulated Friend leukemia cells', *Proc. Natl. Acad. Sci. U.S.A.,* **70**, 2956–2959.
26. Bruce, S. A. (1981). 'Reduced globin gene transcription during bromodeoxyuridine (BrdU) inhibition of erythroleukemic cell differentiation', *J. Cell Biol.,* **91**, 32a, No. 1073.
27. Ashman, C. R., and Davidson, R. L. (1980). 'Inhibition of Friend erythroleukemic cell differentiation by bromodeoxyuridine: correlation with the amount of bromodeoxyuridine in DNA', *J. Cell. Physiol.,* **102**, 45–50.
28. Bick, M. D., and Cullen, B. R. (1976). 'Bromodeoxyuridine inhibition of Friend leukemia cell induction by butyric acid: time course of induction, reversal, and effect of other base analogs', *Somat. Cell Genet.,* **2**, 545–558.
29. Bick, M. D. (1977). 'Bromodeoxyuridine inhibition of Friend leukemia cell induction', *Biochim. Biophys. Acta.,* **476**, 279–286.
30. Preisler, H. D., and Giladi, M. (1975). 'Differentiation of erythroleukemic cells *in vitro*: irreversible induction by dimethyl sulfoxide (DMSO)', *J. Cell. Physiol.,* **85**, 537–545.
31. Gusella, J., Geller, R., Clarke, B., Weeks, V., and Housman, D. (1976). 'Commitment to erythroid differentiation by Friend erythroleukemia cells: a stochastic analysis', *Cell,* **9**, 221–229.
32. Repasky, E., and Eckert, B. S. (1981). 'A reevaluation of the process of enucleation in mammalian erythroid cells', in *The Red Cell: Fifth Ann Arbor Conf., Prog. in Clinical and Biological Res.* (Ed. G. J. Brewer), Alan Liss, Inc., New York, vol. 55, pp. 679–690.
33. Sato, T., Friend, C., and de Harven, E. (1971). 'Ultrastructural changes in Friend erythroleukemia cells treated with dimethyl sulfoxide', *Cancer Res.,* **31**, 1402–1417.
34. Zucker, R. M. (1981). 'Cell cycle dependency of tumor promoter on murine erythroleukemic cells', *Cytometry,* **1**, 373–376.
35. Scher, W. and Waxman, S., (in preparation).
36. Reff, M. E. and Davidson, R. L. (1979). '*In vitro* DNA dependent synthesis of globin RNA sequences from erythroleukemic cell chromatin', *Nucleic Acids Res.,* **6**, 275–287.
37. Nose, K., Tanaka, A., and Okamoto, H. (1981). 'Transcription of globin genes in murine erythroleukemic cell chromatin by RNA polymerase II from mouse cells', *J. Biochem.,* **90**, 103–111.
38. Nose, K., Tanaka, A., and Okamoto, H. (1981). 'Transcriptional activity of globin genes in uninducible variants of Friend leukemic cells', *J. Biochem.,* **89**, 1711–1719.

39. Strätling, W. H. (1976). 'Stimulation of transcription on chromatin by polar organic compounds', *Nucleic Acids Res., 3*, 1203–1213.
40. Nakanishi, S., Adhya, S., Gottesman, M., and Pastan, I. (1974). 'Activation of transcription at specific promoters by glycerol', *J. Biol. Chem., 249*, 4050–4056.
41. Travers, A. (1974). 'On the nature of DNA promotor conformations. The effects of glycerol and dimethyl sulfoxide', *Eur. J. Biochem., 47*, 435–441.
42. Musielski, H., Mann, W., Laue, R., and Michel, S. (1981). 'Influence of dimethylsulfoxide on transcription by bacteriophage T3-induced RNA polymerase', *Z. Allg. Mikrobiol., 21*, 447–456.
43. Weintraub, H., Groudine, M., Weisbrod, S., Riley, D., and Albanese, I. (1979). 'Contral of globin gene expression', in *Cellular and Molecular Regulation of Hemoglobin Switching* (Eds. G. Stamatoyannopoulos and A. W. Nienhuis), Grune and Stratton, Inc., New York, pp. 721–748.
44. Miller, D. M., Turner, P., Nienhuis, A. W., Axelrod, D. E., and Gopala-Krishnan, T. V. (1978). 'Active conformation of the globin genes in uninduced and induced mouse erythroleukemia cells', *Cell, 14*, 511–521.
44a. Sheffery, M., Rifkin, R. A., and Marks, P. A. (1982). 'Murine erythroleukemia cell differentiation: DNAase I hypersensitivity and DNA methylation near the globin genes', *Proc. Natl. Acad. Sci. U.S.A., 79*, 1180–1184.
45. Willing, M. C., Nienhuis, A. W., and Anderson, W. F. (1979). 'Selective activation of human β- but not γ-globin gene in human fibroblast x mouse erythroleukemia cell hybrids', *Nature, 277*, 534–538.
46. Pyati, J., Kucherlapti, R. S., and Skoultchi, A. I. (1980). 'Activation of human β-globin genes from nonerythroid cells by fusion with murine erythroleukemia cells', *Proc. Natl. Acad. Sci. U.S.A., 77*, 3435–3439.
47. Lo, S. C., Aft, R., and Mueller, G. C. (1981). 'Role of nonhemoglobin heme accumulation in the terminal differentiation of Friend erythroleukemia cells', *Cancer Res., 41*, 864–870.
48. Skoultchi, A. I., Pyati, J., Hsiung, N., Warrick, H., Kucherlapati, R., de Riel, J. K., Tuan, D., and Forget, B. G. (1980). 'Introduction and expression of human globin genes in cultured mouse cells', in *In Vivo and In Vitro Erythropoiesis: The Friend System* (Ed. G. B. Rossi), Elsevier/North-Holland Biomedical Press, New York, pp. 403–412.
49. Deisseroth, A., and Hendrick, D. (1979). 'Activation of phenotypic expression of human globin genes from non-erythroid cells by chromosome-dependent transfer to tetraploid mouse erythroleukemia cells', *Proc. Natl. Acad. Sci. U.S.A., 76*, 2185–2189.
50. Axelrod, D. E., Gopalakrishnan, T. V., Willing, M., and Anderson, W. F. (1978). 'Maintenance of hemoglobin inducibility in somatic cell hybrids of tetraploid (2S) mouse erythroleukemia cells with mouse or human fibroblasts', *Somat. Cell Genet., 4*, 157–168.
51. Ross, J., Gielen, J., Packman, S., Ikawa, Y., and Leder, P. (1974). 'Globin gene expression in cultured erythroleukemic cells', *J. Mol. Biol., 87*,. 697–714.
52. Schlegel, R. A., Litwack, A. H., and Phelps, B. M. (1980). 'Nucleosome repeat lengths do not change during *in vitro* differentiation of erythroleukemia cells', *Molec. Biol. Rep., 6*, 115–118.
53. Murphy, R. F., Wallace, R. B., and Boner, J. (1978). 'Altered nucleosome spacing in newly replicated chromatin from Friend leukemia cells', *Proc. Natl. Acad. Sci. U.S.A., 75*, 5903–5907.
54. Terada, M., Fried, J., Nudel, U., Rifkind, R. A., and Marks, P. A. (1977). 'Transient inhibition of initiation of S-phase associated with dimethyl sulfoxide

induction of murine erythroleukemia cells to erythroid differentiation', *Proc. Natl. Acad. Sci., U.S.A.*, **74**, 248–252.

55. Traganos, F., Darzynkiewicz, Z., Sharpless, T. K., and Melamed, M. R. (1979). 'Erythroid differentiation of Friend leukemia cells by acridine orange staining and flow cytometry', *J. Histochem. Cytochem.*, **27**, 382–389.

56. Terada, M., Nudel, U., Fibach, E., Rifkind, R. A., and Marks, P. A. (1978). 'Changes in DNA associated with induction of erythroid differentiation by dimethyl sulfoxide in murine erythroleukemia cells', *Cancer Res.*, **38**, 835–840.

57. Scher, W., and Friend, C. (1978). 'Breakage of DNA and alterations in folded genomes by inducers of differentiation in Friend erythroleukemic cells', *Cancer Res.*, **38**, 841–849.

58. Luchnik, A. N., and Glaser, V. M. (1980). 'Decrease in the number of DNA topological turns during Friend erythroleukemia differentiation', *Molec. Gen. Genet.*, **178**, 459–463.

59. Pantazis, P., Erickson, L. C., and Kohn, K. W. (1981). 'Preservation of DNA integrity in human and mouse leukemic cells induced to terminally differentiate by chemical agents', *Develop. Biol.*, **86**, 55–60.

60. Kohn, K. W., Erickson, L. C., Ewig, R. A. G., and Friedman, C. A. (1976). 'Fractionation of DNA from mammalian cells by alkaline elution', *Biochemistry*, **15**, 4629–4637.

61. Levy, S. B., Leonardson, K. E., Benezra, R., Stollar, B. D., and Lapierre, K. (1980). 'Compositional and structural changes in chromatin related to different malignant states of Friend leukemia cells', in *In Vivo and In Vitro Erythropoiesis: The Friend System* (Ed. G. B. Rossi), Elsevier/North Holland Biomedical Press, New York, pp. 309–322.

62. Leonardson, K. E. and Levy, S. B. (1980). 'Organizational changes in chromatin at different malignant stages of Friend erythroleukemia', *Nucleic Acids Res.*, **8**, 5317–5331.

63. Hanania, J., Shaool, D., Poncy, C., and Harel, J. (1980). 'New gene expression in dimethyl sulfoxide-treated Friend erythroleukemia cells', *Exp. Cell Res.*, **130**, 119–126.

64. Groudine, M., Eisenman, R., and Weintraub H. (1981). 'Chromatin structure of endogenous retroviral genes and activation by an inhibitor of DNA methylation', *Nature*, **292**, 311–317.

65. Groudine, M. and Weintraub, H. (1981). 'Activation of globin genes during chicken development', *Cell*, **24**, 393–401.

66. Van der Ploeg, L. H. T., and Flavell, R. A. (1980). 'DNA methylation in the human γδβ-globin locus in erythroid and nonerythroid tissues', *Cell*, **19**, 947–958.

67. Christman, J. K., Price, P., Pedrinan, L., and Acs, G. (1977). 'Correlation between hypomethylation of DNA and expression of globin genes in Friend erythroleukemia cells', *Eur. J. Biochem.*, **81**, 53–61.

68. Christman, J. K., Weich, N., Schoenbrun, B., Schneiderman, N., and Acs, G. (1980). 'Hypomethylation of DNA during differentiation of Friend erythroleukemia cells', *J. Cell Biol.*, **86**, 366–370.

69. Creusot, F., and Christman, J. K. (1981). 'Localization of DNA methyltransferase in the chromatin of Friend erythroleukemia cells', *Nucleic Acids Res.*, **9**, 5359–5381.

70. Nudel, U., Salmon, J., Fibach, E., Terada, M., Rifkind, R., Marks, P. A., and Bank, A. (1977). 'Accumulation of α- and β-globin messenger RNAs in mouse erythroleukemia cells', *Cell*, **12**, 463–469.

71. Cook, P. R., and Brazell, I. A. (1976). 'Conformational constraints in nuclear DNA', *J. Cell Sci.*, **22**, 287–302.

72. Harris, H. (1965). 'Behavior of differentiated nuclei in heterokaryons of animal cells from different species', *Nature*, **206**, 583–588.
73. Tabuse, Y., Kawamura, M., and Furusawa, M. (1976). 'Induction of haemoglobin synthesis in Friend leukaemia cells without the necessity of mitosis', *Diff.*, **7**, 1–5.
74. Parker, C. C., and Hooper, W. C. (1978). 'Induction of hemoglobin synthesis in dimethyl sulfoxide-treated Friend erythroleukemic cells grown in the presence of cytochalasin B', *Leuk. Res.*, **2**, 295–303.
75. Tsiftsoglou, A. S., and Sartorelli, A. C. (1979). 'Dimethyl sulfoxide-induced differentiation of Friend erythroleukemia cells in the absence of cytokinesis', *Cancer Res.*, **39**, 4058–4063.
76. Terada, M., Fried, J., Nudel, U., Rifkind, R. A., and Marks, P. A. (1977). 'Transient inhibition of initiation of S-phase associated with dimethyl sulfoxide induction of murine erythroleukemia cells to erythroid differentiation', *Proc. Natl. Sci. U.S.A.*, **74**, 248–252.
77. Marks, P. A., Rifkind, R. A., Bank, A., Terada, M., Reuben, R., Fibach, E., Nudel, U., Salmon, J., and Gazitt, Y. (1978). 'Induction of differentiation of murine erythroleukemia cells', in *Cell Differentiation and Neoplasia* (Ed. G. F. Saunders), Raven Press, New York, pp. 453–471.
78. Tsiftsoglou, A. S. and Sarotrelli, A. C. (1981). 'Relationship between cellular replication and erythroid differentiation of murine leukemia cells', *Biochim. Biophys. Acta*, **653**, 226–235.
79. Friend, C., Scher, W., Preisler, H. D., and Holland, J. G. (1973). 'Studies on erythroid differentiation of Friend virus-induced murine leukemic cells', in *Unifying Concepts of Leukemia, Bibl. Haemat.* (Eds. R. M. Dutcher and L. Chieco-Branchi), Karger, Basel, No. 39, pp. 916–923.
80. Friedman, E. A. and Schildkraut, C. L. (1977). 'Terminal differentiation in cultured Friend erythroleukemia cells', *Cell*, **12**, 901–913.
81. Furst, A., Brown, E. H., Braunstein, J. D., and Schildkraut, C. L. (1981). 'α-Globin sequences are located in a region of early-replicating DNA in murine erythroleukemia cells', *Proc. Natl. Acad. Sci. U.S.A.*, **78**, 1023–1027.
82. Epner, E., Rifkind, R. A. and Marks, P. A. (1981). 'Replication of α and β globin DNA sequences occurs during early S phase in murine erythroleukemia cells', *Proc. Natl. Acad. Sci. U.S.A.*, **78**, 3058–3062.
83. Lo, S. C., Ross, J., and Mueller, G. C. (1980). 'Localization of globin gene replication in Friend leukemia cells to a specific interval of the S phase', *Biochim. Biophys. Acta*, **608**, 103–111.
84. Loritz, F., Bernstein, A., and Miller, R. G. (1977). 'Early and late volume changes during erythroid differentiation of cultured Friend leukemic cells', *J. Cell. Physiol.*, **90**, 423–437.
85. Zucker, R. M., Wu, N. C., Mitrani, A., and Silverman, M. (1979). 'Cell volume decrease during Friend leukemia cell differentiation', *J. Histochem. Cytochem.*, **27**, 413–416.
86. Bernstein, A., Boyd, A. S. Crichley, V., and Lamb, V. (1976). 'Induction and inhibition of Friend leukemic cell differentiation; The role of membrane-active compounds', in *Biogenesis and Turnover of Membrane Macromolecules* (Ed. J. S. Cook), Raven Press, New York, pp. 145–159.
87. Friend, C., Scher, W., and Preisler, H. (1974). 'Hemoglobin biosynthesis in murine virus-induced leukemia cells *in vitro*', *Ann. N.Y. Acad. Sci.*, **241**, 582–588.
88. Garbrecht, M., Mertelsmann, R., Hellerschock, G., and Schöch, G. (1974). 'DNA-dependent DNA and RNA polymerases and tRNA-methyl transferases in human leukemia and differentiating Friend virus leukemia cells', in *Modern Trends*

in Human Leukemia (Eds. R. Neth, R. C. Gallo, S. Spiegelmann, and F. Stohlman, Jr.) Grune and Stratton, Inc., New York, pp. 256–269.

89. Lacatena, R. M., Busiello, V., DiGirolamo, A., and DiGirolamo, M. (1981).
'DNA polymerase activities in Friend cells during the differentiation process',
Cell Diff., **10**, 109–116.

90. Giri, J. G., Reuben, R. C., Rifkind, R. A., and Marks, P. A. (1981). 'DNA
polymerase activities during induced differentiation in murine erythroleukemia
cells', *Exp. Cell Res.*, **132**, 137–146.

91. Scher, B. M., Scher, W., Robinson, A., and Waxman, S. (1982). 'DNA ligase
and DNAase activities in mouse erythroleukemia cells during dimethyl
sulfoxide-induced differentiation', *Cancer Res.*, (in press).

92. Long, B. H., Huang, C.-Y., and Pogo, A. O. (1979). 'Isolation and characterization of the nuclear matrix in Friend erythroleukemia cells: Chromatin
and hnRNA interactions with the nuclear matrix', *Cell*, **18**, 1079–1090.

93. Rifkind, R. A., Fibach, E., Maniatis, G., Gambari, R., and Marks, P. A.
(1979). 'Commitment to differentiation of normal and transformed erythroid
precursors', in *Cellular and Molecular Regulation of Hemoglobin Switching*
(eds. G. Stamatoyannopoulos and A. W. Nienhuis), Grune and Stratton, Inc.
New York, pp. 421–436.

94. Muller, M. T., Kajiwara, K., and Mueller, G. C. (1981). 'Role of cytosol
proteins in DNA chain growth and chromatin replication in Friend erythroleukemia cell nuclei', *Biochim. Biophys. Acta*, **653**, 391–407.

95. SöderHäll, S. and Lindahl, T. (1976). 'DNA ligases of eukaryotes', *FEBS
Lett.*, **67**, 1–8.

96. Johnston, L. H. and Nasmyth, K. A. (1978). '*Saccharomyces cervisiae* cell cycle
mutant *cdc9* is defective in DNA ligase', *Nature*, **274**, 891–893.

97. Otto, B. and Reichard, P. (1975). 'Replication of polyoma DNA in isolated
nuclei V. Complementation of *in vitro* DNA replication', *J. Virol.*, **15**,
259–267.

98. Hewish, D. R. and Burgoyne, L. A. (1973). 'The calcium dependent
endonuclease activity of isolated nuclear preparations. Relationships between its
occurrence and the occurrence of other classes of enzymes found in nuclear
preparations', *Biochem. Biophys. Res. Commun.*, **52**, 475–481.

99. Yoshihara, K., Tanigawa, Y., and Koide, S. S. (1974). 'Inhibition of rat liver
Ca^{2+}, Mg^{2+}-dependent endonuclease activity by nicotinamido adenine
dinucleotide and poly (adenosine diphosphate ribose) synthetase', *Biochem.
Biophys. Res. Commun.*, **59**, 658–665.

100. Sheraton, C. C. and Kabat, D. (1976). 'Changes in RNA and protein
metabolism preceding onset of hemoglobin synthesis in cultured Friend leukemia
cells', *Develop. Biol.*, **48**, 118–131.

101. Scher, B. M., Yeh, H., Scher, W., and Waxman, S. (1981). 'Changes in G-actin
and F-actin pools during mouse erythropoiesis', *Blood*, **58, Suppl. 1**, 101a, No. 316.

102. Peterson, J., and McConkey, E. H. (1976). 'Proteins of Friend leukemia cells',
J. Biol. Chem., **251**, 555–558.

103. Neumann, J. R., Housman, D., and Ingram, V. M. (1978). 'Nuclear protein
synthesis and phosphorylation in Friend erythroleukemia cells stimulated with
DMSO', *Exp. Cell Res.*, **111**, 277–284.

104. Lau, A. F., and Ruddon, R. W. (1977). 'Proteins of transcriptionally active and
inactive chromatin from Friend erythroleukemia cells', *Exp. Cell Res.*, **107**,
35–46.

105. Reeves, R., and Cserjesi, P. (1979). 'Sodium butyrate induces new gene
expression in Friend erythroleukemia cells', *J. Biol. Chem.*, **254**, 4283–4290.

106. Candido, E. P. M., Reeves, R., and Davie, J. R. (1978). 'Sodium butyrate inhibits histone deacetylation in cultured cells', *Cell*, **14**, 105–113.
107. Leder, A., and Leder, P. (1975). 'Butyric acid, a potent inducer of erythroid differentiation in cultured erythroleukemic cells', *Cell*, **5**, 319–322.
108. Kameji, R., Obinata, M., Natori, Y., and Ikawa, Y. (1977). 'Induction of globin gene expresion in cultured erythroleukemia cells by butyric acid', *J. Biochem.*, **81**, 1901–1910.
109. Rovera, G. and Surrey, S. (1978). 'Use of resistant or hypersensitive variant clones of Friend cells in analysis of mode of action of inducers', *Cancer Res.*, **38**, 3737–3744.
110. Ebert, P. S., Bonkowsky, H. L., and Deisseroth, A. (1979). 'Evidence for multiple sites of regulation of heme synthesis in murine erythroleukemia cells', *J. Natl. Cancer Inst.*, **62**, 1247–1250.
111. Ono, T., Morioka, K., Komito, K., Nokuo, T., and Ishizawa, M. (1979). 'Comparison of mechanisms for induction of hemoglobin synthesis in Friend leukemic cells by butyrate, dimethyl-sulfoxide, and hexamethylene bisacetamide', in *Oncogenic Viruses and Host Cell Genes* (Eds. Y. Ikawa and T. Okada), Academic Press, New York, pp. 319–326.
112. Housman, D., Levenson, R., Volloch, V., Tsiftsoglou, A., Gusella, J., Parker, D., Kernen, J., Mitrani, A., Weeks, V., Witte, O., and Besmer, P. (1980). 'Control of proliferation and differentiation in cells transformed by Friend virus', *Cold Spring Harbor Symp. Quant. Biol.*, **44**, 1177–1185.
113. Scher, W., Tsuei, D., Sassa, S., Price, P., Gabelman, N., and Friend, C. (1978). 'Inhibition of dimethyl sulfoxide-stimulated Friend cell erythrodifferentiation by hydrocortisone and other steroids', *Proc. Natl, Acad. Sci. U.S.A.*, **75**, 3851–3855.
114. Riggs, M. G., Whittaker, R. G., Neumann, J. R., and Ingram, V. M. (1977). 'n-Butyrate causes histone modification in HeLa and Friend erthroleukemia cells', *Nature*, **268**, 462–464.
115. Boffa, L. C., Vidali, G., Mann, R. S., and Allfrey, V. G. (1978). 'Suppression of histone deacetylation *in vivo* and *in vitro* by sodium butyrate', *J. Biol. Chem.*, **259**, 3364–3366.
116. Sealy, L. and Chalkley, R. (1978). 'The effect of sodium butyrate on histone modification', *Cell*, **14**, 115–121.
117. Cousens, L. S., Gallwitz, D., and Alberts, B. M. (1979). 'Different accessibilities in chromatin to histone acetylase', *J. Biol. Chem.*, **254**, 1716–1723.
118. Ingram, V. M., Hagopian, H. K., Riggs, M. G., Neumann, J. R., Dobson, M. E., Owens, B. B., and Maniatis, G. M. (1979). 'A model for differentiation: modification of chromatin proteins in differentiating erythroid and nonerythroid cells', in *Cellular and Molecular Regulation of Hemoglobin Switching* (Ed. G. Stamatoyannopoulos and A. W. Nienhuis), Grune and Stratton, Inc. New York, pp. 471–489.
119. Reeves, R. and Candido, E. P. M. (1980). 'Partial inhibition of histone deacetylase in active chromatin by HMG14 and HMG17', *Nuc. Acid Res.*, **8**, 1947–1963.
120. Blankstein, L. A. and Levy, S. B. (1976). 'Changes in histone f2a2 associated with proliferation of Friend leukemia cells', *Nature*, **260**, 638–640.
121. Blankstein, L. A., Stollar, B. D., Franklin, S. G., Zweidler, A., and Levy, S. B. (1977). 'Biochemical and immunological characterization of two distinct variants of histone H2A in Friend leukemia', *Biochemistry*, **16**, 4557–4562.
122. Gabrielli, F. (1981). 'Polysomal and nonpolysomal messenger RNA of noninduced and induced Friend erythroleukemic cells. Analysis by cell-free translation', *Diff.*, **19**, 59–64.

123. Morioka, K., Tanaka, K., and Ono, T. (1981). 'Comparison of nuclear proteins of differentiation-induced and uninduced Friend erythroleukemia cells', *J. Biochem.*, **89**, 1633–1638.
124. Morioka, K., Tanaka, K., and Ono, T. (1980). 'Poly(ADP-ribose) and differentiation of Friend erythroleukemia cells', *J. Biochem.*, **88**, 517–524.
125. Triadou, P., Lelong, J.-C., Gros, F., and Crepin, M. (1981). 'Modulation of the initiation of mouse β-globin transcription by non-histone proteins purified from mouse erythropoietic Friend cells', *Biochem. Biophys. Res. Commun.*, **101**, 45–54.
126. Seyedin, S. M., Pehrson, J. R., and Cole, R. D. (1981). 'Loss of chromosomal high mobility group proteins HMG1 and HMG2 when mouse neuroblastoma and Friend erythroleukemia cells become committed to differentiation', *Proc. Natl. Acad. Sci., U.S.A.*, **78**, 5988–5992.
127. Burckard, J., Mazen, A., and Champagne, M. (1975). 'Non-histone chromosomal proteins easily extractable from chick erythrocytes', *Biochim. Biophys. Acta*, **405**, 434–441.
128. Grebanier, A. E. and Pogo, A. O. (1979). 'Cross-linking of proteins in nuclei and DNA-depleted nuclei: from Friend erythroleukemia cells', *Cell*, **18**, 1091–1099.
129. Grebanier, A. E. and Pogo, A. O. (1981). 'Non-histone proteins cross-linked by disulfide bonds to histone H3 in nuclei from Friend erythroleukemia cells', *Biochemistry*, **20**, 1094–1099.
130. Keppel, F., Allet, B., and Eisen, H. (1977). 'Appearance of a chromatin protein during the erythroid differentiation of Friend Virus-transformed cells', *Proc. Natl. Acad. Sci., U.S.A.*, **74**, 653–656.
131. Hayashi, K., Matsutera, E., and Ohba, Y. (1974). 'A theoretical consideration of the abnormal behavior of histones on sodium dodecyl sulfate gel electrophoresis', *Biochim. Biophys. Acta*, **342**, 185–194.
132. DeLange, R. J. (1976). 'Characterization of histones', in *Handbook of Biochemical and Molecular Biology, Proteins*, 3rd Ed. (Ed. G. D. Fasman), CRC Press, Cleveland, Ohio, vol. 2, pp. 293–300.
133. Hunt, L. T., Barker, W. C., McLaughlin, P. J., and Dayhoff, M. O. (1973). 'Protein data section', in *Atlas of Protein Sequence and Structure* (Ed. M. O. Dayhoff), National Biomedical Research Foundation, Washington, D.C., vol. 5, suppl. 1, pp. S-9–S-84.
134. Hunt, L. T., Schwartz, R. M., and Dayhoff, M. O. (1978). 'Nucleic acid-associated proteins', in *Atlas of Protein Sequence and Structure* (Ed. M. O. Dayhoff), National Biomedical Research Foundation, Washington, D.C. vol. 5, suppl. 3, pp. 251–264.
135. Briand, D., Kmiecik, D., Sautiere, P., Wouters, D., Borie-Loy, O., Biserte, G., Mazen, A., and Champagne, M. (1980). 'Chicken erythrocyte histone H5', *FEBS Lett.*, **112**, 147–151.
136. Keppel, F., Allet, B., and Eisen, H. (1979). 'Biochemical properties and localization of the chromosomal protein IP25', *Eur. J. Biochem.*, **96**, 477–482.
137. Gjerset, R., Ibarrando, F., Saragosti, S., and Eisen, H. (1981). 'Distribution of IP25 in chromatin and its possible involvement in chromatin condensation', *Biochem., Biophys. Res. Commun.*, **99**, 349–357.
138. Eisen, H., Hasthorpe, S., Gjerset, R., Nasi, S., and Keppel, F. (1980). 'Distribution and behavior of the chromosomal protein IP25 *in vivo* and tissue culture', in *In Vivo and in Vitro Erythropoiesis: The Friend System* (Ed. G. B. Rossi), Elsevier/North Holland, Biomedical Press, New York, pp. 289–296.

139. Zlatanova, J. S. and Swetly, P. (1980). 'Poly-ADP-ribosylation of nuclear proteins in differentiating Friend cells', *Biochem. Biophys. Res. Commun.*, **92**, 1110–1116.
140. Zlatanova, J. S. (1980). 'Synthesis of histone H1° is not inhibited in hydroxy-urea-treated Friend cells', *FEBS Lett.*, **112**, 199–202.
141. Gusella, J. F., Weil, S. C., Tsiftsoglou, A. S., Volloch, V., Neumann, J. R., Keys, C., and Housman, D. E. (1980). 'Hemin does not cause commitment of murine erythroleukemia (MEL) cells to terminal differentiation', *Blood*, **56**, 481–487.
142. Lowenhaupt, K., and Lingrel, J. B. (1979). 'Synthesis and turnover of globin mRNA in murine erythroleukemia cells induced with hemin', *Proc. Natl. Acad. Sci., U.S.A.*, **76**, 5173–5177.
143. Curtis, P., Finnigan, A. C., and Rovera, G. (1980). 'The β major and β minor globin nuclear transcripts of Friend erythroleukemia cells induced to differentiate in culture', *J. Biol. Chem.*, **255**, 8971–8974.
144. Manduca, P. (1981). 'Isolation and characterization of murine erythroleukemia cell variants nonresponsive to hemin for the expression of globin genes', *Somat. Cell Genet.*, **7**, 11–16.
145. Housman, D, Gusella, J., Geller, R., Levenson, R., and Weil, S. (1978). 'Differentiation of murine erythroleukemia cells: the central role of the commitment event', in *Differentiation of Normal and Neoplastic Hematopoietic Cells, Book A* (Eds., B. Clarkson, P. A. Marks, and J. E. Till), Cold Spring Harbor Press, Cold Spring Harbor, pp. 193–207.
146. Mager, D., and Bernstein, A. (1980). 'Phorbol ester tumor promoters block the transition from the early to the hemedependent late program of Friend cell differentiation', *J. Cell. Physiol.*, **105**,. 519–526.
147. Sassa, S., 'Heme biosynthesis in erythroid cells: the distinctive aspects of the regulatory mechanism', in *The Regulation of Hemoglobin Biosynthesis* (Ed. E. Goldwasser), Elsevier/North Holland, Harvard, MA., (in press).
148. Hugues, B., and Osborne, H. B. (1981). 'Dexamethasone inhibits a heme-independent event necessary for terminal differentiation of murine erythroleukemia cells', *Biochem. Biophys. Res. Commun.*, **102**, 1342–1349.
149. Gusella, J. F., Tsiftsoglou, A. S., Volloch, V., Weil, S. C., Neumann, J., and Housman, D. (1982). 'Dissociation of hemoglobin accumulation and commitment during murine erythroleukemia cell differentiation by treatment with imidazole', *J. Cell. Physiol.*, (in press).
150. D'Anna, J. A., Tobey, R. A., and Gurley, L., R. (1980). 'Concentration-dependent effects of sodium butyrate in Chinese hamster cells: cell-cycle progression, inner-histone acetylation, histone H1 dephosphorylation, and induction of an H1-like protein', *Biochem.*, **19**, 2656–2671.
151. Pieler, C., Adolf, G. R., and Swelty, P. (1981). 'Accumulation of histone H1° during chemically induced differentiation of murine neuroblastoma cells', *Eur. J. Biochem.*, **115**, 329–333.
152. Panyim, S., and Chalkley, R. (1969). 'A new histone found only in mammalian tissues with little cell division', *Biochem. Biophys. Res. Commun.*, **37**, 1042–1049.
153. Smith, B. J., and Johns, E. W. (1980). 'Isolation and characterization of subfractions of nuclear protein H1°', *FEBS Lett.*, **110**, 25–29.
154. Zlatanova, J., Oberhummer, K., and Swetly, P. (1980). 'Expresion of histone H1° during differentiation of erythroleukemic mouse cells', in *In Vivo and in Vitro Erythropoiesis: The Friend System* (Ed. G. B. Rossi), Elsevier/N. Holland Biomedical Press, New York, pp. 297–307.

155. Smith, B. J., Walker, J. M., and Johns, E. W. (1980). 'Structural homology between a mammalian H1° subfraction and avian erythrocyte specific histone H5', *FEBS Lett.*, **112**, 42–44.
156. Smith, B. J., and Johns, E. W. (1980). 'Histone H1°: its location in chromatin', *Nucleic Acids Res.*, **8**, 6069–6079.
157. Mura, C. V., and Stollar, B. D. (1981). 'Serological detection of homologies of H1° with H5 and H1 histones', *J. Biol. Chem.*, **256**, 9767–9769.
158. Pehrson, J. R., and Cole, R. D. (1981). 'Bovine H1° histone subfractions contain an invariant sequence which matches histone H5 rather than H1', *Biochem.*, **20**, 2298–2301.
159. Cary, P. D., Hines, M. L., Bradbury, E. M., Smith, B. J., and Johns, E. W. (1981). 'Conformational studies of histone H1° in comparison with histones H1 and H5', *Eur. J. Biochem.*, **120**, 371–377.
160. Shimada, T., Okihama, Y., Murata, C., and Shukuya, R. (1981). 'Occurrence of H1°-like protein and protein A-24 in the chromatin of bullfrog erythrocytes lacking histone 5', *J. Biol. Chem.*, **256**, 10577–10582.
161. Henderson, L. E., Gilden, R. V., and Oroszlan, S. (1979). 'Amino acid sequence homology between histone H5 and murine leukemia virus phosphoprotein p12', *Science,* **203**, 1346–1348.
162. Lunadei, M., Matteucci, P., Ullu, E., Gambari, R., Rossi, G. B., and Fantoni, (1978). 'Disappearance of a 32000 D chromatin polypeptide during early erythroid differentiation of Friend leukemia cells', *Exp. Cell. Res.*, **114**, 468–471.
163. Gaedicke, G., Abedin, Z., Dube, S. K., Kluge, N., Neth, R., Steinheider, G., Weimann, B. J., and Ostertag, W. (1974). 'Control of globin synthesis during DMSO-induced differentiation of mouse erythroleukemic cells in culture', in *Modern Trends in Human Leukemia* (Eds. R. Neth, R. C. Gallo, S. Speigelman, and F. Stohlman), Grune and Stratton, Inc., New York, pp. 278–287.
164. Harel, L., Lacour, F., Friend, C., Durbin, P., and Semmel, M. (1979). 'Early inhibition of phospholipid synthesis in dimethyl sulfoxide (DMSO) treated Friend erythroleukemia (FL) cells', *J. Cell. Physiol.*, **101**, 25–32.
165. Neumann, J., Whittaker, R., Blanchard, B., and Ingram, V. M. (1978). 'Nucleosome-associated proteins and phosphoproteins of differentiating Friend erythroleukemia cells', *Nucleic Acids Res.*, **5**, 1675–1687.
166. Neumann, J. R., Riggs, M. G., Hagopian, H. K., Whittaker, R. G., and Ingram, V. M. (1978). 'Chromatin changes and DNA synthesis in Friend erythroleukemia and HeLa cells during treatment with DMSO and n-butyrate', in *Differentiation of Normal and Neoplastic Hematopoietic Cells, Book A* (Ed. B. Clarkson, P. A. Marks, and J. E. Till), Cold Spring Harbor Press, Cold Spring Harbor, vol. 5, pp. 261–275.
167. Neumann, J. R., Owens, B. B., and Ingram, V. M. (1979). 'Nucleosome-associated protein kinases in murine erythroleukemia cells', *Arch. Biochem. Biophys.*, **197**, 447–453.
168. Hayaishi, O., and Ueda, K. (1977). 'Poly (ADP-ribose) and ADP-ribosylation of proteins', *Ann. Rev. Biochem.*, **46**, 95–116.
169. Hayaishi, M. O. Ueda, K., Kawaichi, M., Ogata, N., Oka, J., Ikai, K., Ito, S., Shizuta, Y., Kim, H., and Okayama, H. (1979). 'Poly (ADP-ribose) and ADP-ribosylation of proteins', in *From Gene to Protein: Information Transfer in Normal and Abnormal Cells* (Eds. T. R. Russel, K. Brew, H. Faber, and J. Schultz), Academic Press, New York, pp. 545–566.
170. Purnell, M. R., Stone, P. R., and Whish, W. J. D. (1980). 'ADP-ribosylation of nuclear proteins', *Biochem. Soc. Trans.*, **8**, 215–227.
171. Ueda, K., Hayaishi, O., Kawaichi, M., Ogata, N., Ikai, K., Oka, J., and Okayama, H. (1979). 'Poly (ADP-ribose) and ADP-ribosylation of proteins', in

Modulation of Protein Functions (Ed. D. E. Atkinson and C. F. Fox), Academic Press, New York, pp. 47–64.

172. Wong, N. C. W., Poirier, G. G., and Dixon, G. H. (1977). 'Adenosine diphospho-ribosylation of certain basic chromosomal proteins in isolated trout testis nuclei', *Eur. J. Biochem.*, **77**, 11–21.

173. Rastl, E. (1976), in *Poly (ADP-ribose)*, report by M. Smulson and S. Shall, on the fourth Internatl. Workshop, *Nature*, **263**, 14.

174. Rastl, E., and Swetly, P. (1978). 'Expression of poly (adenosine diphosphate-ribose) polymerase activity in erythroleukemic mouse cells during cell cycle and erythropoietic differentiation', *J. Biol. Chem.*, **253**, 4333–4340.

175. Stone, P. R., and Shall, S. (1975). 'Poly (ADP-ribose) polymerase activity during the growth cycle of mouse fibroblasts (LS cells)', *Exp. Cell Res.*, **91**, 95–100.

176. Berger, N. A., Petzold, S. J., and Berger, S. J. (1979). 'Association of poly (ADP-rib) synthesis with cessation of DNA synthesis and DNA fragmentation', *Biochim. Biophys. Acta*, **564**, 90–104.

177. Savard, P., Poirer, G. G., and Sheinin, R. (1981). 'Poly (ADP-ribose) polymerase activity in mouse cells which exhibit temperature-sensitive DNA synthesis', *Biochim. Biophys. Acta*, **653**, 271–275.

178. Morioka, K., Tanaka, K., Nokuo, T., Ishizawa, M., and Ono, T. (1979). 'Erythroid differentiation and poly (ADP-ribose) synthesis in Friend leukemia cells', *Gann.*, **70**, 37–46.

179. Morioka, K., Tanaka, K., and Ono, T. (1980). 'Effect of medium change on poly (ADP-ribose) synthesis in Friend erythroleukemia cells', *Biochem. Biophys. Res. Commun.*, **94**, 592–599.

180. Terada, M., Fujiki, H., Marks, P. A., and Sugimura, T., (1979). 'Induction of erythroid differentiation of murine erythroleukemia cells by nicotinamide and related compounds', *Proc. Natl. Acad. Sci., U.S.A.*, **76**, 6411–6414.

181. Weisenthal, L. M., and Ruddon, R. W. (1973). 'Catabolism of nuclear proteins in control and phytohemagglutinin-stimulated human lymphocytes, leukemic leukocytes, and Burkitt lymphoma cells', *Cancer Res.*, **33**, 2923–2935.

182. Jänne, J., Pösö, H., and Raina, A. (1978). 'Polyamines in rapid growth and cancer', *Biochim. Biophys. Acta.*, **473**, 241–293.

183. Canellakis, E. S., Viceps-Madore, D., Kyriakidis, D. A., and Heller, J. S. (1979). The regulation and function of ornithine decarboxylase and of the polyamines', in *Current Topics in Cellular Regulation*, Academic Press, New York, vol. 15, pp. 155–202.

184. Maudsley, D. V. (1979). 'Regulation of polyamine biosynthesis', *Biochem. Pharmacol.*, **28**, 153–161.

185. Aigner-Held, R., and Daves, G. D., Jr. (1980). 'Polyamine metabolites and conjugates in man and higher animals: a review of the literature', *Physiol. Chem. Phys.*, **12**, 389–400.

186. Heby, O. (1981). 'Role of polyamines in the control of cell proliferation and differentiation', *Diff.*, **19**, 1–20.

187. Abraham, A. K., and Phil, A. (1981). 'Role of polyamines in macromolecular synthesis', *Trends Biochem. Sci.*, 106–107.

188. Ahmed, K., Wilson, M. J., Goueli, S. A., and Williams-Ashman, H. G. (1978). 'Effects of polyamines on prostatic chromatin- and non-histone-protein associated protein kinase rections', *Biochem. J.*, **176**, 739–750.

189. Perrella, F. W., and Lea, M. A. (1978). 'Polyamine induced changes in ADP-ribosylation of nuclear proteins from rat liver', *Biochem. Biophys. Res. Commun.*, **82**, 575–581.

190. Dehlinger, P. J., and Litt, M. (1978). 'Ornithine decarboxylase induction and nucleolar RNA synthesis in Friend leukemia cells', *Biochem. Biophys. Res. Commun.*, **81**, 1054–1057.

191. Tsiftsoglou, A. S., and Kyriakidis, D. A. (1979). 'Early changes in ornithine decarboxylase activity during Friend leukemia cell differentiation', *Biochim. Biophys. Acta*, **588**, 279–283.
192. Gazitt, Y., and Friend, C. (1980). 'Polyamine biosynthesis enzymes in the induction and inhibition of differentiation in Friend erythroleukemia cells', *Cancer Res.*, **40**, 1727–1732.
193. Gazitt, Y., and Friend, C. (1980). 'The possible role of polyamine biosynthetic enzymes in the induction of differentiation in Friend erythroleukemic cells', in *In Vivo and In Vitro Erythropoiesis: The Friend System* (Ed. G. B. Rossi), Elsevier/N. Holland Biomedical Press, New York, pp. 209–218.
194. Gazitt, Y. (1981). 'Inhibition of induced L-ornithine decarboxylase stimulation and erythrodifferentiation in Friend erythroleukemia cells by 2',5'-isoadenylate trimer core', *Cancer Res.*, **41**, 2959–2961.
195. Gazitt, Y. (1981). 'Comparative study of two groups of inducers of Friend erythroleukemia cell differentiation in a chemically defined medium', *Cancer Res.*, **41**, 1184–1186.
196. Ohta, Y., Tanaka, M., Terada, M., Miller, O. J., Bank, A., Marks, P. A., and Rifkind, R. A. (1976). 'Erythroid cell differentiation: Murine erythroleukemia cell variant with unique pattern of induction by polar compounds', *Proc. Natl. Acad. Sci., U.S.A.*, **73**, 1232–1236.
197. Diacumakos, E. G., Killos, L., Lee, L., and Anderson, W. F. (1981). 'Induction of mouse erythroleukemia cells by microinjection of inducing compound', *Exp. Cell Res.*, **131**, 73–77.
198. Scher, W., and Waxman, S. (1980). 'Further evidence that there are different biochemical mechanisms for the induction of hemoglobin synthesis in mouse erythroleukemia cells', *Proc. 18th Cong. Internatl. Soc. Hemat.*, p **358**, No. 80.

Current Concepts in Erythropoiesis
Edited by C. D. R. Dunn
© 1983 John Wiley & Sons Ltd.

CHAPTER 14

Hemoglobin switching in humans

C. Peschle*†, G. Migliaccio†, A. R. Migliaccio†,
A. Covelli†, A. Giuliani*, F. Mavilio*, and
G. Mastroberardino‡

*Istituto Superiore di Sanità, Rome; †Istituto Patologia Medica, IInd Faculty, University of Naples, ‡Istituto Patologia Medica (VI), University of Rome.

Contents

§Correspondence and reprint requests to: Cesare Peschle, M. D.,
Laboratory of Hematology, Istituto Superiore di Sanità, Viale Regina Elena, 299–00161 Roma, Italy.

The hemoglobin (Hb) switch provides a unique model to investigate the regulation of gene expression during development and differentiation of eukaryotic cells. It is not surprising, therefore, that a series of conferences (1–3) and reviews (4–6) have recently focused on this topic.

This chapter is essentially restricted to the human fetal → adult Hb switch. The embryonic → fetal Hb switch is not analyzed in detail in view of present uncertainties on human embryonic Hbs (7). Animal models are discussed only in so far as they reflect on the human Hb switch. It seems appropriate to review selected aspects of the thalassemic syndromes, which may contribute significantly to our understanding of molecular mechanisms underlying the Hb switch.

I. INTRODUCTION

A. The human Hb switches

The Hb switches in different ontogenic stages are depicted in Figure 1 (4,9–12). They entail gradual replacement of a globin chain type(s) by another one(s). In early embryonic life Hb Gower I ($\zeta_2 \varepsilon_2$) is synthesized. Transition from embryonic to fetal Hb takes place at ~5–8 weeks from conception. Embryonic ζ-and ε-chains are gradually replaced by fetal α- and γ-globin respectively: HbF ($\alpha_2 \gamma_2$) is thus synthesized together with Hb Gower II ($\alpha_2 \varepsilon_2$) and Portland ($\zeta_2 \gamma_2$). In fetal life HbF is associated with a small amount of HbA, starting from ~5% and increasing to 20% at the end of gestation. In the perinatal period HbF is rapidly replaced by HbA ($\alpha_2 \beta_2$) and A_2 ($\alpha_2 \delta_2$). In post-natal life > 99% of total Hb is accounted for by HbA (~97%) + A_2 (~2.5%). Interestingly, the residual HbF (<1%) is restricted to <8% of RBC ('F-cells', containing ~14–30% of HbF), and is not detectable in the majority of RBC ('A-cells') (13,14).

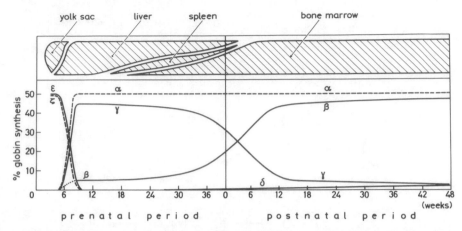

Figure 1. Globin chain synthesis in human ontogenic development. Also indicated are the erythropoietic sites. Modified from (8) and reproduced by permission of Blackwell Scientific Publications Ltd

Two types of γ-chain ($^{G}\gamma, ^{A}\gamma$) exist, which are coded by non-allelic genes (15). They only differ for the amino acid in position 136, i.e., glycine and alanine
respectively. The $^{G}\gamma/^{A}\gamma$ ratio is about 3:1 in fetal life and about 2:3 in the post-natal period (15,16). The normal adult ratio usually ranges between 1:3 and 3:3 (16). The perinatal γ → β switch is thus associated with a $^{G}\gamma \rightarrow ^{A}\gamma$ 'switch' (i.e., a significant decrease of the $^{G}\gamma/^{A}\gamma$ synthetic ratio).

The organization of human globin genes is described in Section III A.

B. Recent advances in erythrocytic differentiation

The genetic program underlying erythrocytic differentiation is expressed *via* prior determination and subsequent maturation of erythrocytic elements. Hematopoietic stem cells are undetermined (i.e., endowed with the potential to feed into a wide spectrum of different cell lineages). They may differentiate into erythrocytic progenitors, *via* gradual restriction of their pluripotential capacity and determination to the erythrocytic lineage. Committed progenitors undergo a multi-step differentiation process (see below). Finally, they give rise to morphologically recognizable precursors or erythroblasts. These initiate their specialization or maturation, *via* synthesis of lineage-specific molecular markers. In ontogenic development, expression of these markers is subject to numerous switches. A typical example of this is represented by the Hb switch.

Recent technology, at both cellular and molecular levels, has allowed an insight to be gained into development and differentiation of the erythron. Selected advances thereon, relevant to the Hb switch, are concisely analyzed here.

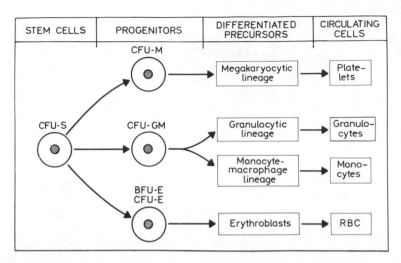

Figure 2. A currently accepted model of hematopoiesis. Reproduced with permission from (22)

1. Cellular aspects (see also 17–22)

a. Clonogenic assays. These permitted identification of hematopoietic stem (23) and progenitor cells (see 17). On the basis of these techniques, studies have been performed to characterize stem elements and erythrocytic progenitors, as well as to investigate their kinetics and control mechanisms.

b. A model of erythropoiesis (Figure 2). Hematopoietic stem cells are capable of extensive self-renewal, and may also differentiate into progenitors. These are 'committed' to either myelocytic or lymphocytic lineages. Progenitors in turn give rise to the respective differentiated cell series.

c. The pluripotential stem cell. This generates both myelocytic and lymphocytic progeny. Its existence has been demonstrated by means of radiation-induced chromosomal aberrations (24). It apparently gives rise to stem elements restricted to either the myelocytic or T-lymphocytic lines (24). It is uncertain whether B-lymphocytes derive from pluripotential and/or myelocytic stem cells (24).

d. The myelocytic stem cell. This gives rise to erythrocytic, granulocytic, macrophage-monocytic, and megakaryocytic lineages (as well as to eosinophilic and mast cell-basophilic series) (Figure 2). The murine stem element (CFU-S) was originally assayed on the basis of its capacity to form macroscopic, mixed colonies in the spleen of lethally irradiated animals (23).

Murine (25) and human (26) stem cells, seeded in semi-solid media*, generate mixed colonies, which contain essentially erythrocytic, granulo-macrophage (GM), and megakaryocytic lineages (Figure 2)†.

e. Erythrocytic progenitors. Two erythrocytic progenitors (BFU-E and CFU-E) have been identified in mammals (28) (Figures 2,3). In this regard, erythrocytic cultures are characterized by sequential hemoglobinization of gradually larger colonies, which take origin from progressively less differentiated progenitors (Figure 3; see 22–24,29–33). Clones undergoing early hemoglobinization are represented by single clusters of erythroblasts, which derive from CFU-E. Later on, large colonies ('bursts') generated by BFU-E become gradually mature. Bursts are essentially composed of multiple CFU-E derived clusters. Finally, mixed colonies of even larger size reach full development (25,26,32). As mentioned above, they derive from stem cells. The growth curves of different types of clones partially overlap (Figure 3a). However, colony recognition is insured by both sequential hemoglobinization and unequivocal morphologic criteria (29–33).

These clonogenic features clearly indicate that the erythrocytic process is of a multi-step type, and basically entails CFU-S → BFU-E → CFU-E → erythroblasts differentiation. BFU-E are closely related to the CFU-S compartment. Thus, BFU-E and CFU-S are characterized by identical cell size and buoyant density (34) although BFU-E show a slightly more elevated cycling activity (see 31) than the slowly-proliferating CFU-S (35). BFU-E → CFU-E differentiation is characterized by a further increase of proliferative rate, as well as of pool amplification, cell size, and buoyant density (see 31).

Cells in the BFU-E and CFU-E pools can be further subdivided. In both humans and mice, Eaves *et al* dissected 'primitive BFU-E' (P-BFU-E) from mature ones (M-BFU-E). The human M-BFU-E is intermediate between P-BFU-E and CFU-E with respect to all above parameters (31) (Figure 3). In human marrow cultures, erythrocytic clusters may be subdivided in two types deriving from 'early' and 'late' CFU-E (19,36) (Figure 3a). It may be conceded that the 'late' one is analogous to the corresponding murine progenitor, and at least in part coincides with the pro-erythroblast.

A continuous spectrum of human erythrocytic progenitors has thus been demonstrated. Their differentiation entails a gradual increase of their number, proliferative activity, cell size, and density. A further differentiation marker is the progressive enhancement of their sensitivity to erythropoietin (EPO), and

---

*Growth of mixed colonies is dependent upon addition not only of erythrocytic (BPA, EPO) but also Gm-specific (CSF) hormones (see below).

†In human cultures, T-lymphocytes are occasionally present upon addition of their specific growth factor (27): this suggests that some mixed colonies may derive from the pluripotential rather than the myelocytic stem cell.

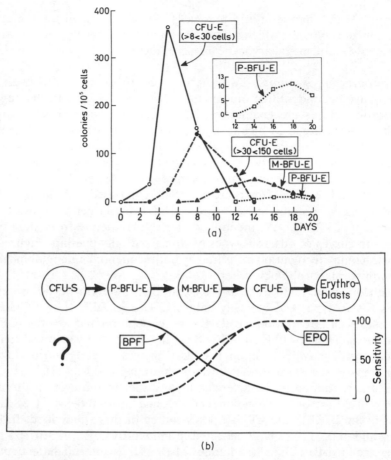

Figure 3(a). Growth curve of four types of human erythrocytic colonies from normal adult marrow (number of colonies/days). For each type the number of cells/colony and the respective progenitor are indicated. From Peschle, C., Migliaccio, A. R., Migliaccio, G. et al.: in vitro regulation of Hb synthesis: Studies in normal subjects and thalassemic patients. In Cao, A., Carcassi, U., and Rowley, P. T. (eds): *Thalassemia: Recent Advances in Defection and Treatment*, New York Alan R. Liss for the March of Dimes Birth Defects Foundation, BD:OAS **18**(7): 131–138,1982

(b) Regulatory role of BPF and EPO in adult erythropcytic differentiation. The relative sensitivity of progenitors and erythroblasts is expressed in arbitrary units. It is still debatable whether or not EPO exerts a significant influence on P-BFU-E (for further discussion see 22). Reproduced with permission from (22)

gradual decrease of their response to 'burst-promoting activity' (BPA) (30–33, Figure 3b).

BFU-E (37) have been demonstrated in the circulating blood of humans and CFU-S (38) and BFU-E (39) in murine blood. The progenitors are apparently confined to the null-lymphocyte fraction (40). Stress erythropoiesis in humans

(36) and mice (41) is associated with marked expansion of the circulating BFU-E pool, thus suggesting an increased traffic of these cells between different erythrocytic areas.

In conclusion, solid evidence allows the postulation of an articulate model of hematopoiesis and erythropoiesis (Figure 2). This model, although universally-accepted, is still clouded by uncertainties. Stem or progenitor cells within the same pool are fairly homogenous when tested by 'cellular' criteria (clonogenic features, size and density, response to hematopoietic hormones, etc.). However, they may prove heterogenous if subjected to molecular analysis. It cannot be excluded that pluripotential and myelocytic stem cells simply represent an emergency reservoir, which plays a limited role in day-by-day hematopoietic differentiation. In this regard, early progenitors of GM-lineage are endowed with self-renewal capacity, if continuously triggered by specific growth hormone(s) (42). The transition between different compartments is considered as strictly unidirectional; this is not necessarily true for stem cell pools, and perhaps not even for those of early progenitors. These uncertainties are emphasized here, in that they reflect on cellular models for the Hb switch (see below).

f. Mechanisms regulating the kinetics of erythropoiesis (Figure 3b). It is well-established that the erythrocytic rate is largely or solely regulated by EPO, a recently purified glycoprotein (molecular weight, $\sim$ 39,000D) (42). EPO specifically induces differentiation of late erythrocytic progenitors into the recognizable erythrocytic compartment (44, Figure 3b). It also provokes an accelerated maturation of erythroblasts (45). In stress erythropoiesis, enhanced EPO activity causes skipping of terminal divisions, and therefore macrocytosis (45). In human cultures, P-BFU-E show little response to EPO, while M-BFU-E and CFU-E are characterized by a gradual increase of their EPO sensitivity (30,31, Figure 3b).

In the fetal period, EPO is derived largely or exclusively from the liver (46), possibly from Kupffer cells (47,48). Kidney EPO production is gradually activated in the perinatal phase (49), and represents the major component of the post-natal hormonal activity (50). Marrow macrophages in the center of erythroblastic islands (51) have received attention recently as a possible, additional source of EPO. No difference has so far been detected between fetal and adult EPO molecules (52,53).

T-lymphocytes and/or macrophages, irradiated or stimulated by lectins or antigens, release *in vitro* a variety of glycoprotein hormones termed 'hematopoietins' (see 17–22). One (or more) of these factors contains an *in vitro* burst-promoting activity (BPA or BPF) (34,54–57)*. A murine BPA of molecular weight $\sim$24,000D has been purified to apparent homogeneity, via a seven-step chromatography procedure (G. Wagemaker, personal communica-

---

*Also described as BEF, BFA, EPA, or EPF.

tion). BPA is clearly distinct from factors stimulating the formation of GM-colonies (CSFs) (57), although massive amounts of pure GM-CSF may in part mimic BPA (55). In cultures of murine and presumably human cells, BPA allows survival of P-BFU-E (56). It also modulates the cycling activity of these progenitors (57), as well as their differentiation to the M-BFU-E and the CFU-E stage (Figure 3b) (56,57,59). It may also stimulate CFU-E growth, particularly in conjunction with EPO (60,61). Although the *in vivo* role of BPA is still uncertain, it is generally conceded that, in the hematopoietic microenvironment, it may play a function similar to that *in vitro*.

Axelrad *et al.* (62) recently suggested that the cycling activity of murine P-BFU-E is also modulated by a protein inhibitor, controlled by the Fv-2 locus (determining susceptibility or resistance to Friend leukemia virus). Thus, BFU-E proliferation would be subject to both a positive and a negative control mechanism.

In long-term cultures of murine cells, regulation of CFU-S kinetics is apparently mediated by the balance between two opposing factors (63); the first one stimulates and the second one inhibits stem cell proliferation. Interestingly, Wagemaker has apparently separated a murine glycoprotein modulating CFU-S cycling, which is identical or closely related to BPA (57).

g. The erythrocytic system in the fetal stage. Human fetal liver contains erythrocytic progenitors generating colonies in semi-solid media (64,65). These progenitors have recently been characterized in methylcellulose cultures (33). Three classes (P-BFU-E, M-BFU-E, CFU-E) have been identified, on the basis of their differential clonogenic characteristics (i.e., colony morphology and number, time–growth curve, differential EPO, and BPA sensitivity, *in vitro* [^{3}H]thymidine suicide index). Differentiation of fetal erythrocytic progenitors (as well as of adult ones, see above) entails gradual amplification of their pool size, progressive decline of BPA response, and gradual enhancement of EPO sensitivity.

These findings are consistent with the concept (see 56) that fetal erythropiesis is largely modulated by EPO. It is also apparent that BPA may play a similar regulatory role in both adult and fetal life.

Marked differences, however, are observed between the features of corresponding fetal and adult erythrocytic progenitors (33). Thus;
1. Differentiation of the adult cells entails a gradual increase of their proliferative rate, while all fetal progenitors are characterized by maximal cycling activity (33). Interestingly, the doubling time of cells in fetal bursts (~19–21 hr, mean value) is distinctly lower than in adult ones (~30–33 hr), while intermediate values are observed in cord blood bursts (~25 hr) (Figure 4) (33). These observations suggest that ontogenic maturation of the erythron is associated with a progressive decline of

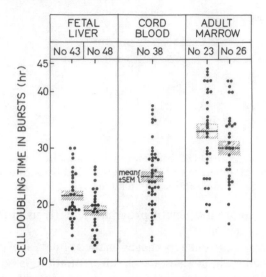

Figure 4. Doubling time (hr) of erythrocytic cells in bursts from fetal liver, cord blood and normal adult marrow. For further details see (33). $p < 0.01$ when comparing all groups. Reproduced with permission from (33)

proliferative activity of early and intermediate erythrocytic progenitors, as well as of cell doubling time in erythrocytic differentiation.

2. Adherent cells apparently play a key role in BPA production in adult marrow cultures (30), but not in fetal liver ones (33). In the adult, the T-lymphocyte–macrophage complex is apparently involved in hematopoietic hormone production (see above). In the fetus, the placenta may release large amounts of the hormonal modulators of early hematopoiesis (66).

3. The sensitivity to added EPO of fetal CFU-E and M-BFU-E is apparently higher than that of corresponding adult progenitors (33,67).

2. Molecular aspects (see 68,69).

Recent development of recombinant DNA technology has allowed the cloning of eukaryotic genes, thus permitting their purification and analysis. This breakthrough has been effectively coupled with introduction of;

1. Restriction endonuclease gene mapping by Southern blot hybridization.
2. Rapid DNA sequencing techniques.
3. *In vitro* gene transcription of cloned genes.
4. Methods for gene insertion into both normal and neoplastic cells (see 68,69).

It is thereby possible, for the first time, to probe the crucial relationship between gene structure and expression in eukaryotic cells. In particular, it now

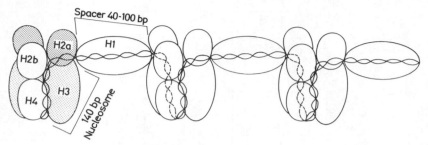

Figure 5. A schematic representation of chromatin structure, including nucleosomes and 'spacer' regions. Modified from (8) and reproduced by permission of Blackwell Scientific Publications Ltd

seems feasible to explore the genetic programs underlying hematopoietic and erythrocytic differentiation.

A detailed review of current hypotheses on the regulation of eukaryotic gene expression, particularly in hematopoietic differentiation, is beyond the scope of this chapter. It may be appropriate, however, to concisely analyze selected aspects of this area, which are relevant to the discussion of molecular mechanisms underlying the human Hb switch.

A crucial advance has been provided by studies on lymphocytic differentiation. In this regard, B-lymphocyte maturation is associated with multiple deletions and rearrangements of DNA sequences in immunoglobin genes. Particularly, the IgM → IgG (or → IgA) switch is associated with complete deletion of the gene coding for the invariant region of IgM (70,71). It cannot be excluded that similar genetic mechanisms, possibly of a more discrete nature, may contribute to modulate gene expression in hematopoietic and erythrocytic differentiation.

Chromatin structure obviously represents a key aspect. In this regard, chromatin is composed of repeated subunits termed nucleosomes (Figure 5) (72). Each of them consists of a protein core, formed by four pairs of histone molecules (H2a,H2b,H3,H4), wrapped by ~140 base pairs (bp) of DNA. Nucleosomes are separated by a 'spacer' region of ~40–100 bp associated with histone H1. Little is known, however, on putative protein modulators of DNA transcription. Indeed, our understanding of the control of DNA transcription is limited by insufficient knowledge of non-histone DNA-associated proteins.

Growing evidence suggests that rearrangements in chromatin structure (73), either localized (74,75) or of higher order (i.e., DNA supercoiling) (77), may represent key regulatory mechanisms of gene activation and repression. In all cases tested so far, active genes are indeed in an altered conformation, as indicated by their hypersensitivity to specific nucleases, particularly the pancreatic DNAase I (see 68,69). Additionally, it is apparent that nucleosomes may be either distributed at random or 'phased' in preferential, specific locations (78). Both hypotheses are supported by suggestive evidence, gathered from different experimental models. In this regard, the possibility that nucleosome phasing is related to regulation of gene expression and/or replication is under active investigation.

It is generally conceded that DNA modifications in eukaryotic cells largely take place in the course of DNA replication (S-phase). Thus, cell determination and maturation (i.e., activation of lineage-specific genes) is apparently linked to active proliferation. In higher eukaryotic cells, methylation is virtually the only post-synthetic modification of DNA (79), which may selectively affect either parental or daughter strand (80).* A growing body of evidence indicates that a low level of DNA methylation is present in active gene sequences, at least in a large number of cases (80–82). This correlation may indeed represent a general phenomenon (84). Particular genes (i.e., avian endogenous retroviral sequences in chicken cells, several X-linked human genes) are derepressed by experimentally-induced demethylation (84,85). This provides evidence for a cause–effect relationship between undermethylation and gene activation, at least in these particular models.

In conclusion, it is generally conceded that a key relationship may exist between gene activation, changes in chromatin structure and DNA undermethylation. The relationship, if any, between the latter two phenomena is still a matter of speculation.

II. CELLULAR ASPECTS OF THE Hb SWITCH

A. Pioneering studies

The perinatal Hb switch was initially interpreted in terms of a *biclonal hypothesis* (86). This concept postulated two clones of stem cells: a 'fetal' one, prevailingly committed to HbF synthesis, and an 'adult' one, programmed to exclusive HbA production. Emergence of the adult clone may underlie the progressive rise of HbA production in the fetal life and the rapid perinatal Hb switch. Adult F-cells might derive from a small pool of fetal stem elements, which escaped the perinatal Hb switch. The last concept, however, is in contrast with two series of observations, which indicate that A- and F-cells originate from a single clone of adult stem elements. In this regard;

1. Polycythemia vera and chronic myelogenous leukemia are admittedly clonal diseases of the stem cell (87): both are constantly associated with presence of F- and A-cells, usually in a normal ratio (88,89).

---

*DNA methylation in eukaryotic DNA occurs at the 5-position of C, mostly in 5'-CpG-3' dinucleotides. The degree of methylation is determined by specific restriction endonucleases, which recognize sequences containing CG depending or not upon C-methylation (see 81). Obviously, these enzymes do not allow the probe of CG sites occurring in sequences not recognized by these enzymes.

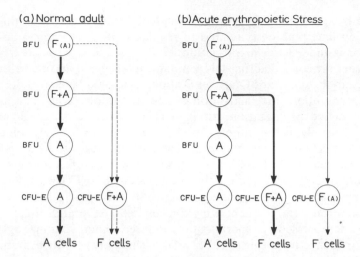

Figure 6. Model for genesis of F-cells by Stamatoyannopoulos and co-workers (92–94). The basic concept is that differentiation of erythrocytic progenitors is linked to gradual obliteration of their Hb F synthetic program (For further details see text). Reproduced by permission of Alan R. Liss, Inc. from (3)

2. Adult red blood cells (RBC) maintain in part some characteristics of fetal elements (i antigen, CAI level): these features are equally expressed in both F- and A-cells (90,91).

Further observations reviewed below are hardly compatible with the biclonal hypothesis; of particular significance is the continuous distribution of HbF and A synthesis in single cord blood bursts (Section II C).

A *monoclonal model* was proposed by Stamatoyannopoulos *et al.* (Figure 6), on the basis of pioneer studies on Hb synthesis in erythrocytic colonies grown in semisolid cultures (92,93). These authors evaluated;

1. *Globin chains synthesis* in the whole erythrocytic population in a culture dish, by means of carboxymethylcellulose chromatography (CMC);
2. Presence of HbF and/or A in single erythrocytic bursts, by means of *immunofluorescence techniques*.

The relative rates of HbF and A synthesis in cultures of fetal liver or cord blood were comparable to corresponding *in vivo* values. On the other hand, γ-chain synthesis in adult-derived cells ($\sim$10–15%) was markedly enhanced over *in vivo* levels ($<$1%). This increase was interpreted in terms of *in vitro* recruitment of fetal-type BFU-E, endowed with a significant program for HbF synthesis. In this regard, immunofluorescence studies apparently indicated that adult-derived bursts contain either HbA + F (F[+] clones), or HbA alone (F[−] clones). More important, F[+] bursts may consist of both F[+] and F[−] subcolonies. These data were interpreted to imply that three types of BFU-E exist;

1. The fetal progenitor, giving rise to fully F^+ bursts.
2. The intermediate one, producing both F^+ and F^- subcolonies.
3. The adult one, generating strictly F^- colonies. (Section II B gives a critical appraisal of these immunofluorescence results.)

It was further postulated that the three types of BFU-E may represent sequential stages of differentiation in the erythrocytic pathway, thus leading to an attractive model for the Hb switch (Figure 6). Accordingly, the stage of differentiation of erythrocytic progenitors is inversely correlated to the expression of HbF in their progeny. In particular, BFU-E of 'fetal' type, committed to predominantly HbF synthesis, would progress rapidly to the CFU-E stage (i.e., skipping the multi-step differentiation of adult BFU-E). The fetal erythroblastic progeny would thus synthesize predominantly HbF. BFU-E of 'adult' type, similarly bipotent for both HbF and A synthesis, would preferentially differentiate *via* a multi-stage process, admittedly linked to progressive obliteration of their HbF synthetic program. Most adult CFU-E would derive from these BFU-E, and be deprived of the program for HbF production; they may give rise to A cells. In contrast, a minority of 'adult' CFU-E would be subject to an asymmetric division. Accordingly, one of the two daughter cells would skip, in part, the adult-type, multi-stage differentiation. The resulting CFU-E would hence maintain the program for some HbF synthesis, thus giving rise to F-cells. In adult stress erythropoiesis, the 'fetal-type' differentiation might become prevalent, thus leading to expansion of the F-cell pool.

Experimental analysis of this complex model was initially hampered by:
1. Incomplete characterization of fetal and adult erythrocytic progenitors.
2. Lack of analysis of globin chain synthesis in single erythrocytic bursts.

Both limitations were gradually overcome. Studies were thus performed to identify and characterize fetal progenitors (33), as compared to adult ones (30) (Section I B). More important, the Italian group developed a technique to analyze ε-, $^G\gamma$, $^A\gamma$- and β-chain production in single erythrocytic bursts, by means of a sensitive isoelectric focusing (IEF) technique (29,95). IEF analysis has been extensively employed by Ogawa *et al.* (96,97), and more recently by Stamatoyannopoulos' group (90). On the other hand, the HbA and F content in single erythrocytic colonies may be evaluated by radioimmunoassay (99,100). These novel techniques have allowed us to probe the Hb synthesis program in erythrocytic progenitors, *via* assay of globin chain production (or content) in their clonal progeny. On this basis, studies were focused on Hb synthesis in single erythrocytic colonies at different stages of development or differentiation. A comparative review of these results is rendered uneasy, due to;
1. The variety of culture methods employed in different laboratories, and even in the same one.
2. The still incomplete understanding of mechanisms regulating erythrocytic kinetics *in vitro* and *in vivo* (see Section I B and Chapter 2).

3. Limitations inherent in different methods for assay of globin chain synthesis (or content).

Nevertheless, a critical review of these studies seems now feasible, and may lead to unifying concepts on the regulation of Hb synthesis, *in vitro* and by extrapolation *in vivo*.

B. The perinatal Hb switch

1. The Hb synthesis program in erythrocytic progenitors during development

Comprehensive studies were carried out by the Italian group to evaluate globin chain production in single bursts from fetal liver, cord blood and adult blood or marrow (29,95,101–108). All colonies were grown in standardized culture conditions. More important, they were analyzed at an advanced hemoglobinization stage, in order to avoid the 'maturation bias' (see Section II C). Ogawa *et al* performed, in parallel, a similar series of studies (96,97,109). These investigators, however, evaluated not only mature but also immature colonies.

Well-hemoglobinized *fetal-derived bursts* show a homogenous synthetic pattern, which is always characterized by low β-globin production (~5–20% of non-α synthesis) (102). Similar results have been reported by the Seattle group (98).

The synthetic pattern in mature *cord blood-derived* bursts is highly heterogenous (95). Indeed, γ/β ratios are spread over a wide, continuous spectrum, ranging from 'fetal' to adult values, and they are correlated directly with the $^G\gamma/^A\gamma$ quotients (Figure 7). The continuous distribution of γ/β synthetic values suggests that a single clone of BFU-E is gradually reprogrammed in the perinatal phase. Conversely, apparent lack of a bi- or tri-modal distribution strongly militates against a bi- or tri-clonal hypothesis. Furthermore, the direct correlation between γ/β and $^G\gamma/^A\gamma$ synthetic ratios indicates that both γ → β and $^G\gamma$ → $^A\gamma$ switches occur simultaneously within each cord blood clone.

These results have been extensively confirmed, both *in vitro* (97,110) and *in vivo* (111). In particular, Vedvick *et al.* (111) showed a gradual and parallel rise of the ratio of γ/β and $^G\gamma/^A\gamma$ content in umbilical RBC populations of increasing age. The different *in vivo* results obtained by Alter (112), suggesting an asynchrony between γ → β and $^G\gamma$ → $^A\gamma$ switches, may derive from analysis of whole blood rather than fractionated RBC.

Of particular interest is that all well-hemoglobinized *adult-derived bursts* produce a relatively small, fairly homogenous amount of γ-chain (i.e., ~5–15% of non-α synthesis) (101)*. Furthermore, all subcolonies from adult

---

*The presence of HbF in all colonies was formally demonstrated by a two-step procedure, including (a) separation of HbF by preparative IEF, (b) analysis of the HbF band by analytical IEF or CMC. In both cases the HbF band showed presence of only α- and γ-chains, in a 1 : 1 ratio.

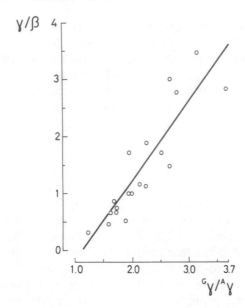

Figure 7. γ/β vs ^{G}γ/^{A}γ synthetic ratios in individual well-hemoglobinized bursts from two cord blood samples. Reproduced by permission of Alan R. Liss. Inc. from (104)

bursts show detectable γ-synthesis. The observed values from subcolonies (~5–45%) were more variable than those of whole bursts, due to the heterogenous hemoglobinization of the analyzed subcolonies ('maturation bias', see Section II C). These results were corroborated by immunofluorescence studies, which indicated the presence of at least some F$^+$ erythroblasts in all well-hemoglobinized bursts and subcolonies.

These observations are in line with those reported by Kidoguchi *et al*. (109). Additionally, Dover and Ogawa (113) evaluted the HbF content in individual cells within adult colonies by a microdensitometric immunodiffusion assay: all bursts and their subcolonies contained a significant number of F$^+$ elements. Stamatoyannopoulos and co-workers also showed the presence of at least some HbF in virtually all adult bursts, when they employed a sensitive HbF assay based on IEF (98,110) or a radioimmune method (101). Both groups observed that adult bursts are characterized by a heterogenous F$^+$ cell number (5–95%) or relative HbF content (0–60%). This heterogeneity is not in contrast with the homogenous pattern reported by the Italian group (101). Indeed, the latter group analyzed exclusively well-hemoglobinized bursts, whereas the former group considered both immature and mature ones. If both types of colonies are analyzed, all agree that the pattern of HbF synthesis or content is highly heterogenous (100,104,109)*.

*In rare adult individuals, the relative γ-synthesis in *well-hemoglobinized* bursts is fairly heterogenous (~5–40%) (101). This unusual pattern is observed essentially in borderline cases between normal adults and patients with hereditary persistence of HbF (HPFH) of heterocellular type (Section IID).

It must also be emphasized that adult mixed colonies, generated by myelocytic stem cells, almost always contain significant levels of HbF (99).

These results conclusively show that all adult bursts and mixed colonies synthesize some HbF. Thereby, doubt is cast on the immunofluorescence studies by the Seattle group, who reported presence of both F^+ and F^- adult bursts, as well as of F^- subcolonies within F^+ bursts (92–94). In this regard, observations of 'F^-' bursts and subcolonies may conceivably be attributed to inadequate sensitivity of the immunofluorescence assay, and/or evaluation of not only mature colonies and subcolonies, but also of immature ones with a very low HbF content. Indeed, erythrocytic cultures are characterized by *asynchronous* hemoglobinization of different bursts in each plate and different subcolonies within each burst (i.e., mature and immature bursts usually coexist in the same plate, and red or pale subcolonies are often simultaneously present in a single burst). It follows that bursts or subcolonies composed essentially of mature erythroblasts (with elevated Hb content) may be scored by immunofluorescence as HbA^+ and F^+. However, bursts or subcolonies containing essentially immature erythroblasts (with low Hb content) might be simultaneously scored as HbA^+ and F^-. This sensitivity bias is rendered more severe if the *in vitro* maturation of erythroblasts is inadequate (i.e., the Hb content/cell is distinctly lower than *in vivo*). It is indeed remarkable that immunofluorescence observations of adult bursts and subcolonies at an advanced stage of hemoglobinization always showed the presence of at least some F^+ cells (101).

More recently, a random distribution of HbF in adult subcolonies was apparently documented by immunofluorescence analysis (94). On the basis of these results, a *stochastic model* was postulated (94). The fetal-type BFU-E would skip the multi-stage differentiation, linked to obliteration of its HbF synthetic program, in a stochastic way. The possibility of this event would be elevated in the fetal age, fairly low in adult stress erythropoiesis, and very low in normal adults. Here again, the possibility cannot be excluded that the stochastic results are due to a random distribution of immature subcolonies in adult bursts.

The uncertainties on the immunofluorescence observations by the Seattle group necessarily reflect on their model (Figure 6) with which it is difficult to reconcile numerous observations. Thus;

1. Adult BFU-E committed only to HbA ($+A_2$) synthesis apparently do not exist, as outlined above.
2. A significant prediction of the model is that differentiation of adult progenitors (P-BFU-E $\rightarrow$ M-BFU-E $\rightarrow$ CFU-E) should be associated with progressive obliteration of their program for HbF synthesis. In this regard, globin chain synthesis was comparatively analyzed in colonies deriving from adult P-BFU-E, M-BFU-E, or 'early-type' CFU-E (103,104). All erythrocytic colonies were grown in the same standardized

cultures, and picked up for labeling at a similar hemoglobinization stage. These studies suggested that, under uniform *in vitro* conditions, the Hb synthesis program remains largely unmodified in the differentiation of adult progenitors. Similarly, no striking modification in the program is observed in the differentiation of corresponding fetal precursors (103).

3. The model also predicts that relative γ-chain synthesis or content should be elevated in adult bursts compared to that in their subcolonies. This postulate, however, conflicts with evidence from two separate studies (101,113).

4. Rowley *et al* indicated that γ-globin gene expression in bursts is not modified by stimulation of growth of P-BFU-E, of both fetal and adult type (114).

In conclusion, studies carried out so far are compatible with the existence of a single clone of BFU-E, and apparently of myelocytic stem cells, which is bipotential for HbF and A synthesis. This clone, endowed with a prevailing HbF program in fetal life, undergoes reprogramming in the perinatal phase, and becomes committed mainly to HbA ($+A_2$) synthesis in the post-natal period. However, all adult BFU-E and stem cells maintain the program for some HbF synthesis (see below).

Under homogenous *in vitro* conditions, differentiation of adult erythrocytic progenitors (P-BFU-E → M-BFU-E → early CFU-E) is not apparently linked with a marked decrease of their HbF synthetic program. A significant decline may (33,115) or may not (33) occur at the level of the late-type CFU-E, which presumably corresponds to the pro-erythroblast.

2. The mechanism(s) underlying the perinatal Hb switch

The results mentioned above do not allow the identification of the perinatal factor(s) modulating the Hb synthesis program in stem cells and BFU-E. Obviously, it is not possible to exclude mechanism(s) of 'extrinsic' type, i.e., long-range hormonal influences or cell–cell interactions in the erythrocytic microenvironment, etc. On the other hand, it seems crucial to elucidate the possible role of factor(s) 'intrinsic' to stem cells and BFU-E. These may include a 'developmental clock' (i.e., reprogramming of BFU-E after a critical number of mitosis) and/or irreversible changes of BFU-E kinetics in the perinatal phase. In any case, the mechanism(s) underlying the perinatal switch is time-programmed; it occurs at about nine months after conception, but not necessarily in the perinatal phase (5). In premature newborns, it takes place after birth, in postmature ones it has already largely occurred.

An extrinsic mechanism has been suggested by Testa and co-workers (116–118). In this regard, cord blood-derived bursts stimulated by 'adult BPA' showed a more elevated β-globin synthesis than those grown in the presence of 'neonatal BPA'*. Hypothetically, a time programmed change of BPA, from a 'fetal' to an 'adult' hormone(s), may underlie the perinatal Hb switch. These intriguing observations, however, are clouded by uncertainties. Thus, the heterogeneity of the globin synthesis pattern in cord blood-derived bursts obscures the significance of the relatively small difference observed between cultures supplemented with neonatal vs adult BPA. Furthermore, the possibility has not been rigorously excluded that bursts from 'adult BPA' cultures were more mature that those from 'neonatal BPA' dishes (maturation bias, Section II C). Further studies are required to clarify these aspects.

Of interest are transplantation studies in the sheep. In the original experiment (119), hematopoietic cells from the fetus were induced to produce adult Hb following transplantation and engraftment in an irradiated adult recipient, unmatched with the donor. Donor and recipient Hb could be differentiated on the basis of their polymorphism at the β-globin locus. The experiment confirmed that fetal stem cells are bipotential for fetal and adult Hb synthesis, thus in line with the monoclonal model suggested above. However, it does not clarify the mechanism(s) mediating reprogramming of the fetal stem cells after transplantation. This may be conceivably attributed to 'extrinsic' factor(s) operating in the adult recipient microenvironment. 'Intrinsic' mechanisms cannot, however, be excluded. Transplanted fetal stem cells conceivably undergo intensive proliferation: this may accelerate their 'developmental clock'. Furthermore, preliminary studies by Wood and Bunch (120) indicate that the post-transplantation Hb switch is not as rapid as previously indicated, thus rendering more uncertain the interpretation of this phenomenon.

Adult erythrocytic progenitor cells, transplanted into fetuses, are never induced to revert to the fetal Hb synthesis program (121). This confirms that the perinatal Hb switch is at least in part irreversible, as indicated by studies in vitro (see above).

Mechanisms underlying the Hb switch may be explored in long-term BFU-E cultures (42), whereby progenitors of fetal, neonatal, or adult type are sampled and cloned at sequential times. However, the long-term survival of human BFU-E is far from satisfactory (see 22). It follows that modifications of the Hb synthetic program in cultured BFU-E may be attributed to their in vitro selection, rather than reprogramming in culture. No striking difference has been reported in preliminary studies on cord blood and adult BFU-E (98,108). Fetal liver experiments occasionally showed an in vitro acceleration of the fetal→adult switch (98). These results, however, are of dubious significance so far, in view of the above remarks.

---

*The crude BPA preparation was medium conditioned by adult or cord blood leucocytes, or by a T-leukemia cell line.

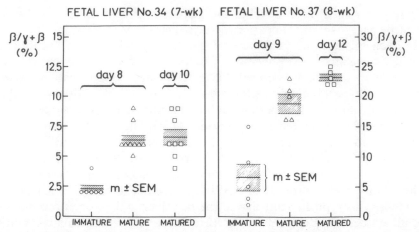

Figure 8. Relative synthesis of β-globin chains, evaluated by IEF, in single fetal liver bursts at different stages of maturation: two representative experiments are shown here. The colonies picked up at day 8 (left panel) or 9 (right panel) were either 'immature' or 'mature'; 'matured' colonies were identified as immature on days 8 and 9, and then allowed to mature in the culture dish until day 10 or 12 respectively. Mean ± s.e.m. values are indicated. $p < 0.01$ when comparing the 'mature' or 'matured' group with the 'immature' one. Modified from (102) by permission of Academic Press, Inc.

C. The asynchrony of HbF and A synthesis in erythroblastic differentiation

In suspension cultures of fetal liver cells, γ- and β-synthesis peak, respectively, at earlier or later times (122). The asynchrony has been confirmed in pooled bursts from cord and adult blood (123). The same phenomenon was independently observed by the Italian group in single bursts from fetal liver, cord blood, normal adult blood, or marrow (102,104,105). More important, the possibility was excluded that the early γ-peak in culture simply reflects an experimental artefact (i.e., preferential expression in early culture phases of erythrocytic clones endowed with greater capacity for γ-chain synthesis) (102,104). Indeed, all erythrocytic clones showed an early γ- and a late β-synthetic peak, irrespective of their proliferation velocity (Figure 8).

These studies have been extensively confirmed *in vitro* (111), and, more important, *in vivo* (124). In normal adults, reticulocytes still show γ-chain synthesis, while production has apparently stopped in late F-normoblasts (124). In adult stress erythropoiesis (Section II E), however, HbF synthesis occurs even in reticulocytes (124).

The γ-/β-mRNA synthetic ratio is more elevated in immature than mature adult bursts (125). This suggests that the asynchrony of HbF and A production is due to a mechanism acting at the transcriptional level.

This 'maturation phenomenon' seems therefore of physiological significance in all stages of development. More important, it may represent the experimental basis for a model of the genesis of F-cells (Section II D), and reconcile a large series of apparently contradictory results (Section II D).

In neonatal (95) and adult-derived bursts (97), γ/β and $^G\gamma/^A\gamma$ ratios, are directly correlated. As previously mentioned, this phenomenon is best expressed in cord blood-derived colonies (Figure 7). Correlation between γ/β and $^G\gamma/^A\gamma$ synthetic ratios may also be observed in adult erythroblastic maturation, particularly in peripheral blood cultures, if very 'immature' bursts are compared with markedly 'red' colonies (104). The early maturation phase, characterized by peak γ-gene expression, is apparently associated with a more elevated $^G\gamma/^A\gamma$ synthetic ratio. The late one is characterized by peak β-chain production and a lower $^G\gamma/^A\gamma$ quotient. This phenomenon is best expressed in hereditary persistence of HbF (HPFH), heterocellular type (Figures 9 and 10) (104). This is presumably due to the fact that, in this condition, the more prominent decline of γ/β ratio in erythroblastic maturation entails a marked decrease of the $^G\gamma/^A\gamma$ quotient. Conversely, if the drop of γ/β values is only small, the corresponding reduction of $^G\gamma/^A\gamma$ ratio is perhaps too fine to be detected by current methods (110).

In summary, the observations available so far indicate that the perinatal $\gamma \rightarrow \beta$ (and also apparently $^G\gamma \rightarrow {}^A\gamma$) switch is in part recapitulated during adult erythroblastic maturation. This suggests that a similar mechanism(s) may underlie this phenomenon in ontogeny and cytogeny (Section II C).

1. The 'maturation bias': a source of apparently contradictory results

The asynchrony of HbF and A synthesis in erythroblastic maturation should always be considered when interpreting studies on Hb synthesis. Differential modulation of early γ- and/or late β-production may reconcile apparent discrepancies on *in vitro* globin chain production reported by different laboratories. The asynchrony may similarly explain the action of various agents on Hb synthesis. As an example, EPO induces an elevation of relative β-globin production in adult cultures (123), *via* acceleration of erythroblast maturation. If fully mature bursts are analyzed, this EPO effect is no longer seen (123).

D. A cellular model for the Hb switch (Figure 9A,B)

1. Ontogenic development (Figure 9A)

As mentioned above, it is apparent that, in fetal life, a single clone of stem cells and BFU-E is programmed for HbF plus some A synthesis. The clone is gradually reprogrammed in the perinatal period, thus leading to an adult population of stem cells and BFU-E. These are committed prevailingly to HbA ($+A_2$) production, but always contain a program for HbF synthesis.

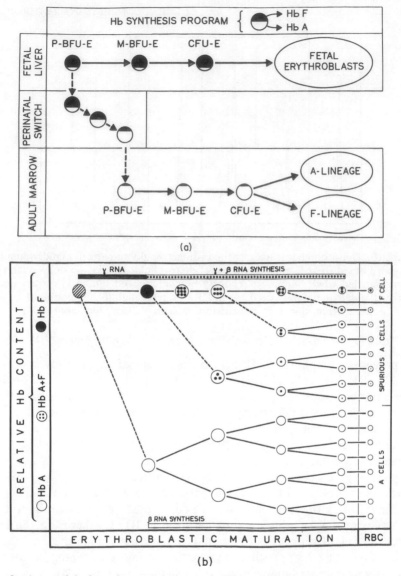

Figure 9. A model for the regulation of Hb synthesis in development and differentiation. This model has been presented in part (104). (a) Hb synthesis program in erythrocytic progenitors in different ontogenic stages (for further details see text). (b) A cellular model for the genesis of F-cells in normal adult erythropoiesis, indicating the relative content of Hb A and F in erythrocytic cells deriving from a very early normoblast (pronormoblast, 'late' CFU-E). The heterogeneity of HbF distribution is essentially explained in terms of hypothetical asymmetric divisions (AD) of erythroblasts, leading to blockade of γ RNA synthesis in one of the two daughter cells (a molecular model for AD is shown in Figure 16a). The span of RNA synthesis is presented for both F-lineages (top) and A-lineages (bottom). The level of RNA synthetic activity is obviously not considered. It is assumed that γ RNA synthesis in F-normoblasts may gradually decrease, perhaps due to mechanisms detailed in Figure 16b Reproduced by permission of Alan R. Liss, Inc.

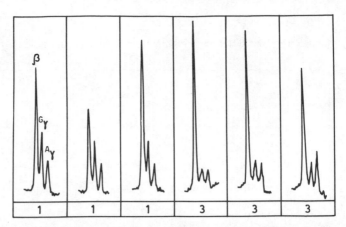

Figure 10. Densitometric tracing of the radioactive globin pattern in individual bursts from cord blood BFU-E of a patient with heterocellular HPFH. Colonies were picked up and labeled when 'immature' (poorly hemoglobinized, grade 1) or 'mature' and 'matured' (well hemoglobinized, grade 3). A representative experiment is shown here. Reproduced by permission of Alan R. Liss, Inc. from (104)

2. Adult erythroblastic differentiation: genesis of F-cells (Figure 9B)

As previously emphasized, HbF in normal adults is apparently confined to <8% of RBC (F-cells) (13,14). Any model for Hb synthesis must obviously cope with these findings.

The mechanism(s) generating F-cells may act at; 1. The progenitor and/or 2. The erythroblastic level.

1. As discussed above, the hypothesis has been entertained (92–94), that, in the differentiation of adult BFU-E, asymmetric divisions may occur, thus generating CFU-E programmed for synthesis of either only HbA or HbA+F. These CFU-E would give rise to A- or F-cells respectively (Figure 6). Criticisms may be raised against the immunofluorescence studies leading to this concept (Section II B). Furthermore, numerous results fail to support it (Section II B). In particular, the Hb synthetic program does not decline markedly during differentiation of adult progenitors under homogenous culture conditions (103,104).

2. Baglioni suggested that HbF synthesis might be related to the stage of *erythroblastic maturation* (126). This hypothesis has found recent support in new experimental results. As mentioned above, a wave of γ-globin production peaks early during adult erythroblastic differentiation. It may be postulated that the γ-synthetic phase is differentially modulated in various erythrocytic clones, thus leading to the heterogenous HbF content in RBC (A- vs F-cells). This mechanism predicts that a very small, so far unmeasurable amount of HbF is present even in A-cells.

Unfortunately, it is not known whether A-cells are strictly F$^-$. They may contain miniscule, currently unmeasurable amounts of HbF. At least a majority of A-cells may be F$^-$, in that the HbF content in RBC can be accounted for solely by the amount of HbF in F-cells (127). On the other hand, A-cells containing HbF may also exist, since the F-cell distribution is not normal, but skewed (128). This may suggest that HbF in some A-cells is lower than the threshold limit of detection of immunofluorescence assays.

If A-cells are not only truly F$^-$ but also in part really F$^+$, emergence of F- vs A-lineage may be explained in terms of a model (104) which includes not only modulation of early γ- and late β-synthesis, but also asymmetric divisions (AD) in early erythroblastic maturation (Figure 9). Each AD would lead to two daughter cells, endowed or not with the capacity for γ-mRNA synthesis, thus leading respectively to the F- vs A-lineage. AD might also occur at later maturation stages in the F-lineage, thus generating 'spurious' A-cells (i.e., A-cells containing miniscule, unmeasurable amounts of HbF). A molecular model for the AD in erythroblastic maturation is proposed below (Section III) (108). An additional factor modulating the HbF level in adult RBC may be represented by skipping of terminal divisions (45). This would clearly dampen the impact of the late β-synthetic phase, thus leading to a moderate rise of the relative HbF content in RBC. Skipping of terminal divisions is typically observed in stress erythropoiesis (45); it is apparent therefore that this mechanism is mainly operative in this condition, as discussed below.

3. Modulation of γ-synthesis in adult erythroblasts

The mechanism modulating the early γ-phase (and/or the hypothetical AD) is still unknown. Under strictly homogenous *in vitro* conditions, the Hb synthesis program remains substantially unmodified in the differentiation of erythrocytic progenitors (Section IIB). On the other hand, if culture conditions are heterogenous, the program may be modulated. In this regard, BFU-E kinetics are largely controlled by BPA. It has been claimed that *in vitro* addition of BPA induces an enhanced γ-chain synthesis in adult-derived bursts. These studies, however, are not conclusive, in that the analysis was not carried out on colonies of corresponding hemoglobinization stage. The Italian group showed, in a retrospective analysis, that when adult-derived bursts were grown in cultures supplemented by different FCS batches, either rich or poor in BPA, single, well-hemoglobinized bursts grown in BPA-rich cultures showed a higher level of relative γ-synthesis (~5–15%) than those in BPA-poor plates (~1–2%) (Figure 11). More important, the latter values are close to those normally observed *in vivo*. Altogether, results available so far are compatible with the concept that BPA levels in the adult may at least contribute to the modulation of *in vivo* levels of γ-synthesis, *via* mechanisms mentioned above. Further studies are obviously required to elucidate these crucial aspects.

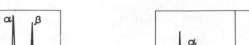

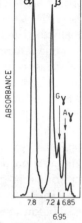

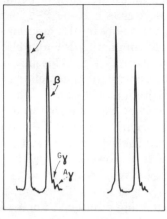

Figure 11. Densitometric tracing of the radioactive globin pattern from single normal adult blood bursts, grown in (a) BPA-rich or (b) BPA-poor FCS and labeled when well-hemoglobinized. Reproduced with permission from *Blood*, **53**, 977–986 (1979)

E. Adult stress erythropoiesis and heterocellular HPFH

A rise of HbF production in the adult is routinely observed in acute erythrocytic expansion (130–132). It is apparent, however, that the degree of this elevation varies considerably among different individuals (133). The variability is amplified in baboons. These primates, challenged with acute hemolytic anemia, show enhanced HbF synthesis, in the range from ~1–2% in low responders and up to 60% in high-responders (134–136)*. The variability in humans has been attributed to a genetic polymorphism of the locus regulating the HbF response to erythrocytic stress in the adult age (137). This locus is apparently linked to the β-gene complex (137).

Considerable light on these aspects has been shed by evaluation of HbA and F in single erythrocytic cells. Elevation of HbF in acute erythrocytic expansion is consistently mediated *via* an increase of the number of F-cells, while the HbF content/cell does not necesarily change (131). Similarly, the rise of γ-synthesis in adult bursts may be attributed to a six- to 50-fold rise in F-cell number, rather than to the discrete elevation of the relative HbF content/cell (113).

It is apparent, therefore, that the rise of HbF production in acute stress erythropoiesis is essentially mediated *via* an amplification of the pool of F-cells. Indeed, a correlation between HbF levels and F-cell number has been

---

*An increase of HbF production may or may not be observed in other miscellaneous conditions, including normal pregnancy, hydatiform mole, various types of leukemia, thyrotoxicosis, etc. (see 8).

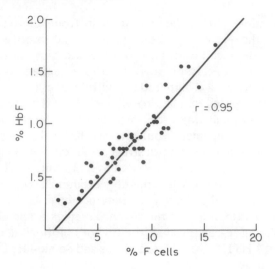

Figure 12. The correlation between %HbF and %F-cells in adult peripheral blood

documented in normal adults (Figure 12) as well as in hereditary or acquired elevations of HbF (14,129). In both humans (137) and baboons (135), a significant correlation exists between the F-cell level in normal, non-anemic parents and the F-cell expansion induced by erythrocytic stress in their offspring (i.e., sickle cell anemia subjects and phenylhydrazine-treated baboons). It may be suggested therefore that the F-cell response in anemia is controlled by the genetic locus regulating the F-cell number in normal conditions (137).

In terms of the model postulated above, an amplification of the F-cell pool can be simply explained in terms of a blockade of the hypothetical AD in erythroblastic maturation (Figure 9B). Alternatively or additionally, enhancement of the early γ-synthesis in numerous F-clones may be postulated. Skipping of terminal divisions may conceivably contribute to enhance the HbF content in RBC.

These observations should be correlated with results in heterocellular HPFH. This condition is characterized by elevation of HbF synthesis due to expansion of the F-cell pool in the peripheral blood (138). The magnitude of this amplification is low in 'Swiss', and more pronounced in 'British' type (138). The latter one is characterized by 50% or 100% F-cells in hetero- or homozygotes respectively (138). In heterozygous HPFH, the rise of HbF content may be accounted for mainly or exclusively by a rise of F-cells (138). If HPFH is associated with mild stress erythropoiesis, i.e., heterozygous β-thalassemia (139), recovery from sideropenic anemia (132), pregnancy (140), the relative HbF content shows a further, marked increase. Once again, this elevation is mainly due to a rise of F-cell number (139).

In vitro observations (104) indicate that bursts from heterozygotes show an enhancement of the early γ-synthetic phase in erythroblastic maturation (Figure 9), i.e., a deranged transition into the late β-production stage. This phenomenon may be conceivably attributed to an enhanced number of F^+ cells within HPFH bursts, as compared to control values (113).

It is tentatively suggested that heterocellular HPFH is caused by a deranged function of the locus regulating F-cell production, in both normal and stress erythropoiesis. The derangement would elevate the level of F-cell number over control levels, in both steady-state and stress condition, *via* enhancement of the erythroblastic mechanisms mentioned above. In line with this unifying concept, gross DNA alterations, and possibly even smaller or point mutations, are not present in the γδβ domain in heterocellular HPFH (Section IIB; 139,141). It is also intriguing that the β-gene complex is apparently linked to the locus regulating F-cell production in both normal adults (137) and heterocellular HPFH (139,141,142; see above and Section III B).

F. Disorders of Hb synthesis

The molecular pathology of these disorders is dealt with in Section III B. From the cellular viewpoint, β-thalassemia syndromes are characterized by marrow selection of erythrocytic clones endowed with a more balanced α/non-α ratio (8). Selection mechanisms may also explain otherwise paradoxic phenomena. In homozygous $(\delta\beta)^\circ$-thalassemia, the $^{G}\gamma/^{A}\gamma$ synthetic ratio is more elevated in red than in pale colonies (33), thus in exact opposition with the normal pattern (see above). This apparent paradox may be due to *in vitro* selection of erythrocytic clones endowed with a more elevated capacity for γ-synthesis, a higher $^{G}\gamma/^{A}\gamma$ ratio, and a more balanced α/non-α synthetic quotient. Similarly, homozygous β-thalassemias show a more elevated $^{G}\gamma/^{A}\gamma$ ratio in peripheral blood than in marrow (143), thus in line with the *in vitro* observations.

III. MOLECULAR ASPECTS OF THE Hb SWITCH

A. Structure and function of globin genes

Human globin genes are organized in two different clusters: the α-like genes, duplicated in $5'\text{-}\zeta_2\text{-}\zeta_1\text{-}\alpha_2\text{-}\alpha_1\text{-}3'$ sequence in chromosome 16, and the β-like ones, clustered $5'\text{-}\varepsilon\text{-}^{G}\gamma\text{-}^{A}\gamma\text{-}\delta\text{-}\beta\text{-}3'$ in the short arm of chromosome 11 (Figure 13; 9). In both cases globin genes are arranged $5' \rightarrow 3'$ in the order of their expression during development. This structure/function relationship is also observed in all other mammalian species studies so far, as well as in the duck (see 144).

The complete nucleotide sequence of the five β-like globin genes and their flanking regions has been determined (145). The full sequence of α_2 gene has

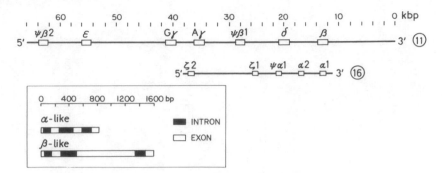

Figure 13. Organization and fine structure of α- and β-like globin genes. The letter ψ denotes pseudogenes

also been established (146). The 'canonical' structure of globin genes is detailed in Figure 13.

A comparison between human and other mammalian globin genes revealed sequence homologies in their 5' flanking regions (9,145). These include:

1. The ATA box (at 29–30 base pairs upstream from Cap site), which probably binds RNA polymerase and initiates transcription.
2. The CCAAT box (70–78 nucleotides upstream from Cap site), the function of which is more uncertain.

In this regard, the human δ-globin gene differs from other β-like genes in regard to both distance between CCAAT and ATA boxes and presence of a C rather than a T in the CCAAT sequence. These differences may relate to the fact that the gene is less efficiently transcribed than other β-like genes, *in vitro* as well as *in vivo*.

Both α- and β-like clusters contain intergenic sequences termed pseudogenes (Figure 13) (9, 147). These display a significant homology to corresponding functional genes. However, they bear mutations in the promoter, splice, or coding sequences, preventing their expression. Each pseudogene might be associated with the gene(s) activated in a particular ontogenic period. Accordingly, pseudogenes may perhaps play key regulatory role(s) (i.e., contribute to establish functional chromatin 'domains', or serve as alternative sites for binding of modulators of gene transcription).

Analysis of intergenic domains revealed the presence of six short repeated sequences, located both 5' to the ε gene and in the flanking regions of $^{G}\gamma^{A}\gamma$ and δβ genes (Figure 14; 9,149). They are members of the 'Alu' family of repeated sequences, which incorporate a site recognized by the restriction endonuclease, Alu I. Alu sequences are reiterated approximately 3×10^5 times in the human genome (150), and also show homology with an abundant class of small nuclear RNAs (151). Interestingly, they contain a sequence homologous to that found near the replication origin of SV40, polyoma, and BK DNA tumor virus (152). Although the functional significance of these repetitive elements

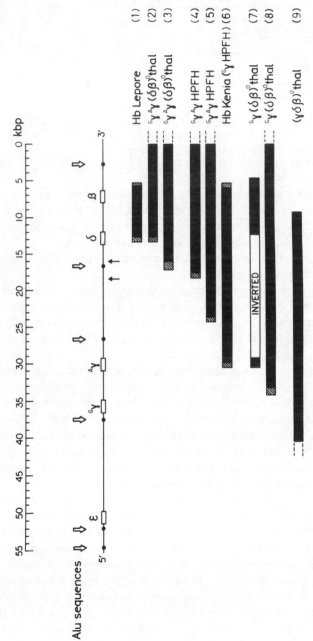

Figure 14. Deletions in various types of disorders of hemoglobin synthesis. Shaded portion in bars represent uncertain deletion areas. Location of Alu sequences is indicated by clear arrow (⇨). The area hypothetically involved in modulation of γ → β perinatal switch (see text) is delimited by black arrows (↑). Reprinted by permission from *Nature*, **291**, 39–44. Copyright © 1981 Macmillan Journals Ltd

in eukaryotic genomes is speculative, they are presently under scrutiny for their hypothetical role in replication of globin genes and control of their expression (see below).

The molecular events underlying the biosynthesis of human globin chains are similar to those of other mammalian proteins (153). They involve essentially:

1. Transcription of structural genes to nuclear RNA precursors.
2. Processing of nuclear RNA to mature mRNA (including splicing of intervening sequences, 'capping', poly-A addition).
3. Cytoplasmic mRNA translation.

It seems established that the basic mechanism(s) controlling globin gene expression operates at the level of DNA transcription. RNA processing and translation play a relatively minor regulatory role, which is essentially restricted to fine-tuning of the α/non-α synthetic balance.

The regulation of human globin gene expression is still poorly understood. Evidence thereon has been largely provided by analysis of patients with deletions in the β-like gene complex, and studies on chromatin structure and methylation in chicken embryo (see below). Both approaches have obvious limitations. The deletions involve large DNA regions, and may obviously affect gene expression *via* different mechanism(s). They provide, therefore, circumstantial rather than direct evidence on regulatory mechanisms of globin gene expression. Nevertheless, the observations reported so far fall neatly into place to suggest, but not prove, the presence of a regulatory locus in the $^A\gamma\,\delta$ intergenic region. On the other hand, any extrapolation from chickens to humans should obviously be considered with caution. However, an impressive series of experimental results suggest that alterations of chromatin conformation and gene undermethylation play a key role to mediate activation of globin genes in the ontogeny of chicken, and perhaps, by extrapolation, of humans as well.

The above remarks emphasize the need for a novel, direct experimental approach, such as microinjection into individual cells (154) of various human DNA fragments, selected to probe regulatory mechanisms of globin gene expression. More generally, it may be conceded that insight into mechanisms regulating eukaryotic gene transcription will largely derive from genetic transformation and *in vitro* transcription experiments.

B. Molecular pathology of the Hb switch: selected aspects of thalassemic syndrome*

The hereditary disorders associated with abnormal expression of the non-α gene cluster may be conveniently classified into three groups (138):

---

*The disorders of α-globin expression are not discussed here, since they do not seem relevant to the $\gamma \to \beta$ perinatal switch.

1. β-thalassemias.
2. δβ-thalassemias and pancellular HPFH.
3. HPFH of heterocellular type.

This classification is based on the difference of γ gene expression in these conditions.

1. In β-thalassemias, synthesis of β-chain is absent or drastically reduced, while γ-chain production is either normal or only slightly increased. The molecular defects underlying β-thalassemias are quite heterogenous, in that they may affect nearly every step of the normal β-chain synthetic process (for a review, see 155). In all cases, except one (156), they are not associated with detectable deletions in the β-globin gene region.

2. δβ-thalassemias and HPFH of pancellular type are characterized by absence or considerable reduction of both δ- and β-chain synthesis, which is more or less efficiently compensated for by persistent expression of the γ-globin genes (138). The degree of compensation differs considerably among these disorders. HbF synthesis is more elevated in HPFHs than in δβ-thalassemias. Thus, the former are not associated with evident hematological and clinical abnormalities, while the latter are usually characterized by moderate to severe anemia (138).

   a. Regulatory sequences in the $^{A}\gamma\delta$ intergenic region. A number of gene deletions and/or major rearrangements within the β-gene cluster are associated with most δβ-thalassemias and pancellular HPFH (Figure 14; 155,157). In all cases the deletion affects, partially or totally, δ and β gene. A strong correlation exists between the extent of the deletion, upstream from the δ gene, and the degree of persistent $^{G}\gamma$ and $^{A}\gamma$ gene activity. As shown in Figure 14, the deletion in Lepore hemoglobinopathy (type No 1) and $^{G}\gamma^{A}\gamma$ (δβ)°-thalassemias (No 2,3) extends for <3 kb from the 5' end of δ gene. On the other hand, HPFH deletions (No 4–6) include further sequences upstream. Particularly, the deletion in HPFH No 4 is apparently <1.0 kb more extended, than in δβ-thalassemia No 3 (157). This <1.0 kb region may be crucial to mediate perinatal repression of fetal genes and activation of adult ones. Indeed, its loss in HPFH (No 4–6) apparently prevents the perinatal switch, i.e., $^{G}\gamma$ and $^{A}\gamma$ gene activity persists virtually at fetal levels. On the other hand, its presence in δβ-thalassemias (No 1–3) may cause a nearly complete repression of δβ genes, which is not associated with activation of the adult ones, due to their partial or total deletion. This critical DNA region includes one of the Alu repetitive sequences interspersed within the β-like gene cluster (Figure 14) (157). Hypothetically, these sequences may play a key role in modulating the fetal → adult Hb switch (see below). In this regard, any putative sequence(s) regulating γ gene expression, wherever located, should operate in *cis*. Heterozygotes with Hb Kenia HPFH (158) and δβ-thalassemia (157) may show polymorphism of the $^A\gamma$ locus (i.e., $^A\gamma^T$ and $^A\gamma^I$): in these cases persistent $^A\gamma$ synthesis is always of the type coded by $^A\gamma$ gene linked to the δβ deletion.

b. Chromatin domains. An intriguing condition is represented by the $^G\gamma$ (δβ)°-thalassemia (type No. 8, Figure 14) (159,160). This disease is associated with thalassemia-like features, possibly because deletion of $^A\gamma$ gene considerably reduces the over-all output of γ-chains, even if the remaining $^G\gamma$ gene is not inactivated*. The (γδβ)°-thalassemia (No 9) (161) also deserves discussion. Hereby, the β gene is inactive, although present together with its nearest 5' and 3' flanking sequences. The possibility of a concomitant β-thalassemia mutation inactivating the β gene cannot be ruled out. However, this condition may more likely indicate that even deletions occurring relatively far from the β gene may result in suppression of its activity via cis-acting mechanism(s).

These conditions can be interpreted in terms of the chromatin 'domains' hypothesis (162). Accordingly, the human non-α gene cluster is organized in two alternative 'domains', which contain fetal $^G\gamma^A\gamma$ and adult δβ genes respectively. Their boundaries are defined by regulatory regions controlling their activation and repression. Each domain would require presence of intact boundaries for its normal function. In both $^G\gamma(\delta\beta)$°-thalassemia and (γδβ)°-thalassemia, structural genes would thus be inactivated by deletions of the boundaries of their chromosomal domains.

3. Heterocellular HPFH (Section II E), of either British or Swiss type, is not associated with abnormalities within the β-like gene cluster, as evaluated by current gene mapping techniques (139,141). Furthermore, even small or point mutations seem unlikely, since they would conceivably affect the whole RBC population, rather than only amplify the F-cell pool. A considerable degree of genetic linkage between heterocellular HPFH and the β gene has been demonstrated in a large number of cases (139,141,142). However, the observed recombination rate appears to be too high to be compatible with a location of the mutation(s) underlying the HPFH within the γδβ gene region, at least without considering the possibility of hot spots of genetic recombination. In conclusion, no evidence indicates alterations of DNA sequences within the non-α gene cluster. This strengthens the possibility that the mechanism suggested above (Section II E) plays a key pathogenetic role in this condition.

---

*A complex rearrangement within the γδβ gene cluster has been recently described in a case of $^G\gamma$-(δβ)°-thalassemia (148). It involves two deletions and, more important, inversion of the entire $^A\gamma$-δ intergenic sequences (No 7). The thalassemic condition may derive here from (1) the $^A\gamma$ deletion and/or (2) the inverted $^A\gamma$-δ intergenic region. If the latter mechanism is indeed operative, it may indicate that presence of any putative regulatory sequence in the inverted region is not sufficient to allow its normal function. It is also mandatory that it maintains both its correct arrangement and relative position with respect to structural genes.

C. Molecular mechanism(s) underlying the Hb switch in ontogeny and cytogeny: a unifying model

1. The globin gene deletion hypothesis

As previously mentioned, globin genes in humans and other mammals are arranged 5' → 3' in the order of their expression in the ontogeny (Figure 13). It was initially suggested that genes may be successively excised during development (as observed in B-lymphocyte differentiation) (70,71,163). In normal ontogeny, large deletions have never been observed in the γδβ domain (164). It cannot be excluded, however, that very small excisions take place, and perhaps underlie the γ → β switch in development and differentiation. This remote possibility should be tested on purified populations of early *vs* late erythroblasts in different ontogenic stages. Less unlikely, deletions might occur in the embryonic gene domain, particularly in adult erythroblasts. This would explain the apparent complete lack of embryonic Hb expression in adult life.

2. Gene activation via chromatin structure rearrangement(s): the chicken embryo model (73,75,76,165–170)

In chicken embryos, nucleated RBC containing only embryonic or 'adult'* Hb can be obtained at four or 14 days of development respectively. In the intact nuclei from these pure RBC populations, embryonic and 'adult' β-globin genes have been tested for their sensitivity to DNAase I. Expressed genes are markedly sensitive to digestion with this nuclease, as compared to control DNA of the ovalbumin gene. The hypersensitivity of active genes apparently depends on binding of non-histone chromosomal proteins, high mobility groups (HMG) 14 and 17, to the nucleosomes packaging them. Furthermore, expressed genes are undermethylated. All these phenomena (marked DNAase I sensitivity upon binding of HMG to nucleosomes, undermethylation) are strictly confined to the active gene sequences. These observations are consistent with the assumption that an altered chromatin conformation underlies the activation of globin genes. Hypothetically, rearrangement of chromatin structure may be in turn linked with gene undermethylation.

In embryonic RBC, adult globin genes show an intermediate level of DNAase I sensitivity† (i.e., lower than that of embryonic genes, but more elevated than of control ovalbumin DNA). This may suggest that adult genes are in a

---

*Chicken erythropoiesis is characterized by a primitive and two definitive cell lines, which sequentially emerge in the early embryonic phase, the late one and the hatching period. The primitive lineage produces only embryonic β-globin. Both definitive lines contain only 'adult' β-chains.

†This was shown by liquid hybridization, but cannot be observed when employing Southern blot analysis.

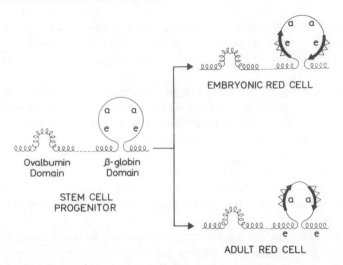

Ovalbumin   β-globin
Domain   Domain

STEM CELL
PROGENITOR

EMBRYONIC RED CELL

ADULT RED CELL

Figure 15. Model for globin gene activation in chicken embryo according to Weintraub and coworkers (75,76). For further explanation see text. Slightly modified from (75,76)

'preactivation' state. Indeed, 'run off' transcription experiments *in vitro* indicated that they are virtually not expressed. In adult RBC, embryonic globin genes loose both hypersensitivity to DNAase I and undermethylation.

Additional findings should be mentioned. Short DNA sequences within the β-globin gene domain are also hypersensitive to DNAase I. Since they are different in embryonic and adult RBC, it is tempting to suggest that they may represent regulatory sites available for attachment of modulators of DNA transcription. Also of interest is that, during mitosis, DNAase I sensitivity and HMG$^+$ nucleosomes selectively segregate with the parental coding DNA strand.

On the basis of these co-ordinated findings, Weintraub *et al* have proposed a model for chromosome structure in terms of 'lampbrush' loops (Figure 15). Accordingly, the β-globin gene domain represents a functional loop of ~50–100 kb. Relaxation of the whole loop causes a moderate rise of DNAase I sensitivity. This presumably occurs in erythrocytic progenitors. Terminal differentiation is associated with additional phenomena: HMG binding to nucleosomes, leading to marked DNAase I sensitivity, and undermethylation. These events would be associated with activation of the globin genes. In embryonic RBC, the adult genes are necessarily 'looped out', while in 'adult' RBC, embryonic genes are possibly 'reeled in'.

Studies in chicken embryos may shed light on the human Hb switch. However, three basic aspects should be emphasized;

1. Human globin genes are linearly arranged $5' \rightarrow 3'$ in the order of their expression in development, whereas chicken globin genes are not.

2. Chickens undergo a single embryonic→adult Hb switch, which is of an all-or-nothing type. Therefore, chicken results may best reflect on the human embryonic→fetal Hb switch, which is apparently of all-or-nothing nature.

3. The fetal→adult Hb switch in men involves a gradual transition from prevalent HbF synthesis to prevailing HbA production. Both γ and δβ genes are hence active in fetal, neonatal and adult erythrocytic tissues. In chick embryo development, either embryonic or 'adult' globin genes are alternatively active.

Thus, mechanisms suggested to underlie the Hb switch in chickens are not sufficient to explain the human perinatal switch. Additional hypotheses are required to elucidate the latter phenomenon (see the model postulated below in Figure 16b).

The above remarks emphasize the urgent need for studies on DNAase I sensitivity and methylation of globin genes in human erythrocytic cells, at different stages of development and differentiation. In this regard, a major obstacle is represented by the difficulty to obtain sufficiently purified human erythrocytic cells. Preliminary studies on mixed hematopoietic populations may suggest that active human globin genes are generally undermethylated (171).

3. Mechanisms underlying the perinatal Hb switch

Any molecular model for the fetal→adult Hb switch must include the following aspects: (1) The switch is, at least to a large extent, irreversible. (2) A small DNA area between $^A\gamma$ and δ gene, deleted in δβ-thalassemias but preserved in pancellular HPFHs, may play a key role to regulate the switch. This area contains an Alu sequence. (3) In each erythrocytic clone γ/β and $^G\gamma/^A\gamma$ synthetic ratios are directly correlated. This is particularly obvious in the perinatal phase. Thus, both γ → β and $^G\gamma → ^A\gamma$ switch occur simultaneously within each erythrocytic clone, thereby suggesting that both are mediated via similar mechanisms.

In the histone gene cluster model, small DNA sequences distant from structural genes may be involved in their regulation (172). Alu sequences, and particularly the one upstream of the δ gene, have been considered as candidates for a similar regulatory function at the level of human β-like globin genes (157,173). Hypothetically, Smithies suggested that Alu sequences may represent the site of origin of the replication fork in the eukaryotic genome, and particularly the human non-α globin domain (173). Genes duplicated from an origin upstream of the leading DNA strand would become active, while those duplicated from an origin downstream would be turned off. In human fetal life DNA replication would proceed from the Alu sequence upstream of the γ domain, in the adult stage, from that upstream of the δ gene. This attractive model, however, does not explain two perinatal phenomena: (1) the decrease of the $^G\gamma/^A\gamma$ ratio and (2) the correlation between γ/β and $^G\gamma/^A\gamma$ synthetic levels.

4. Mechanisms underlying Hb synthesis in adult erythropoiesis

Any hypothesis should cope with the following findings:

1. The heterogeneity of HbF content in adult RBC (F- *vs* A-cells), as well as the rise of the F-cell number in acute stress erythropoiesis.
2. The perinatal $\gamma \rightarrow \beta$ (and possibly $^G\gamma \rightarrow {}^A\gamma$) switch is in part recapitulated in adult erythroblastic maturation.

A cellular model for the genesis of F-cells has been proposed (Figure 10; 104). The novel hypothesis therein is represented by the asymmetric divisions (AD) in the F-lineage, whereby γ-mRNA transcription is blocked in one of the two daughter cells. This mechanism may, at least in part, mediate emergence of a minority of F-cells *vs* a majority of A-cells. Its partial suppression would underlie the increase of F-cell number in stress erythropoiesis.

A molecular model may be proposed to explain these AD (Figure 16; 108). As mentioned above, active globin genes in chicken embryo are both undermethylated and accessible to nucleases due to binding of HMG to the nucleosomes packaging them. During mitosis, DNAase I sensitivity and HMG^+ nucleosomes apparently segregate with the parental leading DNA strand (+). Newly synthesized nucleosomes segregate with the non-coding strand (−). Nucleosome segregation may represent the mechanism underlying AD in F-erythroblast maturation, according to a biphasic phenomenon (Figure 16a).

1. All or a majority of early erythroblasts may synthesize a small amount of γ-chain. This would be due to activation of γ genes, *via* rearrangement of chromatin structure and/or undermethylation.
2. In subsequent mitosis, this mechanism would be switched off. In parallel the β-domain would be activated, again *via* chromatin rearrangement and/or undermethylation. The β-activation mechanism would be maintained for DNA strands synthesized thereafter.

In phase 1 nucleosomes attached to the leading DNA strand (+), with activated γ genes, may segregate to one of the daughter cells (F-lineage). The other one (A-lineage) would receive the parental nonsense DNA strand (−) and newly-synthesized nucleosomes. In phase 2 $\delta\beta$ genes would be activated in both F- and A-lineages, while γ genes might maintain their activity only in the F-line. A series of four AD would hence result in a minority of F-cells ($\sim$6%) *vs* a majority of A-cells, which may or may not contain miniscule, unmeasurable amounts of HbF.

5. Unifying model on the Hb switch in ontogeny and cytogeny

The model described above, although highly hypothetical, may neatly account

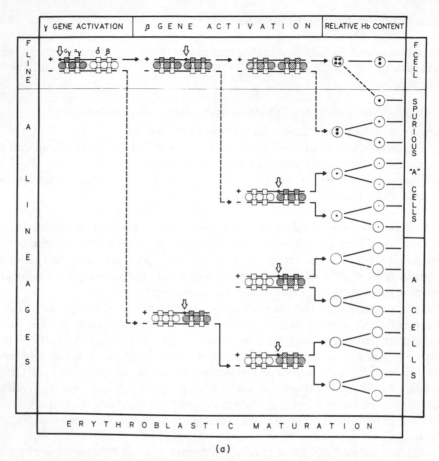

(a)

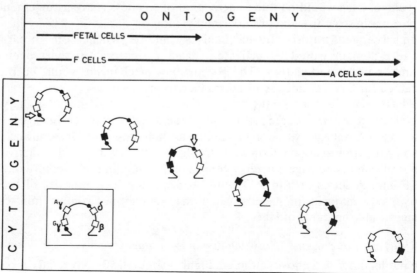

(b)

for most results available so far. In adult stress erythropoiesis, enhanced HbF synthesis and amplification of F-cell pool may be mediated mainly *via* a more prolonged function of the γ-activating mechanism(s), thus abolishing early AD and extending significant γ-synthesis through late maturation stages. In fetal life, prolonged γ-activation and delayed β-activation would underlie prevailing HbF expression.

The model postulated above may be further modified to explain the correlation between γ/β and $^G\gamma/^A\gamma$ synthetic ratios, which is observed in ontogeny, and probably also in adult erythroblastic differentiation (Figure 16b). This correlation is best interpreted in terms of a 'transcriptional wave', which would progress along the non-α gene cluster during cytogeny in both fetal, neonatal, and adult life (104). A similar concept has been independently proposed (144). Thereby, $^G\gamma^A\gamma\delta\beta$ genes would be sequentially transcribed during erythroblastic differentiation (Figure 16b). The initial 'fetal-type' maturation period may involve peak γ-chain synthesis, with an elevated $^G\gamma/^A\gamma$ ratio due to earlier activation of the $^G\gamma$ gene as compared to the $^A\gamma$ one. The final, 'adult' phase of maturation would be associated with peak β-synthesis and rapid decline of γ-production. The $^G\gamma/^A\gamma$ ratio would be lower, due to later inactivation of the $^A\gamma$ gene, as compared with $^G\gamma$. In the fetal age, erythroblastic differentiation would entail essentially the 'fetal-type' maturation. In adult life, it would be characterized by a rapid transition from the 'fetal' to the 'adult-type' maturation, the latter being the only one operating in A-lineages.

In normal adults, synthesis of δ-globin is detected in marrow but not in peripheral reticulocytes (174), i.e., it is apparently complete by the late normoblastic stage. Although this difference might be attributed to a shorter half-life of δ- *vs* β-mRNA (174), this hypothesis is far from demonstrated. Alternatively, this phenomenon may be referred to the asynchrony of

---

Figure 16. (a) A molecular model for the genesis of F-cells in normal adults, based on the cellular hypothesis in Figure 9b. Asymmetric divisions of erythroblasts (---) are explained in terms of a nucleosome segregation mechanism. Genes are represented as either active (—■—) or inactive (—□—) in both + and −DNA strands. Nucleosomes are schematically shown in their activated (—●—) or inactive (—○—) configuration. The activation event is also shown (⇔). Levels of relative or absolute gene expression are not considered. For further details see text. (b) A unifying model for the regulation of Hb synthesis in ontogeny and cytogeny. It combines: (a) the chicken embryo model by Weintraub and co-workers (75,76; Figure 13) and (b) the 'transcriptional wave' hypothesis (104,144), which may explain the direct correlation of γ/β and $^G\gamma/^A\gamma$ synthetic ratios (see Figure 7). ■ = active genes, □ = inactive or low expressed genes. This model is not necessarily incompatible with the hypothesis by Smithies (174), i.e., the activating mechanism(s) (◊) might act at the level of Alu sequences (—●—) upstream from the γ and δβ domains *via* initiation of a DNA replication fork

$HbA_2 \rightarrow A$ synthesis in adult erythropoiesis. This in turn would suggest that δ and β genes are sequentially transcribed in cytogeny, thus in line with the transcriptional wave hypothesis (Figure 16b).

It is thus apparent that the 'transcriptional wave' concept may represent the unifying mechanism underlying globin gene expression in both ontogeny and cytogeny. This model may even be expanded to other species: the $5' \rightarrow 3'$ sequence of globin genes is in order of their expression in both development and differentiation in men, other mammals and the duck (see 144).

In conclusion (Figure 16) the $\gamma\delta\beta$ domain might be in a 'preactivation' state in erythrocytic progenitors. This would be followed by sequential activation of the $^G\gamma^A\gamma\delta\beta$ complex during erythroblastic maturation. Progression of this 'transcriptional wave' would be slow in fetal age and much more rapid in the adult period. Adult stress erythropoiesis would be characterized by a transcriptional wave progressing less rapidly than in normal conditions, and thus associated with partial blockade of asymmetric divisions of erythroblasts.

IV. ACKNOWLEDGMENTS

Supported by Grants from: Volkswagen Foundation, Hannover; EURA-TOM, Bruxelles (No. BI0-C-353-I); CNR, Rome (Progetto Finalizzato 'Controllo della Crescita Neoplastica' No. 80.01615.96, 81.01437.96). We wish to express our appreciation for the excellent secretarial assistance of Ms G. Di-Lauro.

V. REFERENCES

1. Stamatoyannopoulos, G., and Nienhuis, A. W. (Eds.) (1979). *Cellular and Molecular Regulation of Hemoglobin Switching*, Grune and Stratton, New York.
2. Stamatoyannopoulos, G., and Nienhuis, A. W. (Eds.) (1981). *Organization and Expression of Globin Genes*, Alan R. Liss, New York.
3. Stamatoyannopoulos, G., and Nienhuis, A. W. (Eds.) (1981). *Hemoglobins in Development and Differentiation*, Alan R. Liss, New York.
4. Wood, W. G., Clegg, J. B., and Weatherall, D. J. (1977). 'Development biology of human hemoglobins', in *Progress in Hematology* (Ed. D. B. Brow), Grune and Stratton, New York, pp. 43–90.
5. Nienhuis, A. W. (1978). 'Hemoglobin switching. A new experimental model', *J. Lab. Clin. Med.*, **91**, 857–861.
6. Ogawa, M. (1980). 'Human hemoglobin switching in culture', *Am. J. Hemat.,* **9**, 127–135.
7. Fantoni, A., Farace, M. G., and Gambari, R. (1981). 'Embryonic hemoglobin in man and other mammals', *Blood*, **57**, 623–633.
8. Weatherall, D. J., and Clegg, J. B. (1981). *The Thalassemia Syndromes*, (3rd edn), Blackwell, Oxford, pp. 49–84.
9. Maniatis, T., Fritsch, E. F., Laver, J., Larun, R., Proudfoot, N. J., Shander, M. H. M., and Shen, J. C. K. (1981). 'The structure and chromosomal arrangement of human globin genes', in *Organization and Expression of Globin Genes* (Eds. G. Stamatoyannopoulos and A. W. Nienhuis), Alan R. Liss, New York, pp. 12–31.

10. Gale, R. E., Clegg, J. B., and Huehns, E. R. (1979). 'Human embryonic haemoglobins Gower I and Gower II', *Nature*, **280**, 162–164.
11. Kazazian, H. H., Jr. (1974). 'Regulation of fetal hemoglobin production', *Semin. Hematol.*, **11**, 525–548.
12. Hecht, F., Motulsky, A. G., Lemire, R. J., and Shepard, T. E. (1966). 'Predominance of hemoglobin Gower I in early human embryonic development', *Science*, **152**, 91–92.
13. Boyer, S. H., Belding, K., Margolet, L., and Noyes N. (1975). 'Fetal hemoglobin restriction to a few erythrocytes (F cells) in normal human adults', *Science*, **188**, 361–363.
14. Wood, W. G., Stamatoyannopoulos, G., Lim, G., and Nute, P. E. (1975). 'F-cells in the adult: Normal values and levels in individuals with hereditary and acquired elevations of HbF', *Blood*, **46**, 671–682.
15. Huisman, T. H. J., Schroeder, W. A., Efremov, G. D., Duma, H., Mladenovski, B., Hyman, C. B., Rachmilewitz, E. A., Bouver, N. G., Miller, A., Brodie, A. R., Shelton, J. R., and Apel, G. (1974). 'The present status of the heterogeneity of fetal hemoglobin in β-thalassemia: An attempt to unify some observations in thalassemia and related conditions', *Ann. N.Y. Acad. Sci.*, **232**, 107–124.
16. Huisman, T. H. J., and Altay, C. (1981). 'The chemical heterogeneity of the fetal hemoglobin of black newborn babies and adults: A re-evaluation', *Blood*, **58**, 491–500.
17. Metcalf, D. (1977). 'Hemopoietic colonies. *In vitro* cloning of normal and leukemic cells', in *Recent Results in Cancer Research*, Springer, Berlin, pp. 227.
18. Metcalf, D. (1980). 'Hemopoietic colony stimulating factors', in *Tissue Growth Factors* (Ed. R. Baserga), Springer, New York, pp. 99–121.
19. Cline, M. J., and Golde, D. W. (1979). 'Cellular interactions in hematopoiesis', *Nature*, **277**, 177–181.
20. Peschle, C. (1980). 'Erythropoiesis', *Ann. Rev. Med.*, **31**, 303–314.
21. Till, J. E., and McCulloch, E. A. (1980). 'Hemopoietic stem cell differentiation', *Biochim. Biophys. Acta*, **605**, 431–459.
22. Peschle, C. (1982). 'Hemopoietic stem and progenitor cells: Recent advances of physiologic relevance', in *Butterworths International Medical Reviews*, Haematology-Oncology (Ed. M. L. N. Willoughby and S. E. Siegel), Butterworths, London, vol. 1 (in press).
23. Till, J. E., and McCulloch, E. A. (1961). 'A direct measurement of the radiation sensitivity of normal mouse marrow cells', *Radiat. Res.*, **14**, 213–222.
24. Barnes, D. W., Ford, C. E., Gray, S. M., and Loutit, J. F. (1959). 'Spontaneous and induced changes in cell populations in heavily irradiated mice', *Prog. Nucl. Energy (Biol.)*, **2**, 1–10.
25. Metcalf, D., Johnson, G. R., and Mandel, T. E. (1979). 'Colony formation in agar by multipotential hemopoietic cells', *J. Cell. Physiol.*, **98**, 401–420.
26. Fauser, A. A., and Messner, H. A. (1979). 'Granulo-erythropoietic colonies in human bone marrow, peripheral blood and cord blood', *Blood*, **52**, 1243–1248.
27. Messner, H. A., Izaguirre, C. A., and Jamal, N. (1981). 'Identification of T lymphocytes in human mixed hemopoietic colonies', *Blood*, **58**, 402–404.
28. Axelrad, A. A., McLeod, D. L., Shreeve, M. M., and Heath, D. S. (1974). 'Properties of cells that produce erythropoietic colonies *in vitro*', in *Hemopoiesis in Culture* (Ed. W. A. Robinson), GPO, Washington, DC, pp. 226–234.
29. Peschle, C., Migliaccio, A. R., Migliaccio, G., Mastroberardino, G., Gianni, A. M., Comi, P., Ottolenghi, S., and Giglioni, B. (1982). '*In vitro* regulation of Hb synthesis: Studies in normal subjects and thalassemic patients', in *Proceedings of*

the International Symposium on Recent Advances in Thalassemia (Eds: A. Cao and U. Carcassi), March of Dimes, (in press).

30. Eaves, C. J., and Eaves, A. C. (1978). 'Erythropoietin (Ep) dose-response curves for three classes of erythroid progenitors in normal human marrow and in patients with polycythemia vera', *Blood,* **52**, 1196–1210.

31. Eaves, C. J., Humphries,. R. K., and Eaves, A. C. (1979). '*In vitro* characterization of erythroid precursor cells and the erythropoietic differentiation process', in *Cellular and Molecular Regulation of Hemoglobin Switching* (Eds. G. Stamatoyannopoulos and A. W. Nienhuis), Grune and Stratton, New York, pp. 251–273.

32. Humphries, R. K., Eaves, A. C., and Eaves, C. J. (1981). 'Self-renewal of hemopoietic stem cells during mixed colony formation *in vitro*', *Proc. Natl. Acad. Sci., (USA).,* (in press).

33. Peschle, C., Migliaccio, A. R., Migliaccio, G., Ciccariello, R., Lettieri, F., Quattrin, S., Russo, G., and Mastroberardino, G. (1981). 'Identification and characterization of three classes of erythroid progenitors in human fetal liver', *Blood,* **58**, 565–572.

34. Wagemaker, G. (1978). 'Induction of erythropoietin responsiveness in vitro', in *Hemopoietic Cell Differentiation* (Eds. D. W. Golde, D. Metcalf, and C. F. Fox), Academic Press, New York, pp. 109–118.

35. Lajtha, L. G., Pozzi, L. V., Schofield, R., and Fox, M. (1969). 'Kinetic properties of hemopoietic stem cells', *Cell Tissue Kinet.,* **2**, 39–49.

36. Ogawa, M., Grush, O. C., O'Dell, R. F., Hara, H., and MacEachern, M. D. (1977). 'Circulating erythropoietic precursors assessed in culture: Characterization in normal men and patients with hemoglobinopathies', *Blood,* **50**, 1081–1092.

37. Ogawa, M., and Sexton, J. (1976). 'Circulating erythropoietic precursors in human blood', *Clin. Res.,* **24**, 316a (abstract).

38. Rickard, K. A., Rencricca, N. J., Shadduck, R. K., Monette, F. C., Howard, D., Garrity, M., and Stohlman, F., Jr. (1971). 'Myeloid stem cell kinetics during erythropoietic stress', *Brit. J. Haemat.,* **21**, 537–547.

39. Hara, H., and Ogawa, M. (1977). 'Erythropoietic precursors in murine blood', *Exp. Hemat.,* **5**, 159–163.

40. Nathan, D. G., Chess, L., Hillman, D. G., Clarke, B., Breared, J., Merler, E., and Housman, D. E. (1978). 'Human erythroid burst-forming unit: T-cell requirement for proliferation in vitro', *J. Exp. Med.,* **147**, 324–339.

41. Hara, H., and Ogawa, M. (1977). 'Erythropoietic precursors in mice under stimulation and suppression', *Exp. Hemat.,* **5**, 141–148.

42. Dexter, T. M., Garland, J., Scott, D., Scolnick, E., and Metcalf, D. (1980). 'Growth of factor-dependent hemopoietic precursor cell lines', *J. Exp. Med.,* **152**, 1036–1047.

43. Miyake, T., Kung, C. K. H., and Goldwasser, E. (1977). 'Purification of human erythropoietin', *J. Biol. Chem.,* **252**, 5558–5564.

44. Filmanowicz, E., and Gurney, C. W. (1961). 'Studies on erythropoiesis, XVI. Response to a single dose of erythropoietin in the polycythemic mouse', *J. Lab. Clin. Med.,* **75**, 65–72.

45. Stohlman, F., Jr. (1971). 'Control mechanisms in erythropoiesis', in *Regulation of Erythropoiesis* (Eds. A. S. Gordon, M. Condorelli, and C. Peschle), Il Ponte, Milano, pp. 71–88.

46. Schooley, J. C., and Mahlmann, L. J. (1974). 'Extrarenal erythropoietin production by the liver in the weanling rat', *Proc. Soc. Exp. Biol. Med.,* **145**, 1081–1083.

47. Zucali, J. R., Stevens, V., and Mirand, E. A. (1975). 'In vitro production of erythropoietin by mouse fetal liver', *Blood, 46*, 85–90.
48. Peschle, C., Marone, G., Genovese, A., Rappaport, I. A., and Condorelli, M. (1976). 'Increased erythropoietin production in anephric rats with hyperplasia of the reticuloendothelial system induced by colloidal carbon or zymosan', *Blood, 47*, 325–337.
49. Peschle, C., Marone, G., Genovese, A., Magli, M. C., and Condorelli, M. (1976). 'Erythropoietin production in the rat: Additive role of kidney and liver', *Am. J. Physiol., 230*, 845–848.
50. Fried, W. (1972). 'The liver as a source of extrarenal erythropoietin production', *Blood, 40*, 671–677.
51. Bessis, N. (1958). 'L'ilot erythroblastique, unite fonctionelle de la moelle osseuse', *Nouv. Rev. Franc. Hemat., 13*, 8–13.
52. Krantz, S. B., and Jacobson, L. O. (1970). *Erythropoietin and the Regulation of Erythropoiesis*, University of Chicago Press, Illinois, p. 329.
53. Gordon, A. S. (1973). 'Erythropoietin', *Vitamins and Hormones, 31*, 105–174.
54. Iscove, N. N., and Guilbert, L. J. (1978). 'Erythropoietin-independence of early erythropoiesis and a two-regulator model of proliferative control in the hemopoietic system', in *In Vitro Aspects of Erythropoiesis* (Eds. M. J. Murphy, C. Peschle, A. S. Gordon, and E. A. Mirand), Springer-Verlag, New York, pp. 3–7.
55. Wagemaker, G. (1978). 'Cellular and soluble factors influencing the differentiation of primitive erythroid progenitor cells (BFU-e) *in vitro*', in *In Vitro Aspects of Erythropoiesis* (Eds. M. J. Murphy, C. Peschle, A. S. Gordon, and E. A. Mirand), Springer-Verlag, New York, pp. 44–57.
56. Iscove, N. N. (1978). 'Erythropoietin-independent stimulation of early erythropoiesis in adult marrow cultures by conditioned media from lectin-stimulated mouse spleen cells', in *Hemopoietic Cell Differentiation* (Eds. D. W. Golde, M. J. Cline, D. Metcalf, and C. F. Fox), Academic Press, New York, pp. 37–52.
57. Wagemaker, G. (1980). 'Erythropoietin-independent regulation of early erythropoiesis', in *In Vivo and In Vitro Erythropoiesis: The Friend System* (Ed. G. B. Rossi), Elsevier, Amsterdam, pp. 87–96.
58. Metcalf, D., Burgess, A. W., and Johnson, G. R. (1980). 'Stimulation of multipotential and erythroid precursor cells by GM–CSF', in *Experimental Hematology Today* (Eds. S. J. Baum, G. D. Ledney and D. W. van Bekkum), Springer-Verlag, New York, pp. 3–12.
59. Wagemaker, G. (1981). 'Hemopoietic factors required for differentiation of multipotential cells *in vitro*', in *Hemoglobins in Development and Differentiation* (Eds. G. Stamatoyannopoulos and A. W. Nienhuis), Alan R. Liss, New York, pp. 85–92.
60. Lusis, A. J., and Golde, D. W. (1981). 'Human T-lymphocyte derived erythroid-potentiating activity: Partial purification and characterization', in *Hemoglobins in Development and Differentiation* (Eds. G. Stamatoyannopoulos and A. W. Nienhuis), Alan R. Liss, New York, pp. 93–102.
61. Fagg, B. (1981). 'Is erythropoietin the only factor which regulates late erythroid differentiation?', *Nature, 289*, 184–186.
62. Axelrad, A. A., Croizat, H., and Eskinazi, D. (1981). 'A washable macromolecule from Fv2rr marrow negatively regulates DNA synthesis in erythropoietic progenitor cells, BFU-E', *Cell, 26*, 233–244.
63. Toksoz, D., Dexter, T. M., Lord, B. I., Wright, E. G., and Lajtha, L. G. (1980). 'The regulation of hemopoiesis in long-term bone marrow cultures. II. Stimulation and inhibition of stem cell proliferation', *Blood, 55*, 931–936.

64. Rowley, P. T., Olsson, W. B. M., and Farely, B. A. (1978). 'Erythroid colony formation from human fetal liver', *Proc. Natl. Acad. Sci., (USA)*, **75**, 984–988.
65. Hassan, M. W., Lutton, J. D., Levere, R. D., Rieder, R. F., and Cederquist, L. (1979). '*In vitro* culture of erythroid colonies in human fetal liver and umbilical cord blood', *Brit. J. Haemat.*, **41**, 477–484.
66. Burgess, A. W., Wilson, E. M. A., and Metcalf, D. (1977). 'Stimulation by human placental conditioned medium of hemopoietic colony formation by human marrow cells', *Blood,* **49**, 573–583.
67. Rich, I. N., and Kubanek, B. (1976). 'Erythroid colony formation (CFU-e) in fetal liver and adult bone marrow and spleen from the mouse', *Blut*, **33**, 171–180.
68. Abelson, J., and Butz, E. (eds.) (1980) 'Recombinant DNA', *Science,* **209**, 1317–1435.
69. Brown, D. D. (1981). 'Gene expression in eukaryotes', *Science,* **211**, 667–674.
70. Hozumi, N., and Tonegawa, S. (1976). 'Evidence for somatic rearrangement of immunoglobulin genes coding for variable and constant regions', *Proc. Natl. Acad. Sci., (USA)*, **73**, 3628–3632.
71. Seidman, J. G., Leder, A. Naa, N., Norman, B., and Leder, P. (1978). 'Antibody diversity', *Science,* **202**, 11–17.
72. McGhee, J. D., and Felsenfeld, G. (1980). 'Nucleosome structure', *Ann. Rev. Biochem.*, **49**, 1115–1156.
73. Weintraub, H., and Groudine, M. (1976). 'Chromosomal subunits in active genes have an altered conformation', *Science,* **193**, 848–856.
74. Garel, A., and Axel, R. (1976). 'Selective digestion of transcriptionally-active ovalbumin genes from oviduct nuclei', *Proc. Natl. Acad. Sci., (USA)*, **73**, 3966–3977.
75. Groudine, M., Peretz, M., and Weintraub, H. (1981). 'The structure and expression of globin chromatin during hematopoiesis in the chicken embryo', in *Organization and Expression of Globin Genes* (Eds. G. Stamatoyannopoulos and A. W. Nienhuis), Alan R. Liss, New York, pp. 163–173.
76. Weintraub, H., Weisbrod, S., Larsen, A., and Groudine, M. (1981). 'Changes in globin chromatin structure during red cell differentiation in chick embryos', in *Organization and Expression of Globin Genes* (Eds. G. Stamatoyannopoulos and A. W. Nienhuis), Alan R. Liss, New York, pp. 175–190.
77. Smith, G. R. (1981). 'DNA supercoiling: Another level for regulating gene expression', *Cell,* **24**, 599–600.
78. Zachan, H. G., and Igo-Kemenes, T. (1981). 'Face to phase with nucleosomes', *Cell,* **24**, 597–598.
79. Grippo, P., Jaccarino, M., Parisi, E., and Scarano, E. (1968). 'Methylation of DNA in developing sea urchin embryos', *J. Mol. Biol.*, **36**, 195–208.
80. Razin, A., and Riggs, A. D. (1980). 'DNA methylation and gene function', *Science,* **210**, 604–610.
81. Ehrlich, M., and Wang, R. Y. H. (1981). '5-methylcytosine in eukaryotic DNA', *Science,* **212**, 1350–1357.
82. Lindahl, T. (1981). 'DNA methylation and control of gene expression', *Nature,* **290**, 363–364.
83. Naveh-Many, T., and Cedar, H. (1981). 'Active gene sequences are undermethylated', *Proc. Natl. Acad. Sci., (USA)*, **78**, 4244–4250.
84. Groudine, M., Eisenman, R., and Weintraub, H. (1981). 'Chromatin structure of endogenous retroviral genes and activation by an inhibitor of DNA methylation', *Nature,* **292**, 311–317.
85. Mohandas, T., Sparkers, R. S., and Shapiro, L. J. (1981). 'Reactivation of an

inactive human X chromosome: Evidence for X inactivation by DNA methylation', *Science, 211,* 393–396.

86. Weatherall, D. J., Clegg, J. B., and Wood, W. G. (1976). 'A model for the persistence or reactivation of fetal hemoglobin production', *Lancet,* **ii**, 660–663.

87. Fialkow, P. J. (1980). 'Clonal and stem cell origin of blood cell neoplasm', in *Contemporary Hematology/Oncology* (Eds. R. Silver, J. LoBue, and A. S. Gordon), Plenum Publishing Corporation, New York, vol. 1, pp. 1–43.

88. Papayannopoulou, T., and Stamatoyannopoulos, G. (1979). 'On the origin of F-cells in the adult: Clues from studies in clonal hemopathies', in *Cellular and Molecular Regulation of Hemoglobin Switching* (Eds. G. Stamatoyannopoulos and A. W. Nienhuis), Grune and Stratton, New York, pp. 73–84.

89. Bunch, C., Wood, W. G., and Weatherall, D. J. (1979). 'Cellular origins of the fetal-haemoglobin-containing cells of normal adults', *Lancet,* **i**,. 1163–1165.

90. Papayannopoulou, T., Chen, P., Maniatis, A., and Stamatoyannopoulos, G. (1980). 'Simultaneous assessment of i-antigenic expression and fetal hemoglobin in single red cells by immunofluorescence', *Blood,* **55**, 221–232.

91. Boyer, S. H., Dover, G. J., Smith, K. D., and Scott, A. (1981). 'Some interpretations of *in vivo* studies of globin gene switching in man and primates', in *Hemoglobins in Development and Differentiation* (Eds. G. Stamatoyannopoulos and A. W. Nienhuis), Alan R. Liss, New York, pp. 225–241.

92. Papayannopoulou, T., Brice, M., and Stamatoyannopoulos, G. (1977). 'Hemoglobin F synthesis *in vitro*: Evidence for the control at the level of primitive erythroid stem cells', *Proc. Natl. Acad. Sci., (USA),* **74**, 2923–2927.

93. Stamatoyannopoulos, G., and Papayannopoulou, T. (1979). 'Fetal hemoglobin and the erythroid stem cell differentiation process', in *Cellular and Molecular Regulation of Hemoglobin Synthesis* (Eds. G. Stamatoyannopoulos and A. W. Nienhuis), Grune and Stratton, New York, pp. 323–349.

94. Papayannopoulou, T., Nakamoto, B., Kurachi, S., Kurnit, D. and Stamatoyanno-poulos, G. (1981). 'Cell biology of hemoglobin switching. II. Studies on the regulation of fetal hemoglobin synthesis in human adults', in *Hemoglobins in Development and Differentiation* (Eds. G. Stamatoyannopoulos and A. W. Nienhuis), Alan R. Liss, New York, pp. 307–320.

95. Comi, P., Giglioni, B., Ottolenghi, S., Gianni, A. M., Polli, E., Barba, P., Covelli, A., Migliaccio, G., Condorelli, M., and Peschle, C. (1980). 'Globin chain synthesis in single erythroid bursts from cord blood: Studies on $\gamma \to \beta$ and $^{G}\gamma \to ^{A}\gamma$ switches', *Proc. Natl. Acad. Sci., (USA),* **77**, 362–365.

96. Kidoguchi, K., Ogawa, M., Karem, J. D., McNeil, J. S., and Fitch, M. S. (1979). 'Hemoglobin biosynthesis in individual bursts in culture: Studies of human umbilical cord blood', *Blood,* **53**, 519–527.

97. Teresawa, T., and Ogawa, M. (1980). 'Hemoglobin biosynthesis in individual bursts from human adult peripheral and umbilical cord blood: Analysis of the relative rate of synthesis of $^{G}\gamma$ and $^{A}\gamma$ globin chains', *J. Cell. Physiol.,* **105**, 483–488.

98. Stamatoyannopoulos, G., Papayannopoulou, T., Brice, M., Kurachi, S., Nakamoto, B., Lim, G., and Farquhar, M. (1981). 'Cell biology switching I. The switch from fetal to adult hemoglobin formation during ontogeny', in *Hemoglobins in Development and Differentiation* (Eds. G. Stamatoyannopoulos and A. W. Nienhuis), Alan R. Liss, New York, pp. 287–305.

99. Fauser, A. A., and Messner, H. A. (1979). 'Fetal hemoglobin in mixed hemopoietic colonies (CFU-GEMM), erythroid bursts (BFU-E) and erythroid colonies (CFU-E): Assessment by radioimmunoassay and immunofluorescence', *Blood,* **54**, 1384–1394.

100. Dean, A., Schechter, A. N., Papayannopoulou, T., and Stamatoyannopoulos, G.
     (1981). 'Evidence for heterogeneity of erythroid precursors; Radioimmunoassay
     quantitation of hemoglobin in single bursts', in *Hemoglobins in Development and
     Differentiation* (Eds. G. Stamatoyannopoulos and A. W. Nienhuis), Alan R.
     Liss, New York, pp. 351–358.
101. Peschle, C., Migliaccio, G., Covelli, A., Lettieri, F., Migliaccio, A. R.,
     Condorelli, M., Comi, P., Pozzoli, M. L., Giglioni, B., Ottolenghi, S., Cappellini,
     M. D., Polli, E., and Gianni, A. M. (1980). 'Hemoglobin synthesis in individual
     bursts from normal adult blood: All bursts and subcolonies synthesize $^G\gamma$ and $^A\gamma$
     globin chains', *Blood*, **56**, 218–226.
102. Gianni, A. M., Comi, P., Giglioni, B., Ottolenghi, S., Migliaccio, A. R.,
     Migliaccio, G., Lettieri, F., Maguire, Y. P., and Peschle, C. (1980). 'Biosynthe-
     sis of Hb in individual fetal liver bursts', *Exp. Cell Res.*, **130**, 345–352.
103. Comi, P., Giglioni, B., Pozzoli, M. L., Ottolenghi, S., Gianni, A. M., Migliaccio,
     A. R., Migliaccio, G., Lettieri, F., and Peschle, C. (1981). 'Biosynthesis of globin
     chains in fetal liver and adult marrow cultures', *Exp. Cell Res.*, **133**, 347–356.
104. Peschle, C., Migliaccio, A. R., Migliaccio, G., Lettieri, F., Maguire, Y. P.,
     Condorelli, M., Gianni, A. M., Ottolenghi, S., Giglioni, B., Pozzoli, M. L., and
     Comi, P. (1981). 'Regulation of Hb synthesis in ontogenesis and erythropoietic
     differentiation: In vitro studies on fetal liver, cord blood, normal adult blood or
     marrow, and blood from HPFH patients', in *Hemoglobins in Development and
     Differentiation* (Eds. G. Stamatoyannopoulos and A. W. Nienhuis), Alan R. Liss,
     New York, pp. 359–371.
105. Ottolenghi, S., Peschle, C., Comi, P., Giglioni, B., Pozzoli, M. L., Cappellini, M.
     D., Migliaccio, A. R., Lettieri, F., Migliaccio, G., Barba, P., Covelli, A., and
     Gianni, A. M. (1980). 'Hemoglobin synthesis in single erythroid colonies from
     cord blood and adult blood', in *In Vivo and In Vitro Erythropoiesis: The Friend
     System* (Ed. G. B. Rossi), Elsevier, Amsterdam, pp. 41–47.
106. Peschle, C., Migliaccio, A. R., Migliaccio, G., Lettieri, F., Quatrin, S.,
     Condorelli, M., Gianni, A. M., Sciortino, G., Giglioni, B., and Ottolenghi, S.
     (1980). 'Erythroid precursors in human fetal liver and adult marrow: clonal
     analysis and globin chain synthesis in single colonies', in *In Vivo and In Vitro
     Erythropoiesis: The Friend System* (Ed. G. B. Rossi), Elsevier, Amsterdam, pp.
     49–58.
107. Peschle, C., Migliaccio, G., Migliaccio, A. R., Mastroberardino, G., Gianni, A.
     M., Ottolenghi, S., Giglioni, B., and Comi, P. (1982). 'The Hb switches in
     ontogenesis and erythropoietic differentiation: A unifying model', in *Advances in
     Red Blood Cell Biology* (Eds. D. J.Weatherall and G. Fiorelli), Raven Press,
     New York, (in press).
108. Ottolenghi, S., Comi, P., Giglioni, B., Gianni, A. M., Migliaccio, A. R.,
     Migliaccio, G., Lettieri, F., and Peschle, C. (1982). 'Cellular mechanisms for
     regulation of HbF synthesis', in *Expression of Differentiated Functions in Cancer
     Cells* (Eds. R. Revoltella, G. Pontieri, G. Rovera, C. Basilico, R. Gallo, and J.
     Subak-Sharp), Raven Press, New York, (in press).
109. Kidoguchi, K., Ogawa, M.,and Karam, J. D. (1979). 'Hemoglobin biosynthesis in
     individual erythropoietic bursts in culture', *J. Clin. Invest.*, **63**, 804–806.
110. Papayannopoulou, T., Kurachi, S., Brice, M., Nakamoto, B., and Stamatoyanno-
     poulos, G. (1981). 'Asynchronous synthesis of HbF and HbA during erythroblast
     maturation. II. Studies of $^G\gamma$, $^A\gamma$, and chain synthesis in individual erythroid
     clones from neonatal and adult BFU-E cultures', *Blood*, **57**, 531–536.
111. Vedvick, T. S. Wheeler, S. A., and Koenig, H. M. (1980). 'Switching of the non
     allelic forms of fetal hemoglobin during late gestation', *Blood*, **56**, 732–736.

112. Alter, B. P. (1979). 'The $^{G}\gamma{:}^{A}\gamma$ composition of fetal hemoglobin in fetuses and newborns', *Blood,* **54**, 1158–1163.
113. Dover, G. J., and Ogawa, M. (1980). 'Cellular mechanisms for increased fetal hemoglobin production in culture. Evidence for continuous commitment to fetal hemoglobin production during burst formation', *J. Clin. Invest.,* **66**, 1175–1178.
114. Rowley, P. T., Ohlsson-Wilhelm, B. B., Farely, B., and Kosciolek, B. (1981). 'Hemoglobin switching; Does stimulation of in vitro erythropoietic differentiation alter globin gene expression?' in *Hemoglobins in Development and Differentiation* (Eds. G. Stamatoyannopoulos and A. W. Nienhuis), Alan R. Liss, New York, pp. 397–403.
115. Kidoguchi, K., Ogawa, M., Karam, J. D., and Martin, A. G. (1978). 'Augmentation of fetal hemoglobin (HbF) synthesis in culture by human erythropoietic precursors in the marrow and peripheral blood: Studies in sickle cell anemia and nonhemoglobinopathic adults', *Blood,* **52**, 1115–1129.
116. Testa, U., Vainchenker, W., Beuzard, Y., Dubart, A., Breton-Gorius, J., and Rosa, J. (1980). 'Hemoglobin switching in erythroid cultures from human fetuses and neonates', in *In Vivo and In Vitro Erythropoiesis: The Friend System* (Ed. G. B. Rossi), Elsevier, Amsterdam, pp. 69–76.
117. Testa, U., Beuzard, Y., Vainchenker, W., Goossens, M., Dubart, A., Monplaisir, N., Brizard, C. P., Papayannopoulou, T., and Rosa, J. (1979). 'Elevated HbF associated with an unstable hemoglobin, hemoglobin Saint Etienne: Hb synthesis in blood BFU-E in culture', *Blood,* **54**, 334–343.
118. Testa, U., Vainchenker, W., Guerrasio, A. Tsapis, A., Dubart, A., Beuzard, Y., Breton-Gorius, J., Golde, D., and Rosa, J. (1981). 'Influence of burst-promoting activity and culture conditions on the expression of γ and β genes in culture of erythroid precursors during ontogenesis', in *Hemoglobins in Development and Differentiation* (Eds. G. Stamatoyannopoulos and A. W. Nienhuis), Alan R. Liss, New York, pp. 373–387.
119. Zanjani, E. D., McGlave, P. B., Bhakthavathsalen, A., and Stamatoyannopoulos, G. (1979). 'Sheep fetal haematopoietic cells produce adult haemoglobin when transplanted in the adult animal', *Nature,* **280**, 495–496.
120. Wood, W. G., and Bunch, C. (1981). 'The switch from fetal to adult hemoglobin in sheep', in *Proceedings of the International Symposium on Recent Advances in Thalassemia* (Eds. A. Cao and U. Carcassi), March of Dimes, (in press).
121. Zanjani, E. D., Lim, G., McGlave, P. B., Clapp, J. F., Mann, L. I., Norwood, T. H., and Stamatoyannopoulos, G. (1981). 'Hemoglobin phenotypes in genetically AA sheep fetuses transplanted with cells of genetically BB adult animals', in *Hemoglobins in Development and Differentiation* (Eds. G. Stamatoyannopoulos and A. W. Nienhuis), Alan R. Liss, New York, pp. 263–274.
122. Shchory, M., and Weatherall, D. J. (1975). 'Haemoglobin synthesis in human fetal liver maintained in short-term tissue culture', *Brit. J. Haemat.,* **30**, 9–20.
123. Papayannopoulou, T., Kalamantis, T., and Stamatoyannopoulos, G. (1979). 'Cellular regulation of hemoglobin switching: Evidence for inverse relationship between fetal hemoglobin synthesis and degree of maturity of human erythroid cells', *Proc. Natl. Acad. Sci., (USA),* **76**, 6420–6424.
124. Dover, G. J., and Boyer, S. H. (1980). 'Quantitation of hemoglobin within individual red cells: Asynchronous biosynthesis of fetal and adult hemoglobin during erythroid maturation in normal subjects', *Blood,* **56**, 1082–1091.
125. Farquat, M. H., Papayannopoulou, T., Brice, M., and Stamatoyannopoulos, G. (1981). 'Cellular regulation of hemoglobin synthesis in man: Investigation of $^{G}\gamma$ and $^{A}\gamma$ mRNA accumulation in clonal erythroid cultures initiated from erythroid

progenitors from fetuses, neonates and adult individuals', *Develop. Biol.*, (in press).

126. Baglioni, C. (1963). 'Correlations between genetics and chemistry of human hemoglobins', in *Molecular Genetics* (Ed. J .Taylor), Academic Press, New York, pp. 405–475.

127. Boyer, S. H., and Dover, G. J. (1979). '*In vivo* biology of F cells in man', in *Cellular and Molecular Regulation of Hemoglobin Switching* (Eds. G. Stamatoyannopoulos and A. W. Nienhuis), Grune and Stratton, New York, pp. 47–71.

128. Cappellini, M. D., Sampietro, M., Bernini, L. F., and Fiorelli, G. (1982). 'F cell distribution in normals and heterocellular HPFH (Swiss type)', in *Advances in Red Blood Cell Biology* (Eds. D. J. Weatherall and G. Fiorelli), Raven Press, New York, pp. 271–279.

129. Zago, M. A., Wood, W. G., Clegg, J. B., Weatherall, D. J., O'Sullivan, M., and Gunson, H. (1979). 'Genetic control of F-cells in human adults', *Blood,* **53,** 977–986.

130. Alter, B. P. (1979). 'Fetal erythropoiesis in bone marrow failure syndromes', in *Cellular and Molecular Regulation of Hemoglobin Switching* (Eds. G. Stamatoyannopoulos and A. W. Nienhuis), Grune and Stratton, New York, pp. 87–106.

131. Dover, G. J., Boyer, S. H., and Zinkham, W. H. (1979). 'Production of erythrocytes that contain fetal hemoglobin in anemia. Transient *in vivo* changes', *J. Clin. Invest., 63*, 173–176.

132. Papayannopoulou, T., Vichinsky, E., and Stamatoyannopoulos, G. (1980). 'Fetal Hb production during acute erythroid expansion. I. Observations in patients, with transient erythroblastopenia and post-phlebotomy', *Brit. J. Haemat.,* **44,** 535–546.

133. Boyer, S. H., Dover, G. J., Smith, K. D., and Scott, A. (1981). 'Some interpretations of *in vivo* studies of globin gene switching in man and primates', in *Hemoglobins in Development and Differentiation* (Eds. G. Stamatoyannopoulos and A. W. Nienhuis), Alan R. Liss, New York, pp. 225–241.

134. DeSimone, J., Biel, S. I., and Heller, P. (1978). 'Stimulation of fetal hemoglobin synthesis in baboons by hemolysis and hypoxia', *Proc. Natl. Acad. Sci., (USA),* **75,** 2937–2940.

135. DeSimone, J., Heller, P., Amsel, J., and Usman, M. (1980). 'Magnitude of the fetal hemoglobin response to acute hemolytic anemia in baboons is controlled by genetic factors', *J. Clin. Invest.,* **65,** 224–226.

136. DeSimone, J., Heller, P., Zwiers, D., and Koeller, D. (1981). 'Genetic relationship between resting fetal Hb levels and maximal fetal Hb levels attained in baboons after erythropoietic stress', in *Hemoglobins in Development and Differentiation* (Eds. G. Stamatoyannopoulos and A. W. Nienhuis), Alan R. Liss, New York, pp. 275–280.

137. Dover, G. J., Boyer, S. H., and Pembrey, M. E. (1981). 'F-cell production in sickle cell anemia: Regulation by genes linked to β-hemoglobin locus', *Science,* **211,** 1441–1444.

138. Wood, W. J., Clegg, J. B., and Weatherall, D. J. (1979). 'Hereditary persistence of fetal hemoglobin (HPFH) and δβ thalassemia', *Brit. J. Haemat.,* **43,** 509–520.

139. Marinucci, M., Mavilio, F., Gabbianelli, M., Massa, A., Guerriero, R., Giampaolo, A., Giuliani, A., Maffi, D., Chiome, P., Cappellini, M. D., Taramelli, R., and Tentori, L. (1982). 'Cellular mechanisms of increased HbF production in the interaction between HPFH and β-thalassemia', in *Advances in Red Blood Cell Biology* (Eds. D. J. Weatherall and G. Fiorelli), Raven Press, New York, pp. 263–270.

140. Dubart, A., Testa, U., Musumeci, S., Vainchenker, W., Beuzard, Y., Henri, A., Schiliro, G., Romeo, M. A., Russo, G., Rochant, H., and Rosa, J. (1980). 'Elevated HbF associated with β-thalassemia trait: Haemoglobin synthesis in reticulocytes and in blood BFU-E', *Scand. J. Haemat., 25*, 339–346.

141. Wood, W. G., Old, J. M., Darbre, P. D., Clegg, J. B., Weatherall, D. J., and McRae, I. (1982). 'Heterocellular HPFH (British type): Cellular and molecular analysis of increased HbF production', in *Advances in Red Blood Cell Biology* (Eds. D. J .Weatherall and G. Fiorelli), Raven Press, New York, pp. 249–262.

142. Wood, W. G., Weatherall, D. J., and Clegg, J. B. (1976). 'Interaction of heterocellular hereditary persistence of fetal haemoglobin with β-thalassemia and sickle cell anaemia', *Nature, 264*, 247–249.

143. Mazza, U., Camaschella, C., Guerrasio, A., Ciocca-Vasino, M. A., Pich, P. G., Capaldi, A., Trento, M., Ame, C., and Saglio, G. (1982). 'Gγ and ᴬγ globin chain synthesis in the peripheral blood and in the bone marrow of β-thalassemia homozygotes', in *Proceedings of the International Symposium on Recent Advances in Thalassemia* (Eds. A. Cao and U. Carcassi), March of Dimes, (in press).

144. Wood, W. G., and Jones, R. W. (1981). 'Erythropoiesis and hemoglobin production: A unifying model involving sequential gene activation', in *Hemoglobins in Development and Differentiation* (Eds. G. Stamatoyannopoulos and A. W. Nienhuis), Alan R. Liss, New York, pp. 243–261.

145. Efstratiadis, A., Psakony, J. W., Maniatis, T., Lawn, R. M., O'Connell, C., Spritz, R. A., DeRiel, J. K., Forget, B. G., Weissman, S. M., Slightom, J. L., Bleche, A. E., Smithies, O., Baralle, F. E., Shoulders, C. C., and Proudfoot, N. J. (1980). 'The structure and evolution of the human β globin gene family', *Cell, 21*, 653–668.

146. Liebhaber, S. A., Goossens, M. J., and Kan, Y. W. (1980). 'Cloning and complete nucleotide sequence of human 5'-α-globin gene', *Proc. Natl. Acad. Sci., (USA), 77*, 7054–7058.

147. Smithies, O., Bleche, A. E., Shen, S., Slightom, J. L., and Vanin, E. F. (1981). 'Co-evolution and control of globin genes', in *Organization and Expression of Globin Genes* (Eds. G. Stamatoyannopoulos and A. W. Nienhuis), Alan R. Liss, New York, pp. 101–116.

148. Jones, R. W., Old, J. M., Trent, R. J., Clegg, J. B., and Weatherall, D. J. (1981). 'Major rearrangements in the human β-globin gene cluster', *Nature, 291*, 39–44.

149. Fritsch, E. F., Lawn, R. M., and Maniatis, T. (1980). 'Molecular cloning and characterization of the human B-like globin gene cluster', *Cell, 19*, 959–972.

150. Houck, C. M., Rinehart, F. F., and Schmid, C. W. (1979). 'An ubiquitous family of repeated DNA sequences in the human genome', *J. Mol. Biol., 132*, 289–306.

151. Jelinek, W. G., and Leinwand, L. (1978). 'Low molecular weight RNAs hydrogen-bonded to nuclear and cytoplasmic poly-A-terminated RNA from cultures of chinese hamster ovary cells', *Cell, 15*, 205–214.

152. Jelinek, W. G., Toomey, T. P., Leinwand, L., Duncan, C. H., Biro, P. A., Choudary, P. N., Weissman, S. M., Rubin, C. M., Houck, C. M., Deininger, P. L., and Schmid, C. W. (1980). 'Ubiquitous interspersed repeated sequences in mammalian genomes', *Proc. Natl. Acad. Sci., (USA), 77*, 1398–1402.

153. Bank, A., Mears, J. G., and Ramirez, F. (1980). 'Disorders of human hemoglobin', *Science, 207*, 486–493.

154. Anderson, W. F., Kretschmer, P. J., Sanders-Haig, L., Killos, L., and Diacumakos, E. G. (1981). 'Gene transfer and *in vitro* expression', in *Organization and Expression of Globin Genes* (Eds. G. Stamatoyannopoulos and A. W. Nienhuis), Alan R. Liss, New York, pp. 301–312.

155. Maniatis, T., Fritsch, E. F., Laver, J., and Lown, R. M. (1980). 'The molecular genetics of human hemoglobins', *Ann. Rev. Genet.,* pp. 45–178.

156. Orkin, S. H., Old, J. M., Weatherall, D. J., and Nathan, D. G. (1979). 'Partial deletion of β globin gene DNA in certain patients with β₀ thalassemia', *Proc. Natl. Acad. Sci., (USA)*, **76**, 2400–2404.

157. Ottolenghi, S., Giglioni, B., Taramelli, R., Comi, P., Mazza, U., Saglio, G., Camaschella, C., Izzo, R., Cao, A., Galanello, R., Gimferrer, E., Baiget, M., and Gianni, A. M. (1982). 'Molecular comparison of δβ thalassemic and HPFH DNA: Evidence for a regulatory area?' *Proc. Natl. Acad. Sci., (USA)*, (in press).

158. Huisman, T. H. J., Schroeder, W. A., Efrenov, G. D., Duma, H., Mladenowski, B., Hyman, C. B., Rachmilevitz, E. A., Bouver, N., Miller, A., Brodie, A., Shelton, J. B., and Apell, G. (1974). 'The present status of the heterogeneity of fetal hemoglobin in β-thalassemia: An attempt to unify some observations in thalassemia and related conditions', *Ann. N.Y. Acad. Sci.*, **232**, 107–124.

159. Fritsch, E. F., Larn, R. M., and Maniatis, T. (1979). 'Characterization of deletions which affect the expression of fetal globin genes in man', *Nature*, **279**, 598–603.

160. Orkin, S. H., Alter, B. P., and Altay, C. (1979). 'Deletion of the $^{A}\gamma$-globin gene in $^{G}\gamma$-δβ thalassemia', *J. Clin. Invest.*, **64**, 866–869.

161. Van der Ploeg, L. H. T., Konings, A., Oort, M., Roos, D., Bernini, L., and Flavell, R. A. (1980). 'γ-β-thalassemia studies showing that deletion of the γ- and δ-genes influences β-globin gene expression in man', *Nature*, **283**, 637–642.

162. Bernards, R., and Flavell, R. A. (1980). 'Physical mapping of the globin gene deletion in hereditary persistence of fetal haemoglobin (HPFH)', *Nucl. Acid Res.*, **8**, 1521–1534.

163. Kabat, D. (1972). 'Gene selection in hemoglobin and in antibody-synthesizing cell', *Science*, **175**, 134–140.

164. Papayannopoulou, T., Nute, P. E., Stamatoyannopoulos, G., and McGuire, T. C. (1977). 'Hemoglobin ontogenesis: Test of the gene excision hypothesis', *Science*, **197**, 1215–1216.

165. Seidman, M. M., Levien, A. J., and Weintraub, H. (1979). 'The asymmetric segregation of parental nucleosomes during chromosome replication', *Cell*, **18**, 439–449.

166. Stalder, J., Larsen, A., Engel, J. B., Donal, M., Groudine, M., and Weintraub, H. (1980). 'Tissue-specific DNA cleavages in the globin chromatin domain introduced by DNAase I', *Cell*, **20**, 451–460.

167. Stalder, J., Groudine, M., Dogson, J. B., Engel, J. D., and Weintraub, H. (1980). 'Hb switching in chickens', *Cell*, **19**, 973–980.

168. Weisbrod, S., and Weintraub, H. (1981). 'Isolation of actively transcribed nucleosomes using immobilized HMG 14 and 17 and an analysis of γ-globin chromatin', *Cell*, **23**, 391–400.

169. Groudine, M., and Weintraub, H. (1981). 'Activation of globin genes during chicken development', *Cell*, **24**, 393–401.

170. Weintraub, H., Larsen, A., and Groudine, M. (1981). 'α-globin gene switching during the development of chicken embryos; Expression and chromosome structure', *Cell*, **24**, 333–344.

171. Van der Ploeg, L. H. T., and Flavell, R. A. (1980). 'DNA methylation in the human γδβ-globin locus in erythroid and nonerythroid tissues', *Cell*, **19**, 947–958.

172. Grosschede, R., and Birnstiel, M. L. (1980). 'Identification of regulatory sequences in the prelude sequences of an HZA histone gene by the study of specific deletion mutants *in vivo*', *Proc. Natl. Acad. Sci., (USA)*, **77**, 1432–1436.

173. Smithies, O. (1982). 'The control of globin and other eukaryotic genes', *J. Cell. Physiol.*, (in press).
174. Wood, W. G., Old, J. M., Roberts, A. V. S., Clegg, J. B., and Weatherall, D. J. (1978). 'Human globin gene expression: Control of β, δ and δβ chain production', *Cell*, **15**, 437–446.

Current Concepts in Erythropoiesis
Edited by C. D. R. Dunn
© 1983 John Wiley & Sons Ltd.

CHAPTER 15

Genetic engineering and erythropoiesis

KAREN E. MERCOLA
Division of Hematology-Oncology
Department of Medicine
UCLA School of Medicine
Los Angeles

Contents

I. INTRODUCTION

The maturing erythrocytic cell has provided a useful model system for the study of gene regulation and expression. The maturation process reveals well-documented changes in morphology and biosynthetic capabilities of the erythrocytic cell and offers several opportunities for characterizing different aspects of the regulatory process. In the embryonic development of humans and other vertebrate species the site of erythropoiesis changes sequentially, thus affording the opportunity to examine the regulation of cell populations. As the embryo matures, the production of different hemoglobin chains varies. For example, in an organism such as the chick embryo, one has access to the embryo at a time of major change in the pattern of hemoglobin synthesis in the sixth day of embryonic life. This biologic system has been extensively studied in an attempt to determine the regulatory factors involved in the switch from one cell type to another and that cause differential gene expression during erythrocytic maturation. There is considerable evidence that in man and other mammals the regulation of erythropoiesis is mediated in part by the pathway-specific hormone erythropoietin (1); however, this hormone does not appear to be involved during the earliest phase of erythrocytic embryogenesis.

The globin gene products of humans and other species have been extensively characterized, including analyses of primary, secondary, and tertiary molecular structures. More recently, sequences for α-, β, and γ-globin gene messenger RNAs (mRNA) (2–5) and the pathway of globin gene expression from embryo to adult have been analyzed. In mice, at least three gene loci have been identified which, when mutated, cause anemia by different mechanisms (6,7). In humans, structural abnormalities in both α and β genes leading to clinical syndromes of hemoglobinopathies have been characterized with regard to globin gene defects and globin messenger RNA transcripts. The molecular bases for several forms of thalassemia, leading to abnormalities in the rate of globin gene production and various stages of anemia, have recently been elucidated.

Although significant advances have been made in understanding the biology of erythropoiesis, the controls of gene expression in erythrocytic and other eukaryotic cells remain incompletely understood. Advances in this field will allow the application of concepts of genetic engineering to the regulation of erythropoiesis and to the treatment of erythrocytic disorders.

II. TECHNIQUES IN GENETIC ENGINEERING

A. Molecular biological analyses

1. Restriction endonuclease mapping

Restriction endonuclease mapping is a tool that permits precise molecular determination of normal and abnormal globin gene organization. Knowledge of the cleavage sites of various restriction enzymes makes it possible to compare cellular DNA from thalassemia patients with normals and to approach such questions as the extent of defective gene sequences and rearrangement of DNA within or adjacent to globin genes. These results in turn can be correlated with ineffective transcription of DNA, synthesis of non-functional mRNA or synthesis of abnormally unstable mRNA (8–10).

The technique of restriction endonuclease mapping is based on the hybridization of complementary strands of DNA, one of which is highly radioactive. It is based upon a technique originally devised by Southern (11). In this approach, high-molecular-weight DNA is extracted from cells and digested with site-specific endonucleases. The DNA is then separated by electrophoresis on agarose gels and transferred ('blotted') on to a nitrocellulose filter. The filter is hybridized to a radiolabeled probe containing complementary DNA sequences and the location of specific DNA fragments is determined by autoradiography. Hybridization can also be performed on gels *in situ* (12).

2. *Cloning*

Analysis of cellular DNA and individual genes has been aided by the development of cloning techniques using bacteria to amplify selected DNA sequences (13–16). These techniques are applicable to single-copy genes such as β-globin genes, which amount to less than one-millionth of the total cellular DNA. In cloning techniques, gene sequences of interest are inserted into a vector such as a bacterial plasmid or phage which is then introduced into the bacterial host cell. Bacteria, vector and inserted gene all replicate, making available large amounts of the relevant gene. The first globin sequences cloned in bacteria were double-stranded DNA copies (cDNA) or mRNA. These have been used to identify globin genes and flanking sequences (17–21). Complementary DNA (or cDNA) made in this manner has been very useful in understanding the regulation of gene expression. For example, regulation may occur by increasing mRNA concentration or by increasing mRNA translation efficiency. Hybridization of cDNA to mRNA allows quantitation of cellular mRNA and provides information about these alternatives.

B. Gene insertion methods

The transfer of genetic material from the genome of one organism to another has probably occurred since the early stages of evolution. Evolutionary adaptation may have occurred with some frequency *via* genetic elements adapted for shuttling between different regions of genomes (22). Transmission of information between species may be more efficient than mutation in introducing new genetic characteristics that provide a survival advantage. An example of the former mechanism of evolutionary adaptation is the acquisition of resistance to antibiotics by transfer of plasmids between bacteria. Among higher animals there is inferential evidence for the transmission of genetic information *via* viral vectors from rodents to primates (23).

Experiments in interspecies transfer of genetic information occurred as early as 1928 when Griffith demonstrated alteration in microbial structure and function when living attenuated and non-encapsulated type II Pneumococcus were exposed to heat-killed, fully encapsulated, and virulent type III Pneumococcus (24). In the 1970s significant advances in recombinant DNA technology were made, so that it became possible to select and isolate a given sequence of nucleotide base pairs, to modify it by addition or deletion of nucleotide sequences and to introduce such modified DNA into replicating vectors such as bacterial plasmids or viruses for the purpose of cloning, thus providing large quantities of purified genes.

Concomitant with the development of these techniques, a variety of methods were evolved for introducing foreign DNA into animal cells growing in tissue culture. These methods include the use of viruses, cell fusion methods, chromosome-mediated transfer of genetic information, DNA-mediated transformation and the direct injection of new genes into recipient cells.

1. Recombinant viruses

Cloned genes have been introduced into mammalian cells by such vectors as modified papovavirus SV40, in which the regulation of replication and gene expression has been well studied (25,26). In combining prokaryotic or eukaryotic genes with SV40 it is often necessary to employ a helper virus since genes necessary for growth and replication of virus are frequently deleted. Using this approach, important questions concerning transcription and processing of DNA in eukaryotes have been studied (27–30). A recombinant molecule made from covalent linkage of a viral promoter such as SV40, adenovirus or polyoma and a gene such as β-globin may facilitate transcription of the globin gene in host cells. Applicability of these methods to living animals is limited by the infectious nature and transforming properties of the viruses.

2. Cell fusion methods

There are several techniques that involve the physical fusion of cell membranes. Direct treatment of target cells and donor cells with chemicals such as polyethylene glycol or inactivated Sendai virus (31) have been used to effect cell fusion. After nuclear fusion between paired cells, a hybrid cell containing chromosomes from both parents is formed. Somatic cell hybridization has been used to map over 200 mammalian gene loci, including human genes (32,33). Chromosome segregation and loss may be unpredictable in closely related species and the hybrid formed from unrelated species may have only a small amount of the genetic material of one of the parents (34).

In a variation of this approach, artificially constructed lipid vesicles (liposomes) (35,36) or erythrocytes (37) can be loaded with nucleic acids and then fused with target cells. These latter techniques have been more successful utilizing RNA rather than DNA.

Microcells are single chromosomes or small groups of chromosomes contained within a nuclear membrane. They are prepared from tissue culture cells induced to undergo mitotic arrest with colchicine and then subjected to ultracentifugation in the presence of cytochalasin B (25,38). Microcells can be fused to intact cells with Sendai virus and thus affect transfer of a limited amount of donor genetic material. Stable transfer of genetic information can be favored by appropriate selective growth conditions. Murine chromosomes have been successfully transferred into cultured cells of mouse, Chinese hamster and man (31). This technique has been useful for chromosome mapping.

3. Chromosome-mediated transfer of genetic information

The technique of chromosome-mediated gene transfer utilizes isolated metaphase chromosomes as vectors for the transfer of genetic information (39–41). This process typically results in transfer of subchromosomal amounts of genetic material, in a range of sizes up to 1% of the human haploid genome (41). In chromosome-mediated transfer, the 'transgenome' has been shown to be associated with several recipient chromosomes. Each stabilized clone of transformed cells has only a single chromosome associated with only one copy of the transgenome (41). The integration of transferred genes can be stable or unstable. Stable integration may be a rare event occurring in one or a few cells in a population of millions. However, an appropriate selective growth medium can provide an advantage to such a transformed cell, resulting in a stably heritable phenotype with a growth advantage.

4. DNA-mediated gene transfer

In recent years this technique has been used to introduce new genes into mammalian cells growing in culture, yeast, and amphibian oöcytes (42). While cell fusion and other chromosome transfer techniques allow a relatively large amount of genetic information, some of it irrelevant, to be transferred to cells, the cellular endocytosis of calcium microprecipitates of DNA has been used to insert highly purified DNA sequences (43). Since this technique is relatively inefficient, the use of selective techniques favoring the 'transformed' cells becomes important. For example, the transformation of mouse fibroblasts lacking thymidine kinase (Tk^- cells) has been utilized extensively as a model. Tk$^+$ cell clones can be produced using purified Tk genes from Herpes virus when selected for in a medium containing aminopterin, which blocks *de novo* DNA synthesis and allows cells containing the salvage pathway enzyme Tk to grow. The transformed cells have been shown to contain the viral gene sequences and to produce viral enzymes (44–46). High molecular weight DNA from a variety of species has also been used to transfer Tk activity to Tk$^-$ cells. In each instance the Tk produced is that of the DNA donor. For example, mouse Tk$^-$ cells transformed with human DNA were shown to express the human Tk enzyme by isoelectric focusing (47).

The DNA-mediated transformation techniques can also be used to simultaneously insert two or more genes into cells. This process is known as co-transformation. For example, mouse L-cells have been simultaneously transformed with Herpes virus Tk and rabbit β-globin (48). In this experiment the two genes were physically linked together. In other experiments two separate genes are co-precipitated with calcium phosphate and exposed to target cells. In general, cells competent to incorporate exogenous DNA will take up several varieties simultaneously. All types of DNA are, however, not incorporated into the cell's genome and expressed with equal facility. Generally the selective conditions of tissue culture favor cells expressing only one of the incorporated genes, and the other co-transformed genes are not expressed or are expressed poorly. The expressed gene is the one that provides a survival advantage for the recipient cells.

5. Direct injection of new genes into cells

Genetic material can be injected directly into the nucleus of cells. In some instances this material is integrated and expressed. *Drosophila* histone genes have been transcribed in *Xenopus* oöcytes after injection of these genes together with SV40 DNA (49). Jaenisch and Mintz have injected DNA from SV40 into mouse embryos at the blastocyst (42- to 64-cell) stage and reimplanted the blastocysts into foster mothers. Some of the embryos reached full development and carried SV40 DNA sequences one year later (50).

III. UNDERSTANDING THE BIOLOGY OF ERYTHROPOIESIS

A. Controls of gene expression

In vitro methods have been developed in efforts to identify gene sequences responsible for initiation of transcription and other regulatory functions such as binding sites for regulatory proteins. These systems are either whole cell extracts (51) or cytoplasmic extracts with the addition of purified RNA polymerase II (52). Using a whole cell extract of HeLa cells, Proudfoot showed that human embryonic, fetal and adult globin genes were transcribed with equal efficiency (except for δ-globin), indicating that *in vitro* in this system tissue-specific transcription did not occur (53). However, different RNA polymerase II promoters appear to behave differently in the *in vitro* systems. Work is in progress to achieve a better understanding of eukaryotic promoters both *in vitro* and in *in vivo* systems where SV40 vectors (29,54) and DNA-mediated transfer (48,55) are being studied. Generally, cell-free systems have provided the opportunity to study the effects of hormones, nutritional factors, and a recently described leukocyte-derived factor (56) on erythropoiesis.

Another approach to the regulation of globin gene transcription has been the use of hybrid cell lines. Anderson *et al* were able to demonstrate activation of fibroblast globin genes in hybrids made from mouse erythroleukemia and human fibroblasts (57). Several clones were positive for both human and mouse β-globin mRNA after hybridization analysis. Definitive demonstration of human β-globin polypeptide was not shown; however, it appeared a positive regulatory factor could turn on the globin genes of nonerythrocytic chromosomes.

Microinjection has been used to inject rabbit β-globin genes into the nuclei of HeLa cells with both transcription and translation demonstrated (57). This method may allow indirect analysis of regulation provided there is incorporation of foreign DNA into the host genome.

B. Processing of globin mRNA

Recent studies have shed light on the processing and turnover of globin mRNA during erythrocytic maturation. Regulation of the amount of mRNA can occur at several sites between its synthesis in the nucleus and degradation in the cytoplasm. Gene amplification does not appear to be involved in the increased expression of hemoglobin (58–60). Other levels of regulation include steps of intranuclear processing of precursor molecules such as removal of intervening sequences, capping and polyadenylation. Here the efficiency of processing may determine the amount of mRNA finally transported to the cytoplasm. The stability of the mature message may be a function of the rate of degradation of mRNA in the cytoplasm.

Lingrel *et al* have provided evidence that in the induction of erythroleukemia cells, it is the stability of mRNA early in induction which is important in the accumulation of globin mRNA rather than differential processing (61). The mRNA is stable during the period of maximum accumulation.

C. Differential expression of globin genes

Chickens have been used to study erythropoiesis because of the accessibility of actively transcribing erythrocytic cells in the chick embryo. Recombinant

DNA probes are beginning to be used to analyze molecular mechanisms which mediate the differential expression of globin genes. This problem has been approached in the past with the use of antibodies for probes and with immunofluorescence studies. In this manner it has been demonstrated that the decision as to which globins are to be made can occur after the restriction to erythrocytic differentiation (62) and that globin gene switching occurs within a single cell population.

Since primitive erythrocytic cells derive from precursor cells in the mesenchymal cell population, the infection of primary mesenchyme cells with a transforming virus such as avian erythroblastosis virus or Rous sarcoma virus is a method being developed to produce a library of clones that can be used to study the biochemistry of erythrocytic differentiation (63). Infection by virus within the first 24 hr of development inhibits differentiation until the addition of chemical inducers continues the differentiation process. This produces a population of derivatives which differs in stage of differentiation attained before virus attack.

D. Hemoglobinopathies and thalassemic disorders

Over 300 different hemoglobinopathies have been identified that are associated with globin chain structural abnormalities. On the basis of gene sequence analyses, nucleotide sequence analysis of mRNAs and restriction endonuclease digest analyses, many of these have been characterized. They may have amino acid substitutions or deletions, elongation of globin chains or fused globin chains. While many of these disorders do not cause significant clinical disease, sickle cell disease (resulting from the production of sickle hemoglobin which has valine rather than glutamic acid at position 6 on the β chain) causes severe morbidity and is associated with a markedly shortened lifespan.

Many excellent reviews have been written about the inherited disorders of human hemoglobin called the thalassemic syndromes (64–67). α- and β-thalassemia are a heterogeneous group of anemias characterized by reduced or absent synthesis of the α and β polypeptide chains which form the apoprotein portions of normal adult hemoglobin. At least some of these anemias appear to have molecular defects resulting in abnormal regulation of structurally normal hemoglobin genes. With few exceptions, patients with thalassemia produce globin chains having normal amino acid sequences rather than globin chains having altered structure such as that responsible for sickle cell disease.

Both α and β-thalassemias include disorders in which there is complete absence of chain production (α^0 and β^0) or a reduced rate of chain production (α^+ or β^+). There is a further group of β-thalassemias in which there is an associated defect in δ chain synthesis (δβ-thalassemia) including δβ fusion variants such as hemoglobin Lepore.

Since the thalassemias present a variety of malfunctions in the process of erythrocytic gene expression, there are many opportunities to analyze control of gene expression.

IV. THERAPEUTIC POTENTIALS

A. Diagnosis of inherited disorders of erythropoiesis

The study of genetic polymorphisms using restriction endonuclease mapping may be useful in the diagnosis of inherited diseases of erythropoiesis. The association between structural changes in nucleotides remote from globin gene sequences and disordered hemoglobin genes may have some advantage in prenatal diagnosis of inherited disorders in selected populations. For example, in Sardinia, two-thirds of normal β-globin genotypes are associated with 9.3 Kb fragment when Bam HI endonuclease digestion of amniocentesis fibroblasts is done, while one-third of genotypes are associated with a 22Kb fragment (68). In contrast, thalassemia genes are associated with the 9.3 Kb fragment, indicating that in practice, gene mapping will be useful in one-third of pregnancies at risk for $β^0$-thalassemia in Sardinia, since the finding of a 22 Kb fragment would rule it out.

Also useful in prenatal diagnosis is the strong association of the 13.0 Kb HpA I fragment of β-globin with sickle hemoglobin (66,69) which varies from 60% to 87%. This may be due to either a change in the HpA 1 site near the β-globin structural gene or to insertion of additional sequences in this region. In most normal DNA, treatment with the endonuclease HpA 1 yields a 7.6 Kb fragment containing the β-globin gene. However, in a small percentage of normal black individuals (<10%) and other individuals with HbC there is also an association with the 13.0 Kb fragment (70,71).

In view of the presently accumulated data from extensive analysis using a variety of restriction endonuclease treatments of human DNA, it seems probable that there is considerable variation in the coding and non-coding regions of the genome. Much of this variation may have no clinical relevance; however, application of this kind of approach to other inherited diseases is appropriate if specific correlation between genotypes and polymorphisms can be found.

B. Insertion of new genetic information into living animals

Several different approaches have been taken to introduce new genes into animals. SV40 DNA sequences (50) and a cloned Herpes virus Tk gene (72) have been introduced into somatic tissues of mice by injection of blastocysts

(50) or eggs (72). Transmission of foreign DNA by the mouse germ line has been demonstrated with Moloney leukemia virus DNA introduced by viral infection of embryos (73) and by microinjection of cloned rabbit β-globin DNA (74). However, expression of these foreign genes has not been demonstrated.

Pellicer *et al.* have introduced the Herpes Tk gene and human β-globin gene into mouse teratoma cells deficient in thymidine kinase *in vitro* and selected for Tk$^+$ transformants (75). When transformed cells were injected into mice, they formed solid tumors which, in several animals, continued to have both the transformed genes. In a few instances, the viral gene was expressed as the viral thymidine kinase protein.

Recently we performed a series of experiments aimed at inserting new genes into the bone marrow cells of living mice (76,77). Our strategy was based upon the possibility of introducing into hematopoietic stem cells new genes conveying resistance to the cytotoxic agent methotrexate (MTX) and the administration of MTX to the recipient animals, to exert selective pressure favoring proliferation of cells incorporating and expressing the new genes. The DNA-mediated transformation technique was used to introduce the new genes into isolated bone marrow cells. These cells were subsequently returned to irradiated recipient animals where they proliferated and reconstituted hematopoiesis. In one series of experiments (76) high molecular weight DNA from a mouse cell line highly resistant to MTX and containing reiterated sequences of dihydrofolate reductase (DHFR—the enzyme inhibited by MTX) was used; this DHFR was also unusual in that it had a reduced affinity for MTX.

Under the pressure of MTX administration, cells that had incorporated the new DHFR genes became the predominant dividing cells in the marrow population of some animals. Expression of the proliferative advantage of transformed cells usually became apparent within 30–60 days after the reinoculation of the marrow cells into the mice. In some instances, the new DHFR genes could be passed on to secondary recipients when these were irradiated and injected with marrow from primary animals given transformed cells 30–90 days previously. When drug administration was discontinued in order to stop the selective pressure, the predominance of the transformed marrow population was stable in some animals and unstable in others. Animals receiving transformed marrow were alive and clinically well more than one year later. These initial observations suggest that it is feasible to insert new genes into replicating cells of living animals and that in some instances these genes are incorporated and expressed.

A second series of experiments involved insertion of Herpes simplex virus Tk (HSVTk) genes into bone marrow cells of living mice (77). These were also successful but were more complex in interpretation than those experiments involving mouse DHFR. The clearly interpretable points were that Herpes Tk gene sequences were found in the DNA in the spleen of some animals and some made HSVTk protein. An unexpected observation was that some mice expressed the transformed phenotype in the absence of drug selection. This observation suggests that HSVTk may confer a proliferative advantage on some mammalian bone marrow cells, presumably because they extensively utilize the salvage pathway of DNA synthesis.

Transformation of marrow cells with HSVTk was usually unstable, with the transformed phenotype being expressed only transiently. In occasional instances the phenotype was stably expressed and was transferable to secondary and even tertiary recipients. Animals receiving transformed marrow have been observed for periods up to 12 months and have had no detectable abnormalities.

These experiments indicate that it is possible to transform cells of living animals with a small, completely defined gene from another species and that such genes can function to produce a product.

C. Potential applications of gene transplantation in man

A number of problems must be solved before gene transplantation techniques can be considered applicable to man. The most important of these is the still uncertain strategy for controlling the level of expression of the newly inserted gene. Either too little or too much gene product would be undesirable. For example, a transformed reticulocyte making 100-fold more β-globin than a normal cell would be functionally defective. Unfortunately, the area of molecular biology concerned with the controls of gene expression is relatively new and still has many unanswered questions. Consequently, it is not possible to develop a well-founded, long-term strategy for the insertion of a gene with intact controller sequences. For the immediate future the problem will be to get even minimal levels of expression of genes such as β-globin, which do not provide the recipient cell with a proliferative advantage.

Assuming that this problem of control can be overcome, then the first logical application of gene insertion techniques in man will be in patients with genetic disease of the blood such as sickle cell disease and thalassemia major. These will be the logical targets of attack because they reflect isolated defects of single genes or small gene clusters whose expression is limited to blood-forming cells. This limited expression is important for the following reasons. The current technology of transfer of genetic information in mammalian cells requires cells that can replicate in order to spread a gene throughout a cell population. The existing transfer technology is too inefficient (about one successful transfer for every million cells) to consider applying it to fully differentiated end cells. The blood-forming cells of the bone marrow continue to replicate and maintain pools of pluripotential stem cells throughout life.

Organs other than the bone marrow might also eventually be considered for gene transfer. The cells of the gut, skin and mucous membranes also derive from stem cells that continue to replicate throughout adult life. Unfortunately for the purpose of gene transfer, the means of identifying and isolating such stem cells are still very primitive. For the moment, therefore, we are limited to the bone marrow if we wish to consider gene therapy of a genetic disorder involving differentiated tissues of a postnatal individual. Let us consider possible strategies for treating hemoglobinopathies such as sickle cell disease or thalassemia major.

In theory, one should be able to correct the fundamental defect in these disorders if one could transform marrow stem cells with globin genes that are structurally normal and that contain functionally normal controller sequences. Globin genes have already been inserted into animal cells in culture, but their function has been erratic. Because the globin genes themselves should not provide recipient cells with a proliferative advantage, several investigators have used the strategy of combining the globin genes with other genes that do provide such an advantage. Drug resistance genes have been most widely used and drug administration has provided the selective pressure. It is reasonable to if this same strategy can be applied to patients with genetic diseases of the blood.

Based on animal data, one can calculate that there is one pluripotential stem cell for every 10,000 to 100,000 human bone marrow cells. If one uses an optimistic analysis, then about 10^9 marrow cells would be required to insert a new gene into one such stem cell utilizing DNA-mediated transformation. This means a volume of approximately 25 ml of marrow in a normal subject but possibly a smaller volume in a patient with a hyperplastic marrow. The treated marrow would have to be reinfused and 'space' would have to be created in the marrow cavity for the circulating stem cells to 'home' and begin dividing. Once the marrow containing a few transformed stem cells was reinfused, selective pressure from drug administration would presumably be necessary to allow cells carrying the complex of new genes to have a relative proliferative advantage. This experimental approach would appear to be feasible once we have globin genes in a form in which we can control their level of expression.

It is not yet certain whether the controller regions adjacent to the globin structural genes in chromosomes will suffice to allow effective transcription and ultimate translation to β-globin protein in cells transformed with exogenous DNA. Studies of mammalian cells in tissue culture do not appear promising that 'endogenous' mammalian promoter regions will suffice to get adequate levels of expression of β-globin genes. Consequently, alternative strategies are being considered of which the most popular are those involving promoters obtained from viral genes. Such viral promoters can be physically linked to globin structural genes by recombinant DNA technology. However, unless we can find some manner of controlling these viral promoters once inserted into cells, this strategy would appear to have limited applicability to clinical medicine. At present, we simply need more basic information about the normal controls of mammalian gene expression before we can design a rational approach to gene transplantation techniques.

Thus far, we have considered strategies of gene insertion based on selection of cells transformed to drug resistance. It is possible that in certain genetic diseases of blood cells the new genes would themselves provide an advantage to recipient cells in the absence of drug selection. Severe immunodeficiency as a consequence of adenosine deaminase deficiency comes to mind as a candidate for such an approach. It seems likely that in the near future many human genes will be isolated and cloned. Once the corresponding protein is isolated and sequenced, the genes can be identified and cloned by recombinant DNA technology. When such processes become routine, one will be able to consider cloning a variety of genes that are relevant to human diseases.

V. REFERENCES

1. Grabar, S. E., and Krantz, S. B. (1978). 'Erythropoietin and control of red cell production,' *Ann. Rev. Med.,* **29**, 51–66.
2. Proudfoot, N. J. (1977). 'Complete c' non-coding region sequences of rabbit and human beta-globin messenger RNAs', *Cell,* **10**, 559–570.
3. Wilson, J. T., Wilson, L. B., De Riel, J. K., Villa-Komaroff, L., Efstratiatis, A., Forget, B. G., and Weissman, S. M. (1978). 'Insertion of synthetic copies of human globin genes into bacterial plasmids', *Nucleic Acids Res.,* **5**, 563–581.
4. Proudfoot, N. J., Gillam, S., Smith, M., and Longley, J. I. (1977). 'Nucleotide sequence of 3' terminal 3rd of rabbit alpha globin messenger RNA—comparison with human alpha globin messenger RNA', *Cell,* **11**, 807–818.
5. Little, P., Curtis, P., Coutelle, C., Van den Berg, J., Dalgleish F., Malcolm, S., Courtney, M., Westaway, D., and Williamson, R. (1978). 'Isolation and partial sequence of recombinant plasmids containing human alpha-globin, beta-globin and gamma-globin cDNA fragments', *Nature,* **273**, 640–643.
6. McCulloch, E. A., Till, J. E., Russell, E. S., and Bernstein, S. E. (1965). 'Cellular basis of genetically determined hemopoietic defect in anemic mice of genotype SL/SL[d]', *Blood,* **26**, 399–410.
7. Thompson, M. W., McCulloch, E. A., Siminovitch, L., and Till, J. E. (1966). 'Cellular basis for defect in haemopoiesis in flexed-tailed mice. I. Nature and persistence of defect', *Br. J. Haemat.,* **12**, 152–160.
8. Orkin, S. H., and Nathan, D. G. (1980). 'Molecular genetics of thalassemia', in *Contemporary Hematology/Oncology* (Eds. J. Lobue, A. S. Gordon, A. Silber, and F. M. Muggia), Plenum Medical Book Co., New York, vol. 1, pp. 121–147.
9. Benz, E. J., Jr., and Forget, B. G. (1980). 'Pathogenesis of the thalassemia syndromes', *Pathobiol. Ann.,* **10**, 1–33.
10. Weatherall, D. J., and Clegg, J. B. (1979). 'Recent developments in the molecular genetics of human hemoglobin', *Cell,* **16**, 467–479.
11. Southern, E. M. (1975). 'Detection of specific sequences among DNA fragments separated by gel electrophoresis', *J. Mol. Biol.,* **98**, 503–517.
12. Shinnick, T. M., Lund, E., Smithies, O., and Blattner, F. R. (1975). 'Hybridization of labeled RNA to DNA in agarose gels', *Nucleic Acids Res.,* **2**, 1911–1929.
13. Lacy, E., Lawn, R. M., Fritsch, E., Hardison, R. C., Parker, R. C., and Maniatis, T. (1978). 'Isolation and characterization of mammalian globin genes', in *Cellular*

and Molecular Regulation of Hemoglobin Switching (Eds. G. Stamatoyanno-poulos, and A. W. Neinhuis), Grune and Stratton, New York, pp. 501–519.

14. Maniatis, T., Hardison, R. C., Lacy, E., Lauer, J., O'Connell, C., Quon, D., Sim, G. K., and Efstratiatis, A. (1978). 'Isolation of structural genes from libraries of eukaryotic DNA', *Cell*, **15**, 687–701.

15. Maniatis, T., Sim, G. K., Efstratiatis, A., and Kafatos, F. C. (1976). 'Amplification and characterization of a beta-globin gene synthesized *in vitro*', *Cell*, **8**, 163–182.

16. Higuchi, R., Paddock, G. V., Wall, R., and Salser, W. (1976). 'General method for cloning eukaryotic structural gene sequences', *Proc. Natl. Acad. Sci., USA*, **73**, 3146–3150.

17. Efstratiatis, A., Kafatos, F. C., and Maniatis, T. (1977). 'Primary structure of rabbit beta-globin messenger RNA as determined from cloned DNA', *Cell*, **10**, 571–585.

18. Browne, J., Paddock, G. V., Liu, A., Clarke, M., Heindell, M., and Salser, W. (1977). 'Nucleotide sequence from the rabbit beta globin gene inserted into *Escherichia coli* plasmids', *Science*, **195**, 389–391.

19. Jeffreys, A. J., and Flavell, R. A. (1977). 'Physical map of DNA regions flanking rabbit beta globin gene', *Cell*, **12**, 429–439.

20. Tilghman, S. M., Tiemeier, D. C., Polsky, F., Edgell, M. H., Seidman, J. C., Leder, A., Enquist, L. W., Norman, B., and Leder, P. (1977). 'Cloning specific segments of mammalian genome-bacteriophage-lambda containing mouse globin and surrounding gene sequences', *Proc. Natl. Acad. Sci., USA*, **74**, 4406–4410.

21. Tilghman, S. M., Curtis, P. J., Tiemeier, D. C., Leder, P., and Weissman, C. (1978). 'Intervening sequence of a mouse beta-globin gene is transcribed within 15S beta-globin messenger RNA precursor', *Proc. Natl. Acad. Sci., USA*, **75**, 1309–1313.

22. Cohen, S. N., and Shapiro, J. A. (1980). 'Transposable genetic elements', *Scientific American*, **242**, 40–49.

23. Benveniste, R. E., Callahan, R., Sherr, C. J., Chapman, V., and Todaro, G. J. (1977). 'Two distinct endogenous type C viruses isolated from Asian rodent *mus cervicolor*—conservation of virogene sequences in related rodent species', *J. Virol.*, **21**, 849–862.

24. Griffith, F. (1928). 'The significance of pneumococcal types', *J. Hyg. Cambridge, England*, **27**, 113–159.

25. Ege, T., and Ringertz, N. R. (1974). 'Preparation of microcells by enucleation of micronucleate cells', *Exptl. Cell Res.*, **87**, 378–382.

26. Wigler, M. H., Neugut, A. I., and Weinstein, I. B. (1976). 'Enucleation of mammalian cells in suspension', *Methods in Cell Biol.*, **14**, 87–93.

27. Mulligan, R. C., Howard, B. H., and Berg, P. (1979). 'Synthesis of rabbit β-globin in cultured monkey kidney cells following infection with a SV40 β-globin recombinant genome', *Nature*, **277**, 108–114.

28. Hamer, D. H., and Leder, P. (1979). 'SV40 recombinants carrying a functional RNA splice junction and polyadenylation site from the chromosomal mouse beta-maj globin gene', *Cell*, **17**, 737–747.

29. Hamer, D. H., and Leder, P. (1979). 'Expression of the chromosomal mouse β^{maj}-globin gene cloned in SV40', *Nature*, **281**, 35–40.

30. Upcroft, P., Skolnik, H., Upcroft, J. A., Solomon, D., Khoury, G., Hamer, D. H., and Fareer, G. C. (1978). 'Transduction of a bacterial gene into mammalian cells', *Proc. Natl. Acad. Sci., USA*, **75**, 2117–2121.

31. Fournier, R. E. K., and Ruddle, F. H. (1977). 'Microcell mediated transfer of murine chromosomes into mouse, Chinese hamster and human somatic cells', *Proc. Natl. Acad. Sci., USA*, **74**, 319–323.

32. Ruddle, F. H., and Creagan, R. P. (1975). 'Parasexual approaches to the genetics of man', *Ann. Rev. Genet.*, **9**, 407–486.
33. McKusick, V. A., and Ruddle, F. H. (1977). 'Status of gene map of human chromosomes', *Science*, 390–405.
34. Fournier, R. E. K., and Ruddle, F. M. (1977). *Molecular Human Cytogenetics, ICN-UCLA Symposia on Molecular and Cell Biology*, **7**, 189–199.
35. Ostro, M. J., Giacomoni, D., Lavelle, D., Paxton, W., and Dray, S. (1978). 'Evidence for translation of rabbit beta globin messenger RNA after liposome-mediated insertion into a human cell line', *Nature*, **274**, 921–923.
36. Dimitriadis, G. J. (1978). 'Translation of rabbit globin messenger RNA introduced by liposomes into mouse lymphocytes', *Nature*, **274**, 923–924.
37. Rechsteiner, M. (1978). 'Red cell-mediated microinjection', *Natl. Cancer Inst., Monogr.*, **48**, 57–64.
38. Wigler, M. H., Neugut, A. I., and Weinstein, I. B. (1976). 'Enucleation of mammalian cells in suspension', *Methods in Cell Biol.*, **14**, 87–93.
39. McBride, O. W., and Ozer, M. H. (1973). 'Transfer of genetic information by purified metaphase chromosomes', *Proc. Natl. Acad. Sci., USA*, **70**, 1258–1262.
40. Degnen, G. E., Miller, I. L., Adelberg, E. A., and Eisenstadt, J. M. (1976). 'Chromosome mediated gene transfer between closely related strains of cultured mouse cells', *Proc. Natl. Acad. Sci., USA*, **73**, 2838–2842.
41. Klobutcher, L. A., and Ruddle, F. M. (1979). 'Phenotype stabilization and integration of transferred material in chromosome-mediated gene transfer', *Nature*, **280**, 657–660.
42. Beggs, J. D., Van den Berg, J., Van Ooyen, A., and Weissman, C. (1980). 'Abnormal expression of chromosomal rabbit beta globin gene in *Saccharomyces cerevisiae*', *Nature*, **283**, 835–837.
43. Graham, F. L., and Van der Eb, A. J. (1973). 'A new technique for the assay of infectivity of human adenovirus 5 DNA', *Virology*, **52**, 456–467.
44. Maitland, N. J., and McDougall, J. K. (1977). 'Biochemical transformation of mouse cells by fragments of herpes simplex virus DNA', *Cell*, **11**, 233–241.
45. Wigler, M., Sweet, R., Sim, G. K., Wold, B., Pellicer, A., Lacy, E., Maniatis, T., Silverstein, S., and Axel, R. (1979). 'Transformation of mammalian cells with genes from procaryotes and eukaryotes', *Cell*, **16**, 777–785.
46. Pellicer, A., Wigler, M., Axel, R., and Silverstein, S. (1978). 'The transfer and stable integration of the HSV thymidine kinase gene into mouse cells', *Cell*, **14**, 133–141.
47. Wigler, M., Pellicer, A., Silverstein, S., and Axel, R. (1978). 'Biochemical transfer of single copy eukaryotic genes using total cellular DNA as donor', *Cell*, **14**, 725–731.
48. Mantei, N., Boll, W., and Weissman, C. (1979). 'Rabbit β-globin mRNA production in mouse L cells transformed with cloned rabbit β-globin chromosomal DNA', *Nature*, **281**, 40–46.
49. Mertz, J. E., and Gurdon, J. B. (1977). 'Purified DNAs are transcribed after microinjection into *Xenopus* oocytes', *Proc. Natl. Acad. Sci., USA*, **74**, 1502–1506.
50. Jaenisch, R., and Mintz, B. (1974). 'Simian virus 40 DNA sequences in DNA of healthy adult mice derived from preimplantation blastocysts injected with viral DNA', *Proc. Natl. Acad. Sci., USA*, **71**, 1250–1254.
51. Manley, J. L., Fire, A., Cano, A., Sharp, P. A., and Gefter, M. L. (1980). 'DNA-dependent transcription of adenovirus genes in a soluble whole cell extract', *Proc. Natl. Acad. Sci., USA*, **77**, 3855–3859.
52. Weil, P. A., Luse, D. S., Segall, J., and Roeder, R. G. (1979). 'Selective and accurate initiation of transcription at the AD2 major late promoter in a soluble system dependent on purified RNA polymerase II and DNA', *Cell*, **18**, 469–84.

53. Proudfoot, N. J., Shander, M. H. M., Manley, J. L., Geftler, M. L., and Maniatis, T. (1980). 'Structure and *in vitro* transcription of human globin genes', *Science*, **209**, 1329–1336.
54. Mulligan, R. C., and Berg, P. (1980). 'Expression of a bacterial gene in mammalian cells', *Science*, **209**, 1422–1427.
55. Pellicer, A., Robins, D., Wold, B., Sweet, R., Jackson, J., Lowy, I., Roberts, J. M., Sim, G. K., Silverstein, S., and Axel, R. (1980). 'Altering genotype and phenotype by DNA-mediated gene transfer', *Science*, **209**, 1414–1422.
56. Aye, M. T. (1977). 'Erythroid colony formation in cultures of human marrow—effect of leukocyte conditioned medium', *J. Cell. Physiol.*, **91**, 69–77.
57. Anderson, W. F., Willing, M. C., Axelrod, D. E., Gopalkrishnan, T. V., and Diacumakos, E. G. (1979). 'A new approach in the search for globin gene regulatory factors', in *Cellular and Molecular Regulation of Hemoglobin Switching* (Eds. G. Stamatoyannopoulos and A. W. Neinhuis), Grune and Stratton, New York, pp. 779–792.
58. Harrison, P. R., Hell, A., Birnie, G. D., and Paul, J. (1972). 'Evidence for single copies of globin genes in the mouse genome', *Nature*, **239**, 219–21.
59. Ross, J., Gielen, J., Packman, S., Ikawa, Y., and Leder, P. (1974). 'Globin gene expression in cultured erythroleukemic cells', *J. Molec. Biol.*, **87**, 697–714.
60. Bishop, J. O., and Rosbash, M. (1973). 'Reiteration frequency of duck haemoglobin genes', *Nature New Biol.*, **241**, 204–207.
61. Lingrel, J. B., Lowenhaupt, K., Haynes, J. R., Rosteck, P., Kalb, V. F., and Smith, K. (1979). 'Processing and turnover of globin mRNA during erythroid maturation', in *Cellular and Molecular Regulation of Hemoglobin Switching* (Eds. G. Stamatoyannopoulos and A. W. Neinhuis), Grune and Stratton, New York, pp. 675–689.
62. Tobin, A. J., Chapman, B. S., Hansen, D. A., Lasky, L., and Selvig, S. E. (1970). 'Regulation of embryonic and adult hemoglobin synthesis in chickens', in *Cellular and Molecular Regulation of Hemoglobin Switching* (Eds. G. Stamatoyannopoulos and A. W. Neinhuis), Grune and Stratton, New York, pp. 205–211.
63. Ingram, V. M., Keane, R. W., and Lindblad, P. C. (1979). 'Determination and differentiation in early embryonic erythropoiesis: a new experimental approach', in *Cellular and Molecular Regulation of Hemoglobin Switching* (Eds. G. Stamatoyannopoulos and A. W. Neinhuis), Grune and Stratton, New York, pp. 198–203.
64. Weatherall, D. J., and Clegg, J. B. (1979). 'Recent developments in molecular genetics of human hemoglobin', *Cell*, **16**, 467–479.
65. Forget, B. G. (1979). 'Molecular genetics of human hemoglobin synthesis', *Ann. Int. Med.*, **91**, 605–616.
66. Bank, A., Mears, G., and Ramirez, B. (1980). 'Disorders of human hemoglobin', *Science*, **207**, 486–492.
67. Benz, E. J., Jr., and Forget, B. G. (1980). 'Pathogenesis of the thalassemia syndromes', *Pathobiol. Ann.*, **10**, 1–33.
68. Seale, T. W., and Rennert, O. M. (1980). 'Prenatal diagnosis of thalassemias and hemoglobinopathies', *Ann. Clin. Lab. Sci.*, **10**, 383–394.
69. Kan, Y. W., and Dozy, A. M. (1978). 'Polymorphism of DNA sequence adjacent to human β globin structural gene: relationship to sickle mutation', *Proc. Natl. Acad. Sci., USA*, **75**, 6531–6535.
70. Feldenzer, J., Mears, J. G., Burns, A. L., Natta, C., and Bank, A. (1979). 'Heterogeneity of DNA fragments associated with the sickle-globin gene', *J. Clin. Invest.*, **64**, 751–755.

71. Chang, J. C., Temple, G. F., Trecartin, R. F., and Kan, Y. W. (1979). 'Beta thalassemia-nonsense mutation in man and its correction', *Clin. Res.*, **27**, 457 (abstr.)
72. Constantini, F., and Lacy, E. (1982). 'Genetic transformation of mouse embryos by microinjection of purified DNA', *Nature*, (in press).
73. Jähner, D., and Jaenisch, R. (1980). 'Integration of Moloney leukemia virus into the germ line of mice—correlation between site of integration and virus activation', *Nature*, **287**, 456–458.
74. Constantini, F., and Lacy, E. (1981). 'Introduction of a rabbit β-globin gene into the mouse germ line', *Nature*, **294**, 92–94.
75. Pellicer, A., Wagner, E. F., El Kareh, A., Dewey, M. J., Reuser, A. J., Silverstein, S., Axel, R., and Mintz, B. (1980). 'Introduction of a viral thymidine kinase gene and the human beta globin gene into developmentally multipotential mouse teratocarcinoma cells', *Proc. Natl. Acad. Sci., USA*, **77**, 2098–2102.
76. Cline, M. J., Stang, H., Mercola, K., Morse, L., Ruprecht, R., Browne, J., and Salser, W. (1980). 'Gene transfer in intact animals', *Nature*, **284**, 422–425.
77. Mercola, K. E., Stang, H. D., Browne, J., Salser, W., and Cline, M. J. (1980). 'Insertion of a new gene of viral origin into bone marrow cells of mice', *Science*, **208**, 1033–1035.

Index